Scully's Handbook of
MEDICAL PROBLEMS
IN DENTISTRY

Scully's Handbook of
MEDICAL PROBLEMS
IN DENTISTRY

Professor Crispian Scully CBE

MD, PhD, MDS, MRCS, BSc, FDSRCS, FDSRCPS, FFDRCSI, FDSRCSE, FRCPath, FMedSci, FHEA, FUCL, DSc, DChD, DMed (HC), Dr.hc

Co-Director, WHO Collaborating Centre for Oral Health-General Health; and Emeritus Professor, UCL (London, UK)

ELSEVIER

Edinburgh   London   New York   Oxford   Philadelphia   St Louis   Sydney   Toronto   2016

ELSEVIER

ISBN   978-0-7020-4648-3

Notices

Knowledge and best practice in this field are constantly changing. As new research and experience broaden our understanding, changes in research methods, professional practices, or medical treatment may become necessary.

Practitioners and researchers must always rely on their own experience and knowledge in evaluating and using any information, methods, compounds, or experiments described herein. In using such information or methods they should be mindful of their own safety and the safety of others, including parties for whom they have a professional responsibility.

With respect to any drug or pharmaceutical products identified, readers are advised to check the most current information provided (i) on procedures featured or (ii) by the manufacturer of each product to be administered, to verify the recommended dose or formula, the method and duration of administration, and contraindications. It is the responsibility of practitioners, relying on their own experience and knowledge of their patients, to make diagnoses, to determine dosages and the best treatment for each individual patient, and to take all appropriate safety precautions.

To the fullest extent of the law, neither the Publisher nor the authors, contributors, or editors, assume any liability for any injury and/or damage to persons or property as a matter of products liability, negligence or otherwise, or from any use or operation of any methods, products, instructions, or ideas contained in the material herein.

ELSEVIER your source for books, journals and multimedia in the health sciences

www.elsevierhealth.com

  Working together to grow libraries in developing countries

www.elsevier.com • www.bookaid.org

Content Strategist: Alison Taylor
Content Development Specialist: Lynn Watt and Carole McMurray
Project Manager: Julie Taylor
Designer: Christian J. Bilbow
Illustration Manager: Emily Costantino

The publisher's policy is to use paper manufactured from sustainable forests

Last digit is the print number: 9   8   7   6   5   4   3   2   1

Contents

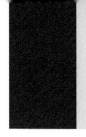

Preface

The aim of this book is to highlight the main points and relevance in oral healthcare of human diseases (clinical medical sciences) in a practical way, indicating their aetiopathogenesis, clinical features, diagnosis and management. The book should prove of value to the whole dental healthcare team, to students, and to trainees and is not a replacement for *Medical Problems in Dentistry* – which contains far more detail. However, with increasing use of the internet, this represents a spin-off of smaller size and is intended to be more user-friendly.

Improved social and medical care has increased the life span of many people, including those with previously life-threatening disorders. Many of these people are vulnerable and require special attention in healthcare, and operative intervention can produce major problems. It is thus important that adequate attention is paid both to medical, drug and social history. It is important to apply preventive programmes and educate patients and parents in hygiene to minimize the risk of infections.

The book aims to cover the curriculum as outlined in the UK General Dental Council (GDC) document 'Preparing for practice; Dental team learning outcomes for registration'. It attempts particularly to cover areas that are of especial concern, and other important conditions, which are mainly the problems associated with providing care to people with:

- Allergies
- Bleeding tendencies
- Cardiac diseases
- Drug use and abuse
- Endocrine disorders, especially diabetes
- Fits, faints, behavioural and neuropsychiatric conditions
- Gravid (pregnant) patients
- Hepatitis and other transmissible diseases including HIV/AIDS
- Iatrogenic issues (immunosuppressive treatment; malignant disease such as cancers)

By affording substantial space to these and some other conditions, less space is committed to less significant disorders and rare conditions cannot be included.

The wide coverage is achieved by presenting material in 10 sections; the first discusses health; the second section summarizes aspects of healthcare such as medical history, preoperative assessment, preoperative planning, analgesia and behaviour management, consent, culture, and gender issues. Section 3 covers the main emergencies (others appear elsewhere in the book), while Section 4 discusses age and gender. Section 5 summarizes organ disorders presented alphabetically. Section 6 deals with issues related to trauma; Section 7 covers infections; Section 8 covers chemical dependence; Section 9 discusses therapeutic modalities; Section 10 deals with disability and impairment.

All categorizations are open to criticism; Aristotle advised:

'To avoid criticism say nothing, do nothing, be nothing.'

Conscious of the quote by Mark Twain:

'I didn't have time to write a short letter, so I wrote a long one instead',

I have endeavoured to be concise.

A risk analysis (risk–benefit analysis) is prudent before dental treatment with any patient and medical advice should be obtained if there is any concern about the medical history. Risks are generally greatest when GA or sedation are used and procedures involve haemorrhage and/or are prolonged. Defer elective care until the patient has been medically stabilized. Emergency dental care should be conservative – principally analgesics and antibiotics.

Update the medical history at every appointment. Well-managed medical conditions generally present no or few problems. Ready access to medical help, oxygen and nitroglycerin is vital. Standard infection control measures are necessary. Guidance on oral hygiene and diet are essential.

Valid consent is crucial. All patient information must be kept in a secure location, and discussing patients' medical status should only occur in a private, closed office to ensure confidentiality.

Short, stress-free appointments are recommended; it is important to avoid anxiety, stress and pain. If LA, analgesics, sedative drugs or antibiotics are contraindicated, this is highlighted below. The behaviour, conscious level, pulse, blood pressure and respiratory rate of all patients should be monitored before starting and periodically during treatment, checking with the patient that they feel well. High-risk patients should be offered dental treatment in hospital.

Drug doses must always be checked before administration. Doses must be reduced for children. Doses may need to be reduced in older people or in some medical conditions. Contraindications must always be checked and the patient warned of any possible adverse effects. Informed patient consent is crucial. The information in this book has been carefully checked, but neither the author nor publisher can accept any legal responsibility for any errors or omissions that may be made. Neither the authors nor publisher makes any warranty, expressed or implied, with respect to material herein.

More detail can be found elsewhere about medical topics (Scully C [2014] *Medical problems in dentistry*, 7e, Elsevier Churchill Livingstone, Edinburgh) and orofacial aspects (Scully C [2013] *Oral and maxillofacial medicine*, 3e, Elsevier, Edinburgh). The book does not attempt to include all dental treatment modifications, which are discussed elsewhere (Scully C et al. [2007] *Special care in dentistry: handbook of oral healthcare*. Churchill Livingstone Elsevier, Edinburgh), but includes considerations of risk assessment, pain and anxiety control, patient access and positioning, treatment modification and drug use. The book is applicable to the whole healthcare team. The aims and objectives are to educate and inspire each member of the dental team, whether in-training or post-qualification.

I warmly acknowledge the guidance and help of Dr Tony Brooke (UK), Professor Mark Griffiths (UK), Professor Oslei paes de Almeida (Brazil), Professor Jose Bagan (Spain), Professor Pedro Diz Dios (Spain), Dr Navdeep Kumar (UK), Dr Eleni Georgakopoulou (Greece), Dr Yazan Hassona (Jordan), Dr Dimitris Malamos (Greece), Professor Adalberto Mosqueda-Taylor (Mexico), Dr Rachel Cowie (UK) and Dr Andrew Robinson (Singapore), and the support of Professor Justin Stebbing (UK) and Sister Jane Dean (UK). My sincere thanks also to Zoe and Frances without whose patience the work would not have been possible.

C.S.
2016

1 Health

Health hazards

Causes of disease are genetic (inherited) or acquired – environmental (e.g. from trauma, infection, chemical or irradiation) or due to lifestyle (e.g. lack of exercise, poor diet, habits – tobacco, alcohol, drugs, betel and other habits) – often combinations of these factors. Since disease arises from interactions of genetic, environmental and lifestyle factors, it may be minimized by avoiding or minimizing these factors. Already genetic diseases like haemophilia effects can be minimized by providing the missing protein (blood clotting factor VIII). Genetic manipulation ('gene therapy') is increasingly possible, and the genetic basis for drug actions and reactions is being elucidated.

Health promotion

We all aspire to health. The World Health Organization (WHO) definition of health is *Health is a state of complete physical, mental and social well-being and not merely the absence of disease or infirmity*. Health includes the ability to undertake normally, activities such as communication, excretion, feeding, recreation, sexual activity, sleep and work, and have no physical suffering, mental suffering or dependency on others.

The leading causes of death (mortality) differ between genders, change with age and vary between and within countries and even cities – determined mainly by social inequalities and factors such as climate and disease (morbidity). For example, in men in the UK, though heart disease, cancers, chronic respiratory diseases, and diabetes consistently rank as top diseases, once a man hits midlife many of these threats have been years in the making, attributable largely to lifestyle choices (Table 1.1). The quality of life (QoL) is as important as, or more important than, its duration.

Disease can be more readily prevented by avoiding certain lifestyle and environmental factors, or minimizing them. Apart from a lifestyle designed to improve or maintain good health by avoiding violence (Section 6) and infections (Section 7), the three most important measures are regular exercise, a healthy diet, and avoiding chemical dependence (Section 8).

Exercise

Physical inactivity often occurs together with an unhealthy diet, contributing to obesity, diabetes, heart disease and cancers. When exercise is combined with a proper diet, weight can be controlled, and obesity – a major risk factor for many diseases – prevented. Other health benefits from exercise, may include for example, some protection against depression and anxiety, osteoporosis, hypertension and Alzheimer disease.

1

Table 1.1 Five main causes of male deaths in US adults (adapted from www.health.harvard.edu)

	Age					
	35–44	45–54	55–64	65–74	75–84	85+
1	Unintentional injuries	Heart disease	Cancer	Heart disease		
2	Heart disease	Cancer	Heart disease	Cancer		
3	Cancer	Un-intentional injuries		Chronic lung diseases		Stroke
4	Suicide		Chronic lung diseases	Stroke		Chronic lung diseases
5	Murder	Chronic liver disease	Diabetes			Alzheimer disease

Healthy diet

A healthy diet – eating the right amount of food for the activity undertaken and eating a range of foods to ensure a balanced diet (fruit and vegetables; wholegrain bread, pasta and rice; some protein-rich foods such as meat, fish, eggs and lentils; and some dairy foods; but low in fat (especially saturated fat), salt and sugar) is important. Carbohydrates as wholegrain unrefined products may help protect against colon cancer, diverticulitis and dental caries. Generous amounts of vegetables and fruit daily appear to protect against cancers of stomach, colon and lung, and possibly against cancers of the mouth, larynx, cervix, bladder and breast. A high-fibre diet may also offer some protection against hypertension and ischaemic heart disease (IHD). Minimizing the intake of saturated fats (especially those from dairy sources) and partially halogenated vegetable fats may lower the risk of heart disease and some cancers.

See www.healthierus.gov/dietaryguidelines and US Department of Agriculture's food guidance system (My Pyramid; www.mypyramid.gov).

Chemical avoidance

Chemical dependence is defined as self-administration without any medical indication and despite adverse medical and social consequences, and in a manner that is harmful. This is discussed in Section 8.

Tobacco use is a major cause worldwide of illness and death, particularly linked to atherosclerotic heart disease, hypertension, stroke and their consequent major adverse cardiac/cerebrovascular events (MACE), and chronic obstructive pulmonary disease (COPD). In addition to nicotine, cigarette smoke is primarily composed of a dozen gases (mainly carbon monoxide) and tar, but also about 4000 other compounds, including nitrosamines and aromatic amines, which are known carcinogens. Cancers of the mouth, larynx, oesophagus, lung, and bladder in particular are linked to tobacco. Secondhand smoke (passive smoking) causes lung cancer in adults and greatly increases the risk of respiratory illnesses in children and also sudden infant death. Pregnant women who smoke cigarettes run a greater risk of having stillborn or premature infants, sudden infant death, infants with low birthweight or children with conduct disorders.

Table 1.2 Prevention of disease			
Environmental		**Lifestyle**	
Trauma	Avoid alcohol, accidents, aggression and dangerous environments, activities and sports	Exercise	Take regular daily exercise for 30 min minimum
Infections	Avoid needlestick injuries. Use latex protection (condoms, gloves, rubber dam). Be vaccinated with routine advised vaccines and hepatitis B (Section 7).	Diet	Eat a balanced diet with at least 5 portions of fruit/vegetables daily, minimize sugar and avoid food fads
Chemical	Label and take care with use of and exposure to toxic agents	Substance dependence	Abstain from use of alcohol, betel, recreational drugs, tobacco. Safe storage and adhere to COSHH (Control Of Substances Hazardous to Health) regulations
Irradiation	Minimize exposure (to radon, sun, X-rays, lasers, damaging lights, etc.) and use safety measures such as protective eyewear and screens		Adhere to IRMER (Ionizing Radiation Medical Exposure Regulations)

Alcohol or use of illegal drugs is damaging to social interactions, and may cause violence/trauma, mental health issues, liver disease and many other issues. Injected illegal drugs can also easily lead to infections. Alcohol consumed by pregnant mothers can cause foetal alcohol syndrome (Section 8).

*Environmental chemical*s exposure should also be minimized; particular dangers are associated for example with asbestos (mesothelioma), benzene (leukaemias), lead and mercury (neurotoxicity). See www.hse.gov.uk/chemicals/ and www.osha.gov/SLTC/hazardoustoxicsubstances/

Advising on good lifestyles and safe environments, and offering access to smoking cessation and other support groups is an important function of all healthcare professionals, including dental.

Detecting most diseases including cancers early, usually means fewer complications and that treatment is more likely to be successful (Table 1.2).

Further reading

Control of substances hazardous to health. Health and Safety Executive. Available at: <http://www.hse.gov.uk/coshh/> (accessed 15.08.15.).
Grogono, A.W., Woodgate, D.J., 1971. Index for measuring health. Lancet 2, 1024–1026.
Health promotion and health education. Available at: <http://phpartners.org/hpro.html> (accessed 15.08.15.).

Health promotion and lifestyles. Available at: <http://www.patient.co.uk/showdoc/16/> (accessed 15.08.15.).

Healthy lives, healthy people. Our strategy for public health in England. HM Government. Available at: <http://www.dh.gov.uk/en/Publichealth/Healthimprovement/Healthyliving/index.htm> (accessed 15.08.15.).

Medical Problems in Dentistry. Elsevier. Available at: <http://www.equip.nhs.uk/topics/Healthtopics/healthyliving.aspx> (accessed 15.08.15.).

Ten ways to boost your health. NHS Choices. Available at: <http://www.nhs.uk/Livewell/healthy-living/Pages/Ten-ways-to-boost-your-health.aspx> (accessed 15.08.15.).

The regulatory requirements for medical exposure to ionizing radiation. Health and Safety Executive. Available at: <http://www.hse.gov.uk/pUbns/priced/hsg223.pdf> (accessed 15.08.15.).

Wellness and Lifestyle. National Institutes of Health. Available at: <http://health.nih.gov/category/WellnessLifestyle> (accessed 15.08.15.).

2 Healthcare

Essential points from the outset of a patient's consultation with a dental clinician as with any other Health Care Professional (HCP) are to:
1. determine what the patient requires and wants;
2. obtain an accurate medical (including drug [medication]), family, social, and sometimes dental, travel or developmental history;
3. perform a risk–benefit analysis related to treatment intents;
4. obtain informed consent to any investigations or procedures that may be needed, from the patient or their legally responsible representative;
5. obtain informed consent to the resulting treatment plan from the patient or their legally responsible representative.

Medical history

A medical history is essential in order to:
- assess the fitness of the patient for the procedure
- decide on the type of behaviour and pain control required
- decide how treatment may need to be modified
- warn of any possible emergencies that could arise
- warn of any possible risk to staff or other patients or visitors.

Some clinicians also use questionnaires completed by the patient (Table 2.1). Relevant systemic disease is generally more common in old people, those with other disabilities, and hospital in-patients.

Preoperative risk assessment

An arbitrary guideline for patient selection for treatment may be based on the classification of Physical Status of the American Society of Anesthesiology (ASA) (Table 2.2). A fairly high percentage of the population aged 65–74 (23.9%) and >75 (34.9%) have ASA scores of III or IV.

Risks increase when the patient is not completely healthy (if the patient has ASA score of III or IV) and any procedure contemplated is invasive, or staff attempt anything overambitious in terms of their skill, knowledge or available facilities. Current guidelines suggest that *surgical* treatment such as oral and maxillofacial, endodontic or periodontal or implant surgery must be significantly modified if the patient has ASA score of III or IV.

The history must particularly be reviewed before any treatment changes, surgical procedure, general anaesthetic, conscious sedation or local anaesthetic is given. Do not assume

Table 2.1 Simple medical questionnaire example for dental patients to complete

		Yes	No	Do not know	Details
1	Have you had any operation or general anaesthetic?				
2	Have you had any problems with anaesthetics?				
3	Have any of your relatives had any problems with anaesthetics?				
4	Are you taking any drugs or other medications (anticoagulants, inhalers, Pill)?				
5	If female, are you or could you be pregnant?				
6	Have you had any corticosteroid drugs in the past? If yes, when?				
7	Have you any allergies (drugs/plasters/latex/antiseptics/foodstuffs)?				
8	Do you have heart disease or have you had a heart attack?				
9	Do you ever have to take antibiotics routinely prior to dental surgery?				
10	Do you get chest pains, indigestion, or acid in the throat?				
11	Do you have a hiatus hernia?				
12	Do you have high blood pressure?				
13	Do you get breathless walking, climbing stairs or lying flat?				
14	Do you have asthma, bronchitis, or chest disease?				
15	Have you ever had a convulsion or a fit?				
16	Do you have arthritis or muscle disease?				
17	Do you have anaemia or other blood disorder?				
18	Do you know your sickle status (if relevant)?				
19	Have you ever had liver disease or been jaundiced?				
20	Have you ever had kidney disease?				
21	Do you have diabetes?				
22	Do you smoke tobacco? If yes, how many a day (also last six months)?				
23	Do you take recreational drugs or drink alcohol? If yes, how many units per week?				
24	Do you have any infection?				
25	Is there anything else you think the doctor should know?				

Table 2.2 American Society of Anesthesiology (ASA) classification of physical status

	Definition	Treatment modifications
I	Normal, healthy patient	None
II	Patient with mild systemic disease, e.g. controlled diabetes, anticoagulation, asthma, hypertension, epilepsy, pregnancy, anxiety.	Medical advice may be helpful. Often few treatment modifications needed, unless GA or major surgery needed.
III	Patient with severe systemic disease limiting activity but not incapacitating, e.g. chronic renal failure, epilepsy with frequent seizures, uncontrolled hypertension, recent myocardial infarct, uncontrolled diabetes.	Medical advice is helpful. Patients are often best treated surgically in a hospital based clinic where expert medical support is available.
IV	Severe asthma, stroke, patient with incapacitating disease that is a constant threat to life, e.g. cancer, unstable angina or recent MI, arrhythmia, recent CVA, end-stage renal disease, liver failure.	Medical advice is indicated. Patients are often best treated surgically in a hospital-based clinic where expert medical support is available.
V	Moribund patient not expected to live more than 24 hours with or without treatment.	Medical advice is essential. Patients are often best treated surgically in a hospital based clinic where expert medical support is available.

normal function has been established after treatment of any condition. Further, many patients with life-threatening diseases now survive as a result of advances in surgical and medical care. An apparently fit patient coming for treatment, can have a serious systemic disease and be under treatment with significant medications. Either or both can significantly affect management or even the fate of the patient. These problems may be compounded if the patient is seen briefly and support is lacking. Morbidity is minimal when local anaesthesia (LA) is used. Conscious sedation (CS) is more hazardous than LA, and must be carried out by adequately trained personnel and with due consideration of the possible risks. General anaesthesia (GA), whether intravenous or inhalational, leads to impaired control of vital functions and is thus only carried out by a qualified anaesthetist, and permitted in a hospital with appropriate facilities.

Preoperative planning

Good preoperative assessment and organization endeavour to anticipate and prevent any issues (Table 2.3).

Pre-treatment issues
- Access
- Anaesthetic

Table 2.3 Example of dental clinic appointment schedule

		Date hour	Date hour	Date hour
Patient	Last name First name Date of birth Unit number Telephones E-mail			
Systemic disease	Main problems			
Communication difficulties	Main problems			
Appointment		**Date hour**	**Date hour**	**Date hour**
Treatment planned				
Support required	Transport Disabled parking Special seating Caregiver present Additional staff, e.g. chaperone, interpreter Other			
Appropriate operative care	Antibiotic prophylaxis Bleeding test BP (blood pressure) monitoring Cardiac monitoring Medical assessment Others			
Drugs to avoid				
Behaviour control	No restraints Drugs, medications or others LA CS GA Others			

- Chaperoning
- Communication
- Co-morbidities
- Consent
- Factor replacement, haemoglobin (Hb) level, International Normalized Ratio (INR)
- Materials, procedures or medication considerations.

At treatment

- Appointment timing and duration
- Chaperoning
- Devices to consider
- Facilities required

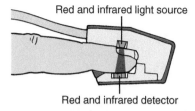
Red and infrared light source

Red and infrared detector

Figure 2.1 Pulse oximeter for measuring oxygen saturation levels.

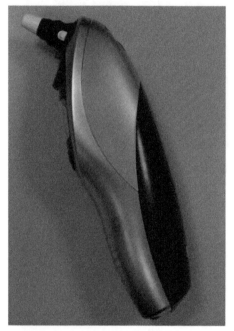

Figure 2.2 Thermometer (aural use).

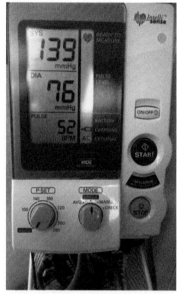

Figure 2.3 IntelliSense sphygmomanometer (Omron, Shiokoji Horikawa, Shimogyo-ku, Kyoto 600-8530 Japan).

- Haemostatics
- Patient posture
- Surgical considerations
- Monitor; vital signs – pulse, BP, respiration, oxygen saturation.

Post-treatment

- Accompanying responsible person
- Care at home
- Dietary considerations
- Hygiene
- Postoperative care
- Recall.

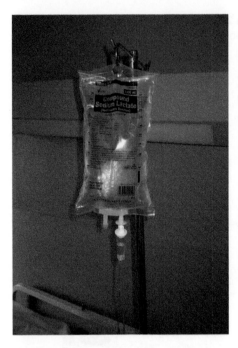

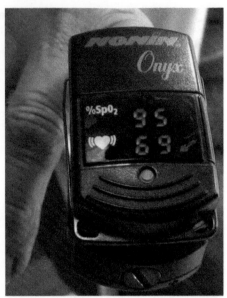

Figure 2.5 Nonin Onyx – pulse monitor.

Figure 2.4 Compound sodium lactate
– intravenous drip bag.

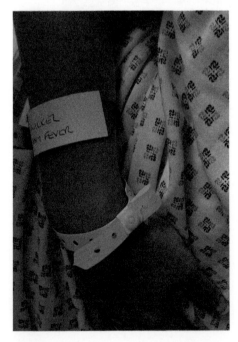

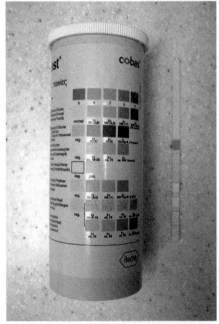

Figure 2.6 Patient identity and medical alert wrist tags.

Figure 2.7 Urinalysis dip sticks (Cobas® Roche).

Consent

In general a patient must give valid consent for any procedure (any touching), otherwise the healthcare professional is liable under UK common law, of battery. This means that a competent person can refuse any treatment, however dire the consequences. Within common law there are defences to battery other than consent: if a patient is not competent to give or withhold consent, and if treatment is in their best interests, then treatment may be undertaken under 'necessity'. The defence of 'emergency' is to allow restraint where you must act quickly to prevent the patient from harming themselves or others (or committing a crime). Emergency treatment to save life or to prevent serious harm to the patient must always be given, over-riding all the safeguards below if the patient is unable to give consent, e.g. owing to unconsciousness. Another example is that of a patient running amok, whom you could restrain – before you have the chance to fully assess the situation. The UK Mental Health Act enables treatment of someone suffering from a mental disorder for that mental disorder under certain circumstances and sets down some conditions for consent for treating in certain circumstances; consent is required and a second opinion is needed. Under all other circumstances, it is vital to obtain the patient's informed consent (valid consent) to any investigations and treatment plan. For a person 'to be competent' or 'to have the capacity to consent' they must be able to reason and weigh the risks and benefits and consequences of their decision. Adults can usually be presumed to have capacity to consent to treatment and, at age 16 years (18 in Australia), a young person is regarded as an adult and can be presumed to have capacity to consent to treatment. Where a child is under 16 years old and has the ability to understand the nature, purpose and possible consequences of the proposed investigation or treatment, as well as the consequences of non-treatment, they can be presumed to have the capacity to consent to treatment. Generally however, formal assent to treatment from a legal parent or guardian is sought for treatment of all children under 16 years.

Some patients with mental health issues, no matter how well the facts about treatment are explained to them, are incapable of understanding them or the implications of the treatment decision they are being asked to make. Such patients are regarded as *not* competent to give consent. Further, if a patient is unable to communicate adequately either by language, gesture or behaviour, they are regarded as not competent to give consent to treatment. Where a child under 16 years old is deemed not competent to consent, a person with parental responsibility (e.g. their mother or guardian) may authorize investigations or treatment, which are in the child's best interests. If a health professional believes a patient lacks the capacity to consent they cannot give or withhold consent to treatment on behalf of that patient, but they may carry out an investigation or treatment judged to be in that patient's best interest. *Principle of best interest*: in deciding what actually is in the patient's best interests the healthcare professional should take into account:

- any evidence of the patient's previous preferences
- knowledge of the patient's background
- treatment option
- views of family members and legal representatives.

Culture

Culture guides decisions and actions of a group through time and can be defined as: the sum total of the way of living; includes values, beliefs, standards, language, thinking patterns, behavioural norms, communications styles, etc. It may involve obvious aspects such as: religion, ethnicity (race), national origin (language), gender, and less obvious things (e.g. age, educational status and mobility (including impairments/handicaps).

Health belief systems may differ from the culture of Western medicine (Table 2.4). Therefore, it is important to LEARN:

Listen to the patient's perception of the problem.

Explain your perception of the problem.

Acknowledge and discuss differences/similarities.

Recommend treatment.

Negotiate treatment; modify treatment if required.

Many people with medical or dental conditions are amenable to treatment in primary care, but some people require special facilities or an escort to facilitate treatment or provide after care. Preventive healthcare, and the avoidance of non-essential surgery, other invasive procedures and operative intervention are particularly important in patients who are medically compromised. Special problems that may be encountered include:

- modifying routine treatment procedures;
- accommodating a person who is deaf or blind;
- treating a person who uses a wheelchair;
- managing/accommodating the behaviour of a resistant patient;
- ensuring airway patency;
- referring for treatment and consultation by specialists.

Treatment modifications depend not only upon the skill and experience of the team(s) involved, but also on the type and severity of the disease, its treatment and complications. Clearly the risks to the patient are greater:

- the more invasive and prolonged the operative interference;
- the more severe the medical condition;
- depending on the type of pain-control or behaviour management needed;
- depending on the extent of interference with airway or feeding, etc. postoperatively.

Table 2.4 Comparison of typical endeavours of Western with some non-Western medicine

Western medicine	Non-Western medicine
Make things better	Accept with grace
Control nature	Balance/harmony with nature
Do something	Wait and see
Intervene now	Cautious deliberation
Strong measures	Gentle approach
Plan ahead	Take life as it comes
Standardize – treat everyone the same.	Individualize – recognize differences.

Communication with other care providers

This can be crucial and ensures optimal care, particularly important in relation to:
- mental competency;
- use of sedation or general anaesthesia;
- control of bleeding tendency;
- potential drug interactions;
- antibiotic prophylaxis;
- timing and sequencing of care in a multi-disciplinary team setting such as in cancer care (e.g. nurses, social workers, support coordinators, oncologists, pathologists, psychologists, physicians, radiologists and surgeons may need to be involved).

Summary: comments that apply to the rest of this book

A risk analysis (risk–benefit analysis) is prudent before dental treatment with any patient and medical advice should be obtained if there is any concern about the medical history. Risks are generally greatest when GA or sedation are used and procedures involve haemorrhage and/or are prolonged. Defer elective care until the patient has been medically stabilized. Emergency dental care should be conservative – principally analgesics and antibiotics.

Update the medical history at every appointment. Well-managed medical conditions generally present no or few problems. Ready access to medical help, oxygen and nitroglycerin is vital. Standard infection control measures are necessary. Guidance on oral hygiene and diet are essential.

Valid consent is crucial. All patient information must be kept in a secure location, and discussing patients' medical status should only occur in a private, closed office to ensure confidentiality.

Short, stress-free appointments are recommended; it is important to avoid anxiety, stress and pain. If LA, analgesics, sedative drugs or antibiotics are contraindicated, this is highlighted in the questionnaire. The behaviour, conscious level, pulse, blood pressure and respiratory rate of all patients should be monitored before starting and periodically during treatment, checking with the patient that they feel well. High risk patients should be offered dental treatment in hospital.

3 Main emergencies

Emergencies are usually a cause for anxiety for all those involved. Therefore it is important to identify patients at risk of emergencies, assess the severity of those risks and, where necessary, recognize the need for help and be able to seek advice from a colleague with special competence in the relevant fields. All clinical staff have an obligation to be conversant with the current Resuscitation Council (UK) guidelines adapted from the 2015 European Guidelines (2015), put patients' interests first, and act to protect them. Central to this responsibility is the need to ensure that health professionals are able to deal effectively with medical emergencies that may arise.

All members of the team need to know their roles in the event of emergency. Staff who employ, manage or lead a team should make sure that:

- there are arrangements for at least two people to be available to deal with medical emergencies;
- all members of staff, not just the registered team members, know their role if a patient collapses or there is another kind of medical emergency;
- all members of staff who might be involved in dealing with a medical emergency are trained and prepared to deal with such an emergency at any time, and regularly practise simulated emergencies together.

Confidence and satisfactory management of emergencies can be improved by the following:

- Repeatedly assessing the patient whilst undertaking any treatment, noting any changes in appearance or behaviour.
- Never practising dentistry without another competent adult in the room.
- Always having accessible the telephone numbers for the emergency services and nearest hospital accident and emergency department.
- Training staff in emergency service contact protocols and emergency procedures: this should be repeated annually.
- All clinics should have a defined protocol for how the emergency services are to be alerted: the protocol should include clear directions for the emergency services to locate and access the clinic and, in a large building, a member of the team should meet the emergency services at the main entrance.
- Having readily accessible emergency box and equipment checked on a *weekly* basis (Table 3.1).
- Taking a careful medical history, assessment of disease severity, careful treatment scheduling and planning and, in some cases, administration of medication prior to treatment.
- Using the simple intervention of laying the patient supine prior to venipuncture or giving injections (e.g. dental local analgesia/anaesthesia [LA]) will prevent virtually all simple faints.
- Ensuring diabetic patients have had their normal meals, appropriately administered medication, and are treated early in the morning session or immediately after lunch is likely to prevent most hypoglycaemic collapses.

Table 3.1 Suggested minimal equipment and drugs for emergency use in dentistry (after Resuscitation Council, 2012)

Equipment	General comments	Detail
Oxygen (O$_2$) delivery	Portable apparatus for administering oxygen Oxygen face (non-rebreathe type) mask with tube Basic set of oropharyngeal airways (sizes 1, 2, 3 and 4) Pocket mask with oxygen port Self-inflating bag valve mask (BVM; 1-L size bag), where staff have been appropriately trained Variety of well-fitting adult and child face masks for attaching to self-inflating bag	Two portable oxygen cylinders* (D size) with pressure reduction valves and flow meters. Cylinders should be of sufficient size to be easily portable but also allow for adequate flow rates (e.g. 10 L/min, until the arrival of an ambulance or the patient fully recovers
Portable suction	Portable suction with appropriate suction catheters and tubing (e.g. the Yankauer sucker)	
Spacer device for inhalation of bronchodilators		
Automated external defibrillator (AED)	All clinical areas should have immediate access to an AED (Collapse to shock time less than 3 minutes)	
Automated blood glucose measuring device		
Equipment for administering drugs intramuscularly	Single-use sterile syringes (2-mL and 10-mL sizes) and needles (19 and 21 sizes)	Drugs as below

Emergency	Drugs required	Dosages for adults
Anaphylaxis	Adrenaline (epinephrine) injection 1:1000, 1 mg/mL	Intramuscular adrenaline (0.5 mL of 1 in 1000 solution) Repeat at 5 minutes if needed
Hypoglycaemia	Oral glucose solution/tablets/gel/powder [e.g. 'GlucoGel®' formerly known as 'Hypostop®' gel (40% dextrose)] Glucagon injection 1 mg (e.g. GlucaGen HypoKit)	Proprietary non-diet drink or 5 g glucose powder in water Intramuscular glucagon 1 mg
Acute exacerbation of asthma	(Beta-2 agonist) Salbutamol aerosol inhaler 100 mcg/activation	Salbutamol aerosol Activations directly or up to six into a spacer
Status epilepticus	Buccal or intranasal midazolam 10 mg/mL	Midazolam 10 mg
Angina**	Glyceryl trinitrate spray 400 mcg/metered activation	Glyceryl trinitrate, two sprays
Myocardial infarct	Dispersible aspirin 300 mg	Dispersible aspirin 300 mg (chewed)

*Where possible, all emergency equipment should be single use and latex free. The kit does not include any intravenous injections.
**Do not use nitrates to relieve an angina attack if the patient has recently taken sildenafil as there may be a precipitous fall in BP; analgesics should be used.

All this is even more important when conscious sedation (CS) is used, when there are invasive or painful procedures, or when medically complex individuals are being treated. 'Forewarned is forearmed', and health professionals must ensure that medical and drug histories are updated at each visit. It is suggested disease severity should be assessed using a risk stratification system, for example the American Society of Anesthesiologists (ASA) classification (see Table 2.2) as this may help identify high-risk individuals.

Few emergencies can be treated definitively in the clinic: the role of the team is one of support and considered intervention using algorithms that can 'do no harm'. The other agents (e.g. flumazenil) and equipment (e.g. a pulse oximeter) are needed if CS is administered.

General anaesthesia (GA) must only be undertaken by anaesthetists and where advanced life support (ALS) is available.

For all medical emergencies, a structured approach to assessment and reassessment prevents any symptoms and signs being missed and any incorrect diagnoses being made. 'Doctors' ABC' highlights the sequence:

- **D**anger (recognizing an emergency).
- **R**espiration (establishing an airway).
- **S**hout for help.
- **A**irway, **B**reathing, **C**irculation.

People who collapse should be put in the 'recovery position' to maintain a clear airway, UNLESS there could be a neck injury such as after a fall, or after a road traffic accident, when the neck must be protected.

Emergency procedure

- Call for local assistance.
- Assess patient – ABCDE (Table 3.2) – and give oxygen if appropriate.
- Use acronym MOVE (see below).

Table 3.2	ABCDE Assessment in emergencies
Airway	Identify any foreign body obstruction and stridor
Breathing	Document respiratory rate; use of accessory muscles; presence of wheeze or cyanosis
Circulation	Assess skin colour and temperature; estimate capillary refill time (normally, this is 2 seconds with hand above heart); assess rate of pulse (normal is 60–100 beats/min)
Disability	Assay blood glucose. Assess conscious level by AVPU: **A**lert responds to **V**oice responds to **P**ainful stimulus **U**nresponsive
Exposure	Respecting the patient's dignity, try to elicit the cause of acute deterioration (e.g. rash, or signs of recreational drug use)

ADULT BASIC LIFE SUPPORT   **Figure 3.1** Adult basic life support (BLS).

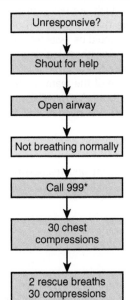

The 'ABCDE' approach to the sick patient

The 'ABCDE' approach to the sick patient in www.resus.org.uk/pages/medental.pdf by the UK Resuscitation Council (2015) cannot be bettered. Specific emergencies are discussed here.

Early recognition of the 'sick' patient is to be encouraged. Pre-empting any medical emergency by recognizing an abnormal breathing pattern, an abnormal patient colour or abnormal pulse rate, allows appropriate help (e.g., ambulance) to be summoned, prior to any collapse.

The patient brought in with an emergency

A systematic approach to recognizing the acutely ill patient based on 'ABCDE' principles is recommended. Accurate documentation of the patient's medical history should further allow those 'at risk' of certain medical emergencies to be identified in advance of any proposed intervention. The elective nature of most procedures allows time for discussion of medical problems. In certain circumstances this may lead to a postponement of the treatment indicated or a recommendation that such treatment be undertaken in hospital.

1. Follow the **A**irway, **B**reathing, **C**irculation, **D**isability, and **E**xposure approach (ABCDE) to assessment and treatment.
2. Treat life-threatening problems as they are identified before moving to the next part of the assessment.
3. Continually re-assess starting with Airway if there is further deterioration.
4. Assess the effects of any treatment given.
5. *Recognize when you need extra help and call for help early.* This may mean dialling 999 for an ambulance. In all circumstances of doubt it is advisable to call for medical assistance as soon as possible.

6. Clearly establish a team leader, organize your team and communicate effectively.
7. Use all members of your team: this allows you to do several things at once, e.g. collect emergency drugs and equipment; dial 999.
8. The aims of initial treatment are to keep the patient alive, achieve some clinical improvement and buy time for further treatment whilst waiting for help.
9. Remember – it can take a few minutes for treatment to work.
10. The ABCDE approach can be used irrespective of your training and experience in clinical assessment or treatment. Individual experience and training will determine which treatments you can give. *Often simple measures only, such as laying the patient down or giving oxygen are needed. Then **MOVE**:*
    Monitor – reassess ABCDE regularly, attach an AED (Automated External Defibrillator) if appropriate.
    Oxygen – 15 L/min through a non-rebreathe mask.
    Verify emergency services are coming.
    Emergency action – correct positioning and drug administration.

An emergency in the dental setting

First steps

In an emergency, stay calm. Ensure that you and your staff are safe.

Look at the patient generally to see if they 'look unwell'. In an awake patient ask, 'How are you?' If the patient is unresponsive, shake them and ask, 'Are you all right?' If they respond normally, they have a clear airway, are breathing and have brain perfusion. If they speak only in short sentences, they may have breathing problems.

Failure of the patient to respond suggests that they are unwell. If they are not breathing and have no pulse or signs of life, start CPR according to current resuscitation guidelines.

Airway (A)

Airway obstruction is an emergency.
1. Look for signs of airway obstruction: Airway obstruction causes 'paradoxical' chest and abdominal movements ('see-saw' respirations) and the use of the accessory muscles of respiration, e.g., neck muscles. Central cyanosis (blue lips and tongue) is a late sign of airway obstruction. In complete airway obstruction, there are no breath sounds at the mouth or nose. In partial airway obstruction, air entry is diminished and usually noisy:
   * *Inspiratory 'stridor'* is caused by obstruction at the laryngeal level or above.
   * *Expiratory 'wheeze'* suggests obstruction of the lower airways, which tend to collapse and obstruct during expiration. This is most commonly seen in patients with asthma or chronic obstructive pulmonary disease.
   * *Gurgling* suggests there is liquid or semi-solid foreign material in the upper airway.
   * *Snoring* arises when the pharynx is partially occluded by the tongue or palate.
2. Airway obstruction is an emergency: In most cases, only simple methods of airway clearance are needed:
   * *Airway opening manoeuvres* – head tilt/chin lift or jaw thrust.
   * *Remove visible foreign bodies*, debris or blood from the airway (use suction or forceps as necessary). Do not perform a blind airway sweep.
   * *Consider simple airway adjuncts*, e.g. oropharyngeal airway. Note that fully conscious patients will not tolerate such adjuncts and insertion is likely to

precipitate gagging or vomiting. Their use is however invaluable in patients with a reduced conscious level.

3. *Give oxygen* initially at a high inspired concentration: Use a mask with an oxygen (O_2) reservoir. Ensure that the oxygen flow is sufficient (15 litres per minute) to prevent collapse of the reservoir during inspiration. If you have a pulse oximeter, titrate the oxygen delivery aiming for normal oxygen saturation levels (94–98%). In very sick patients this may not be possible and a lower oxygen saturation (more than 90%) is acceptable for a short period of time. Note that under normal circumstances it is usual for patients with chronic obstructive pulmonary disease (COPD) to maintain saturations of 88–92%. However, any critically ill patient, including those with COPD, should be treated immediately with high concentration oxygen. Once the condition of the patient has become more stable, the oxygen prescription can be reassessed according to risk of hypercapnic respiratory failure. Using high flow O_2 in patients with COPD is perfectly justified in the initial treatment of an emergency.

Breathing (B)

During the immediate assessment of breathing, it is vital to diagnose and treat immediately life-threatening breathing problems, e.g., acute severe asthma.

1. *Look, listen and feel for the general signs of respiratory distress*: sweating, central cyanosis (blue lips and tongue), use of the accessory muscles of respiration (muscles of the neck) and abdominal breathing.
2. *Count the respiratory rate*. The normal adult rate is 12 to 20 breaths per minute and a child's rate is between 20 and 30 breaths per minute. A high, or increasing, respiratory rate is a marker of illness and a warning that the patient may deteriorate and further medical help is needed.
3. *Assess each breath* depth, the pattern (rhythm) of respiration and whether chest expansion is equal and normal on both sides.
4. *Listen to the patient's breath sounds* a short distance from their face. Gurgling airway noises indicate airway secretions, usually because the patient cannot cough or take a deep breath. Stridor or wheeze suggests partial, but important, airway obstruction.
5. *Use bag and mask (if trained) or pocket mask ventilation with supplemental oxygen* while calling urgently for an ambulance if the patient's breathing is of inadequate depth or rate, or you cannot detect any breathing. 'Agonal' breaths may sound laboured or gasping in nature, are common after cardiac arrest, and should not be confused with normal breathing.
6. Hyperventilation and panic attacks are relatively common and typically resolve with simple reassurance.

Circulation (C)

Simple faints or vasovagal episodes are the most likely cause of circulation problems, which will usually respond to laying the patient flat and if necessary raising the legs. The systematic ABCDE approach to all patients will ensure that other causes are not missed.

1. Look at the colour of the hands and fingers: are they blue, pink, pale or mottled?
2. Assess the limb temperature by feeling the patient's hands: are they cool or warm?
3. Measure the capillary refill time. Apply cutaneous pressure for five seconds on a fingertip held at heart level (or just above) with enough pressure to cause blanching. Time how long it takes for the skin to return to the colour of the surrounding skin after releasing the pressure. The normal refill time is less than two seconds. A prolonged time suggests poor peripheral perfusion. Other factors (e.g. cold

surroundings, old age) can also prolong the capillary refill time therefore a central capillary refill time, obtained by applying similar cutaneous pressure to the skin over the upper chest, is preferable if accessible.

4. Count the patient's pulse rate. It may be easier to feel a central pulse (i.e. carotid pulse) than the radial pulse. Do not however delay starting resuscitation to assess the pulse if the patient is not breathing or displaying any other signs of life.
5. Weak pulses in a patient with a decreased conscious level and slow capillary refill time suggest a low BP. Laying the patient down and raising the legs may be helpful. In patients who do not respond to simple measures, urgent help is needed and an ambulance should be summoned.
6. Cardiac chest pain typically presents as a heaviness, tightness or indigestion-like discomfort in the chest. The pain or discomfort often radiates into the neck or throat, into one or both arms (more commonly the left) and into the back or stomach area. Some patients experience the discomfort in one of these areas more than in the chest. Sometimes pain may be accompanied by belching, which can be misinterpreted as evidence of indigestion as the cause. The patient may have known stable angina and carry their own glyceryl trinitrate (GTN) spray or tablets. If they take these, the episode may resolve. If the patient has sustained chest pain, give GTN spray if the patient has not already taken some. The patient may feel better and should be encouraged to sit upright if possible. Give a single dose of aspirin and consider the use of oxygen.

Disability (D)

Common causes of unconsciousness include profound hypoxia (low oxygen levels), hypercapnia (raised carbon dioxide levels), cerebral hypoperfusion (low BP), or the recent administration of sedatives or analgesic drugs.

1. Review and treat the ABCs: exclude hypoxia and low BP.
2. Check the patient's drug record for reversible drug-induced causes of depressed consciousness.
3. Examine the pupils (size, equality and reaction to light).
4. Make a rapid initial assessment of the patient's conscious level using the **AVPU** method (**A**lert, responds to **V**ocal stimuli, responds to **P**ainful stimuli or **U**nresponsive to all stimuli).
5. Measure the blood glucose to exclude hypoglycaemia, using a glucose meter. If below 3.0 mmol per litre give the patient a glucose containing drink to raise the blood sugar (e.g. *Glucogel; Dextrogel; GSF-syrup* or *Rapilose* gel) or glucose by other means.
6. Nurse unconscious patients in the recovery position if their airway is not protected.

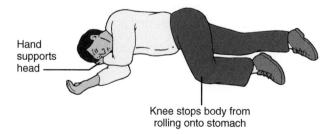

Hand supports head

Knee stops body from rolling onto stomach

Figure 3.2 Recovery position.

Exposure (E)

To assess and treat the patient properly loosening or removal of some of the patient's clothes may be necessary. Respect the patient's culture and dignity and minimize heat loss. This will allow you to see any rashes or perform procedures (e.g. defibrillation).

Cardiopulmonary resuscitation (CPR)

Healthcare staff should all be trained in basic CPR so that, in the event of cardiac arrest, they should be able to:

- recognize cardiac arrest (heart stops beating)
- summon immediate help (dial for the emergency services)
- initiate CPR according to current resuscitation guidelines
- ventilate with high-concentration oxygen via a bag and mask
- apply an AED as soon as possible after collapse. Follow the machine prompts and administer a shock if indicated.

Hands only CPR is now recommended by the British Heart Foundation:

- Call the emergency services.
- Push hard and fast in the centre of the chest to double a person's chances of survival ('Stayin' Alive' music has the right beat for Hands-Only CPR).
- The method of delivering chest compressions remains the same, as does the rate (at 100–120 beats per minute, to a depth of 5–6 cm). Resuscitation Council guidelines recommend a 30 chest compression: 2 breath ratio during CPR. They no longer recommend 2 rescue breaths before starting the chest compressions however. There is a drive to deliver uninterrupted compressions and ideally this is done alongside independent ventilation when an advanced airway is in position. Continuous compressions are better than inadequate breaths in between compressions, so if in doubt, or if there is debris in the mouth with no barrier protection, then just doing compressions is fine. The official guidelines do recommend 30:2 though.

Management of the more common emergencies in dentistry

The most common medical emergency is the simple faint. Apart from that are anaphylaxis, seizures (fitting) in an epileptic patient, asthma, angina pectoris (ischaemic chest pain), and hypoglycaemia in a diabetic patient. Myocardial infarction and cardiopulmonary arrest are more immediately dangerous. *If the patient does not respond to the immediate emergency care outlined below, treatment then the priority is to transfer the patient to hospital as an emergency*. If the patient is unconscious, secure their airway and place in the recovery position and give oxygen.

Anaphylaxis (see also Section 5)

Anaphylaxis is a severe, life-threatening, generalized or systemic type 1 hypersensitivity reaction, characterized by rapidly developing problems threatening the airway and/or breathing and/or circulation usually associated with skin and mucosal changes.

- Always detail known allergies and the severity of any previous hypersensitivity reactions.

- Avoid possible allergens and, when this is not possible, refer for specialist assessment.
- Life-threatening anaphylaxis may occur despite no previous history of allergen exposure.
- The causal agents may include:
  - penicillins – the most common cause, but also other antimicrobials (cephalosporins, sulfonamides, tetracyclines, vancomycin)
  - latex
  - muscle relaxants
  - non-steroidal anti-inflammatory drugs (NSAIDs)
  - opiates
  - radiographic contrast media
  - others – vaccines, immunoglobulins, various foods and insect bites.
- Anaphylactic reactions may follow the administration of a drug or contact with substances such as latex in surgical gloves. Anaphylactic reactions may also be associated with *additives* and *excipients* in medicines. It is wise therefore to check the full formulation of preparations which may contain allergenic fats or oils (including those for topical application).
- Strict avoidance of the causal agent is essential.

Symptoms and signs

Symptoms and signs can develop within minutes:

- Anaphylaxis is the most severe allergic response and manifests with tachycardia (heart rate >110 per minute) and increased respiratory rate, acute hypotension, bronchospasm (stridor and wheezing), urticarial rash and angioedema.
- Vasodilation causes relative hypovolaemia leading to low BP and collapse. This can cause cardiac arrest.
- Marked upper airway (laryngeal) oedema and bronchospasm may develop, causing stridor, wheezing and/or a hoarse voice. Respiratory arrest leading to cardiac arrest.
- Flushing is common, but pallor may also occur, as may urticaria, erythema, rhinitis or conjunctivitis.
- Abdominal pain, vomiting, diarrhoea and a sense of impending doom.
- The lack of any consistent clinical manifestation and a wide range of possible presentations can cause diagnostic difficulty.
- Eventual loss of consciousness.

Treatment

In general, the more rapid the onset of the reaction, the more serious it will be. Early, effective treatment may be life-saving. Patients having an anaphylactic reaction in any setting should expect the following as a minimum:

- Recognition that they are seriously unwell. Initial treatments should not be delayed by the lack of a complete history or definite diagnosis.
- An early call for help.
- Initial assessment and treatments based on an ABCDE approach.
- Treat the greatest threat to life first.
- Remove any obvious allergen exposure.
- First-line treatment includes managing the airway and breathing and restoration of BP (laying the patient flat, raising the feet) and the administration of oxygen (15 litres per minute).

- Adrenaline should be given intramuscularly (anterolateral aspect of the middle third of the thigh) in a dose for adults of 500 micrograms (0.5 mL adrenaline injection of 1:1000); an autoinjector preparation delivering a dose of 300 micrograms (0.3 mL adrenaline injection 1:1000) is available for immediate *self-administration* by those patients known to have severe reactions. This is an acceptable alternative if immediately available. The dose is repeated if necessary at 5 minute intervals according to BP, pulse and respiratory function. The paediatric adrenaline dose is based on the child's approximate age or weight.
- All patients treated for an anaphylactic reaction should then be sent to hospital by ambulance for further assessment, irrespective of any initial recovery. Further treatment may involve use of antihistamines (10 mg i.m. chlorphenamine), steroids (200 mg i.m. hydrocortisone) and IV fluids, but these will be administered by ambulance personnel if necessary.
- Where there is a previous history of anaphylaxis, the patient should thereafter always carry an i.m. injection device, for example EpiPen® (ALK-Abelló, Hungerford, Berkshire, UK), Jext (ALK-Abelló Ltd: 1 Manor Park, Manor Farm Road, Reading, Berkshire, RG2 0NA), Emerade (iMed Systems Ltd;5 Walker Close, London N11 1AQ, UK) or Twinject® (Verus Pharmaceuticals, San Diego, California, USA) (or less commonly epinephrine aerosol, such as MedihalerEpi) for self-administration.

www.resus.org.uk/pages/reaction.pdf.

Angina (see also Section 5)

Angina is characterized by paroxysms of severe chest pain caused by ischaemia and myocardial oxygen demands in coronary atherosclerosis. Mortality rate from myocardial infarction (MI) is about 4% per year.

Emotion (especially anger or anxiety), stress, fear or pain, lead to adrenal catecholamine (adrenaline and noradrenaline) release and consequent tachycardia, vasoconstriction and raised BP which can induce angina.

Symptoms and signs

Central chest pain, or pressure, described as a sense of strangling or choking, or tightness, heaviness, compression or constriction of the chest, sometimes radiating to the neck, left arm or jaw, and possibly nausea or sweating. The pain is brought on more typically by physical exertion, particularly in cold weather, and is relieved by rest.

Treatment

If there is a history of angina, the patient will probably carry glyceryl trinitrate spray or tablets (or isosorbide dinitrate tablets) and they should be allowed to use them.

- Assess the patient.
- Give oxygen and glyceryl trinitrate (GTN) spray or tablets which may offer relief. The patient may feel better and should be encouraged to sit upright if possible.
- If pain does not abate, consider myocardial infarction, give a single dose of aspirin (300 mg) and continue oxygen.
- Where symptoms are mild and resolve rapidly with the patient's own medication, hospital admission is not normally necessary.

Asthma (see also Section 5)

Anxiety, infection, or exposure to an allergen or drugs may precipitate asthma. High-risk asthmatics include those individuals:

- taking oral medication in addition to inhaled β_2 agonists and corticosteroids;
- who regularly use a nebulizer at home;
- who have required oral steroids for their asthma within the last year;
- who have been admitted to hospital with asthma within the last year.

Symptoms and signs

Diagnostic features are:

- Breathlessness.
- Expiratory wheeze.
- Use of accessory muscles – shrugging shoulders with each respiratory cycle with increased severity.
- Rapid pulse (usually over 110/min) with increasing severity but this may slow in life-threatening exacerbation.

Clinical features of **acute severe asthma** in adults include:

- Inability to complete sentences in one breath.
- Respiratory rate >25 per minute.
- Tachycardia (heart rate >110 per minute).

Clinical features of **life-threatening asthma** in adults include:

- Cyanosis or respiratory rate <8 per minute.
- Bradycardia (heart rate <50 per minute).
- Exhaustion, confusion, decreased conscious level.

Treatment

- Oxygen (15 litres per minute) should be given; sit patient upright.
- Most attacks will respond to a few 'activations' of the patient's own short-acting beta2-adrenoceptor stimulant inhaler such as salbutamol (100 micrograms/actuation). Repeat doses may be necessary.
- If the patient does not respond rapidly, or if the patient develops tachycardia, becomes distressed or cyanosed, or cannot complete a sentence in 1 breath, severe asthma is present, and an ambulance should be summoned.
- Up to 10 activations from the salbutamol inhaler should be given using a large-volume spacer device and repeated every 10 minutes if necessary until an ambulance arrives. All emergency ambulances carry nebulizers, oxygen and appropriate drugs.
- If bronchospasm is part of a more generalized anaphylactic reaction and there are 'life-threatening' signs, an intramuscular injection of adrenaline should be given.

www.brit-thoracic.org.uk/guidelines/asthma-guidelines.aspx

Choking (Foreign body respiratory obstruction)

The treatment of the choking patient involves removing any visible foreign bodies from the mouth and pharynx

- In cases of aspiration, encourage the patient to cough vigorously if conscious. If they are unable to cough but remain conscious then sharp back blows should be delivered.

- These can be followed by abdominal thrusts (Heimlich manoeuvre) if the foreign body has not been dislodged.
- Where the patient is symptomatic following aspiration or if foreign material has been or may have been, aspirated they should be referred to hospital as an emergency for a chest radiography and possible removal.
- If the patient becomes unconscious, CPR should be started. This will not only provide circulatory support but the pressure generated within the chest by performing chest compressions may help to dislodge the foreign body.

Collapse (see also Section 5)

Collapse is a universal colloquialism that refers to a person who has had an abrupt loss of postural tone. Often this is a transient loss of consciousness ('blackout'), the most important causes being syncope, epilepsy and psychogenic blackouts. Determining the correct cause is important to ensure treatment is correct but challenging, owing to the heterogeneous nature of causes, ranging from benign neurocardiogenic syncope to potentially fatal cardiac arrhythmias and pulmonary embolism.

The cause may be suggested by the medical history, which may be collapse:

- at the sight of a needle or during an injection is likely to be a simple faint;
- following some minutes after an injection of a drug such as penicillin; this is more likely to be due to anaphylaxis;
- of a diabetic at lunchtime, for example, is likely to be caused by hypoglycaemia;
- of a patient with angina or previous myocardial infarction, which may be caused by a new or further myocardial infarction.

The clinical features of the episode may also aid diagnosis; for example, severe chest pain suggests a cardiac cause.

Other causes of sudden loss of consciousness include:

- Situational syncope provoked by coughing, micturition or postural change.
- Cardiac syncope due to arrhythmia or circulatory obstruction – typically in older people.
- Orthostatic hypotension.
- Neurological disorders.
- Very rarely – *malignant vasovagal syncope* with recurrent, severe and otherwise unexplained syncope.

The principles of the *chain of survival*, which applies to emergencies where the patient is not breathing and has no pulse, involve four stages:

- early recognition and call for help;
- early CPR;
- early defibrillation; and
- early basic life support.

The cause of collapse may not be immediately clear and assessment and treatment should follow the ABCDE approach as outlined previously. Further investigation including full neurological and cardiovascular examination will be required. This may include looking for a postural BP drop (a fall of ≥20 mmHg, or a fall to <90 mmHg after standing for at least 3 minutes), a displaced apex beat, signs of cardiac failure or carotid bruits, or a ventricular pause of >3 seconds precipitated by carotid sinus massage (testing for carotid sinus hypersensitivity). An ECG is warranted.

Epileptic seizure (see also Section 5)

Fits (convulsions) are usually seen in people known to suffer epilepsy. Fits may also affect people with no history of epilepsy, especially following hypoxia from a faint or loss of consciousness for other reasons, or in hypoglycaemia.

Various factors may precipitate a fit in a person who suffers epilepsy, including not eating, cessation of anticonvulsant therapy (patients with epilepsy should continue their normal dosage of anticonvulsant drugs before attending for other treatment), menstruation and some drugs (e.g. alcohol, flumazenil, recreational drugs or tricyclic antidepressants).

Symptoms and signs of a tonic-clonic (grand mal) seizure

- There may be a brief warning or 'aura'.
- Sudden loss of consciousness.
- The patient becomes rigid, falls, may give a cry, and becomes cyanosed (tonic phase).
- After seconds, the limbs jerk repeatedly; the tongue or lip may be bitten (clonic phase).
- There may be frothing from the mouth and urinary incontinence.
- A seizure typically lasts a few minutes; the patient may become floppy but remain unconscious.
- After a variable time the patient regains consciousness but may remain confused.

Treatment

During a seizure, try to ensure that the patient is not at risk from injury but make no attempt to put anything in the mouth or between the teeth (in the mistaken belief this will protect the tongue). Do not attempt to insert an oropharyngeal airway or other airway adjunct while the patient is actively fitting.

- Summon help.
- Clear the airway
- Do *not* attempt to force a spoon or tongue depressor or other hard object between the teeth because you can cause more damage than you are trying to prevent. Clear the area of equipment, furniture or other objects that may cause injury during the seizure. Do not attempt to restrain or hold the person down during the seizure.
- Turn the person onto the side into the 'head-injury position' and protect from aspiration (inhaling) of mucus or vomit.
- If the person having seizures stops breathing or becomes cyanotic, check the airway and prevent the tongue from obstructing it.
- In an uncomplicated seizure no other treatment is necessary. CPR or mouth-to-mouth breathing cannot be performed during a seizure and is rarely needed after seizures.
- Breathing usually recommences spontaneously once the seizure terminates.
- If the patient remains unresponsive check for 'signs of life' (breathing and circulation) and start CPR in the absence of signs of life or normal breathing (ignore occasional 'gasps'). Check for the presence of a very slow heart rate (<40 per minute) which may drop the BP.
- Fitting may be a presenting sign of *hypoglycaemia* and should be considered in all patients, especially known diabetics and children. An early blood glucose

measurement is essential in all actively fitting patients (including known epileptics). Check blood glucose level to exclude hypoglycaemia. If blood glucose <3.0 mmol per litre or hypoglycaemia is clinically suspected, give oral/buccal glucose (e.g. *Glucogel; Dextrogel; GSF-syrup* or *Rapilose* gel), or glucagon (see above and *Hypoglycaemia* below).

- Medication should be given if seizures are prolonged (convulsive movements lasting 5 minutes or longer – *status epilepticus*) or recur in quick succession. In this situation an ambulance should be summoned urgently. If a patient continues to fit after an ambulance has been called, the emergency administration of buccal midazolam to assist in terminating the seizure is warranted in a single 10 mg dose for adults. For children the dose is age-dependent: (child 1–5 years 5 mg, child 5–10 years 7.5 mg, above 10 years 10 mg). Buccolam is available as a 5 mg/mL solution for use in children up to 17 years old. Its use in adults is 'off licence' but the recommended dose is the same as that for the older child, i.e. 10 mg (2 mL). This 'off licence' use is justified in an emergency situation. With prolonged or recurrent seizures, ambulance personnel will often administer i.v. diazepam which is usually rapidly effective in stopping any seizure.

Midazolam is a schedule 3 controlled drug (CD). This means that:

- prescriptions or requisitions for midazolam must comply with the full CD regulations;
- records of midazolam usage do not need to be kept in a CD register;
- invoices for midazolam need to be retained for 2 years;
- midazolam (as other schedule 3 drugs) should be denatured before being placed in waste containers.
- midazolam is exempt from the safe custody requirements and will not legally require storage in a CD cabinet.

In both the 'licensed' and 'off licensed' setting, midazolam does not need to have been prescribed to the patient when used in an emergency. It should however be administered by (or under the supervision of) a healthcare practitioner.

It may not always be necessary to transfer to hospital unless the convulsion was atypical, prolonged (or repeated), or if injury occurred. The National Institute for Health and Clinical Excellence (NICE) guidelines suggest indications for sending a seizure patient to hospital are:

- Status epilepticus.
- High risk of recurrence.
- First episode.
- Difficulty monitoring the individual's condition.

After the seizure the patient may be confused ('post-ictal confusion') and may need reassurance and sympathy. The patient should not be sent home until fully recovered and they should be accompanied by a responsible adult.

Faint

Fainting (syncope) is the most common cause of sudden loss of consciousness. Inadequate cerebral perfusion (and oxygenation) results in hypoxia and loss of consciousness. This most commonly occurs with low BP caused by vagal overactivity (a vasovagal or vasodepressor attack, simple faint, or syncope). This in turn may follow emotional stress or pain. Pressure on the vagus nerve may also cause a faint. Some patients are more prone to this and have a history of repeated faints. Young, fit, adult males in particular are prone to faint, especially before, during and after injections. Predisposing factors include: anxiety, pain, fatigue, fasting (rarely), high temperature and relative humidity.

Symptoms and signs
- Patient feels faint/dizzy/light headed.
- Slow pulse rate.
- Low BP.
- Pallor and cold clammy skin.
- Nausea and vomiting.
- Loss of consciousness.

The diagnosis rests on the history, upright posture, an emotional or painful stimulus, gradual not sudden fading of consciousness, sweating, nausea, pallor, other manifestations of autonomic activity, and rapid recovery on lying down.

Treatment
- Lay the patient flat as soon as possible and raise the legs to improve venous return. People who have fainted recover quickly and spontaneously.
- Loosen tight clothing, especially around the neck and give oxygen (15 litres per minute).
- If a patient becomes unresponsive, always check for 'signs of life' (breathing, circulation) and start CPR in the absence of normal pulse or breathing (ignore occasional 'gasps').

The simple precaution of laying patients flat *before* giving injections may prevent fainting.

Hypoglycaemia (see also Section 5)

Hypoglycaemia (low blood sugar) is dangerous because the brain becomes starved of glucose.

Diabetics treated with insulin, those with poor blood glucose control or poor awareness of their hypoglycaemic episodes have a greater chance of losing consciousness.

Symptoms and signs
- Hypoglycaemia may present as a deepening drowsiness, disorientation, excitability or aggressiveness, especially if it is known that a meal has been missed.
- Patients may recognize the symptoms themselves and will usually respond quickly to glucose. Children may not have such obvious features but may appear lethargic.
- Shaking and trembling.
- Sweating.
- Headache.
- Difficulty in concentration/vagueness.
- Slurring of speech.
- Aggression and confusion.
- Fitting/seizures.
- Unconsciousness.

Treatment

- Try to confirm the diagnosis by measuring the blood glucose. Remember a diabetic person may collapse for other reasons – for example a faint or myocardial infarction. Ischaemic heart disease is common in long-standing diabetes.
- *In early stages – where the patient is co-operative* and conscious with an intact gag reflex, give oral glucose (sugar [sucrose], milk with added sugar, glucose tablets or gel [e.g. *Glucogel; Dextrogel; GSF-syrup* or *Rapilose* gel]). If necessary this may be repeated in 10–15 minutes.
- *In more severe cases – where the patient has impaired consciousness, is uncooperative or is unable to swallow safely*, give oxygen, and buccal glucose gel and IM glucagon (1 mg in adults and children >8 years old or >25 kg, 0.5 mg if <8 years old or <25 kg). Remember it may take 5–10 minutes for glucagon to work and it requires the patient to have adequate glucose stores, and thus may be ineffective in anorexic, alcoholic or non-diabetic patients.
- The patient's mental status should improve within 10 minutes: re-check the blood glucose to ensure it has risen to at least 5.0 mmol per litre.
- If the patient does not respond or any difficulty is experienced, the ambulance service should be summoned immediately.
- If any patient becomes unconscious, always check for 'signs of life' (breathing and circulation) and start CPR in the absence of signs of life or normal breathing (ignore occasional 'gasps').
- It is important, especially in patients who have been given glucagon that, once they are alert and able to swallow, they are given a drink containing glucose and if possible some food high in carbohydrate. The patient may go home if fully recovered and they are accompanied by a responsible adult. They should not drive themselves.

Myocardial infarction (see also Section 5)

The pain of myocardial infarction is similar to that of angina, but generally more severe and prolonged and there may only be a partial or no response to GTN.

Symptoms and signs

- Progressive onset of severe, persistent, crushing pain in the centre and across the front of chest. The pain may radiate to the shoulders and down the arms (more commonly the left), into the neck and jaw or through to the back.
- Nausea and vomiting are common.
- Pulse may be weak and BP may fall.
- Dyspnoea.
- Skin becomes pale and clammy.

Treatment

- Call an ambulance immediately.
- Give sublingual GTN spray if this has not already been given.
- Allow the patient to rest in the position that feels most comfortable; in the presence of breathlessness this is likely to be the sitting position. Patients who faint or feel faint should be laid flat; often an intermediate position (dictated by the patient) will be most appropriate.

- Reassure the patient as far as possible to relieve further anxiety.
- Give aspirin in a single dose of 300 mg orally, crushed or chewed.
- Give high flow oxygen (15 litres per minute) particularly if the patient is cyanosed (blue lips) or conscious level deteriorates.
- If the patient becomes unresponsive, always check for 'signs of life' (breathing and circulation), and start CPR in the absence of signs of life or normal breathing (ignore occasional 'gasps').

Ambulance staff and hospital should be made aware aspirin has been given. Many ambulance services administer thrombolytics before hospital admission.

Cardiac arrest (see also Section 5)

Ventricular fibrillation accounts for most sudden cardiac arrests. Cardiac arrest is more likely in those with a history of ischaemic heart disease, diabetics and older people, but can occur in a patient with no previous history of cardiac problems and causes may include hypoxia, drug overdose, anaphylaxis, severe infection or severe hypotension. Resuscitation Council algorithms refer to the '4 Hs and 4 Ts' when considering possible reversible causes of cardiac arrest: Hypoxia, hypovolaemia, hypothermia, hypo/hyperkalaemia and other metabolic disturbance, thrombosis, tamponade (cardiac), toxins and tension pneumothorax.

Symptoms and signs

Collapse, loss of consciousness, no breathing, no pulse, no BP. Pupil dilatation is a late sign.

Treatment

Defibrillate. Give oxygen. Summon an ambulance. BLS needs to be initiated immediately to maintain adequate cerebral perfusion until the underlying cause is identified and reversed, and comprises:

- initial assessment;
- airway maintenance;
- chest compression (CPR);
- ventilation.

Stroke (see also Section 5)

Stroke may rarely occur in apparently healthy patients, but is more common in older and hypertensive individuals especially with a stroke history.

Diagnosis varies with the amount and site of brain damage but typically includes:

- facial palsy;
- arm or leg unilateral weakness;
- speech loss;
- loss of consciousness.

Treatment

Call ambulance, give oxygen and urgently admit to a stroke unit or hospital. FAST is the acronym covering this – Facial palsy; Arm weakness, Speech disturbance and Time (Get immediately to hospital) (Table 3.3).

Table 3.3 Common emergencies

Emergency	Features	Actions; reassure patient and accompanying people, and		
		1. give oxygen 15 L/min	2. other main actions	3. alert emergency services
Anaphylaxis	Acute Collapse Rash Angioedema Wheezing	Yes	Raise legs Adrenaline 500 micrograms for adult i.m. (0.5 mL of 1 in 1000 adrenaline)	Yes
Angina	Severe chest pain, responding to GTN*	Yes	GTN 2 puffs sublingually	Only if no spontaneous recovery after (2)
Asthma exacerbation	Breathless Wheeze Speechless Possible cyanosis	Yes	Sit patient up and forwards, salbutamol 2 × 100 microgram puffs for adult via spacer	If no spontaneous recovery after (2)
Cardiac arrest	Severe chest pain, not responding to GTN Collapse Pallor Breathlessness Sweating	Yes	GTN 2 puffs and aspirin 300 mg sublingually CPR	Yes
Choking	Inhaled foreign material, Coughing choking	Yes	Back slap 5 times, then abdominal thrust 5 times	Only if no spontaneous recovery after (2)
Epileptic fit	Collapse Seizures Maybe incontinent	Yes	Protect patient from harm Consider midazolam 10 mg for adult in buccal mucosa (or i.m.or sublingually)	Only if no spontaneous or other recovery after 5 minutes, persistent altered conscious state or the fit characteristics differ to previous
Faint	Collapse, responding to laying flat Pallor Slow pulse Sweating No chest pain	No**	Lay patient flat Give glucose orally	Only if no spontaneous recovery after (2)

Table 3.3 Common emergencies—cont'd

Emergency	Features	Actions; reassure patient and accompanying people, and		
		1. give oxygen 15 L/min	2. other main actions	3. alert emergency services
Hypoglycaemia	Confused or aggressive, often known diabetic Shake or tremor Collapse	Yes	Blood glucose assay. Give glucose drink, gel or tablets. If unconscious, glucagon 1 mg IM.	Only if no spontaneous recovery after (2)
Stroke	Face weakness Arm weakness Speech difficulties Test all above	Yes	–	Yes

*GTN = glyceryl trinitrate (nitroglycerine).
**But oxygen will do no harm. NB. Ensure the supply of oxygen will enable adequate flow rates (15 litres/minute) to be maintained until the arrival of the ambulance or the patient recovers (at least 30 minutes supply). A full size D cylinder contains nominally 340 litres of oxygen and therefore should provide oxygen for up to ~22 minutes; a full size CD cylinder contains nominally 460 litres of oxygen and therefore should provide oxygen for up to ~30 minutes; a full size E cylinder contains nominally 680 litres of oxygen and therefore should provide oxygen for up to ~45 minutes. Pre-filled adrenaline syringes are convenient in an emergency due to their ease of use, but those provided for patient use (e.g. Epi-Pens® etc.) may contain less adrenaline than recommended for the management of medical emergencies.

Further reading

Molzen, G.W., Suter, R.E., Whitson, R., American College of Emergency Physicians, 2001. Clinical Policy: critical issues in the evaluation and management of patients presenting with syncope. Ann. Emerg. Med. 37, 771–776. 776. [PubMed]. 9.

Reed, M.J., Gray, A., 2006. Collapse query cause: the management of adult syncope in the emergency department. Emerg. Med. J. 23 (8), 589–594. Review.

Websites

Advanced Life Support Group, Available at: <www.alsg.org> (accessed 12.08.15).

Buttaravoli & Stair: Common Simple Emergencies. Available at: <www.ncemi.org/cse/contents.htm> (accessed 12.08.15.).

Dental Sedation Teachers Group, Available at: <www.dstg.co.uk> (accessed 12.08.15.).

European Resuscitation Council, Resuscitation Guidelines. Available at: <www.erc.edu> (accessed 12.08.15.).

Government Dental Chart Form: Drug Prescribing for Dentistry. Available at: <www.wales.nhs.uk/sites3/> (accessed 12.08.15.).

Healthcare and Emergency Training. Available at: <www.atoetrainingandsolutions.co.uk> (accessed 12.08.15.).

Medical Emergencies in the Dental Practice: Walsall Healthcare NHS Trust. Available at: <www.walsallhealthcare.nhs.uk/media/133096/walsallmedicalposter.pdf> (accessed 12.08.15.).

Preparing for Medical Emergencies: the essential drugs and equipment for the dental office. J. Am. Dent. Assoc. Available at: <http://jada.ada.org/content/141/suppl_1/14S.full> (accessed 12.08.15.).

<https://www.resus.org.uk/resuscitation-guidelines/>

4   Age and gender

CHILDREN

In the UK, people up to the age of 16 years are regarded as children.

Premature babies

At birth the neonate is classified as premature or preterm (<37 weeks' gestation), full-term (37–42 weeks' gestation), or post-dates (born after 42 weeks' gestation). Premature babies are at particular risk from a number of problems. Up to 10% of all births are preterm usually with a low birthweight (<2500 g). Low birthweight may result from intra-uterine growth retardation; these babies may go on to have lower IQs (intelligence quotients) and smaller stature. Preterm babies are less able to maintain body temperature and haemostasis, and are prone to several health consequences. Up to a half suffer long-term sequelae including low IQ, behavioural disorders, co-ordination problems, respiratory and feeding problems. In about 40% the cause of prematurity is unknown, but known causes include multiple pregnancy, infection, maternal smoking, pre-eclampsia, severe anaemia, and heart and renal disease. Periodontal disease in the mother has been suggested to be one causal factor.

Neonates

A neonate is a newborn infant up to 1 month old.

During the neonatal period, most congenital defects (e.g. congenital heart disease) are detected. The consequences of congenital infections (e.g. TORCH syndrome – defects arising from Toxoplasmosis, Rubella, Cytomegalovirus or Herpes simplex virus infections) may manifest. Immunological immaturity predisposes to candidosis, including oral: infections may be transmitted by parents or carers, or from the environment; even tongue spatulas can be a source of infection.

This is a period of rapid growth and development. Facial, skull, jaw and tooth development can be impaired by radiotherapy, by chemotherapy, and by some immunosuppressants during this period.

Infants

The first year of life is infancy.

Child from 1 year (pre-school child)

Young children strive constantly for independence, creating special safety concerns, and also discipline challenges and may be traumatized with orofacial damage from accident or abuse.

Child aged 5–12 years (schoolchild)

The attention span increases from about 15 minutes in 5-year-olds to about an hour by the age of 10. By about 10 years old, most children can follow five commands in a row. Reduced attention may herald attention deficit hyperactivity syndrome (ADHS).

Puberty

Puberty refers to the physical and psychological changes during maturation into an adult capable of reproduction. Manifest by the development of secondary sexual characteristics, it begins between 9 and 16 years of age, but children vary as to when. On average, girls enter puberty 2 years earlier than boys.

The hypothalamus and pituitary gland hormones that control growth and maturation trigger rapid growth at puberty, with increases in height and weight, the appearance of secondary sexual characteristics and increased sexual interest ('sex drive'). Interest in their teeth and oral health may increase over this period.

Adolescence

Adolescence is the transition from child to adult, between 13–19 years of age. As well as sexual maturation, there are emotional, behavioural and social changes. Specific health concerns may include:

- Accidental injuries (leading cause (70%) of death – from motor vehicle accidents, drowning or poisoning [usually drug or alcohol-related]).
- Assaults (often gang-related).
- Pregnancy.
- Sexually transmitted diseases.
- Stress, depression, eating disorders.
- Substance abuse.
- Suicide (third leading cause of death).
- Unlawful killing, often gang-related (second leading cause of death).

Main dental considerations

Care of children is discussed fully in textbooks of paediatric dentistry. Premature infants may have enamel hypoplasia, caused by birth trauma, infections, metabolic or nutritional disorders. Disturbed orofacial development and odontogenesis in childhood can result from a range of causes, including radiotherapy, chemotherapy, drugs, infections or toxins.

Important issues include consent; trauma, caries, and malocclusion; and issues related to anaesthesia and sedation. Informed consent can be difficult to ensure in children too young to understand, but conversely may be possible in some children under age 16 (Gillick competence). Children may present behavioural challenges in dental treatment: relative analgesia and local anaesthesia (LA) may be difficult or impossible to administer to some. Drug doses must be lowered and sugar-free preparations used, some drugs are contra-indicated and children may have unusual reactions to drugs, such as diazepam and intra-venous anaesthetics. Preventive dental care and dietary counselling are of crucial importance. Oral health may suffer if adolescents are away from parental guidance and change to a cariogenic diet.

Children of all ages rely on parents for guidance, protection from harm, and for disci-pline. Accidents are the major cause of morbidity and mortality: children are at increased risk because of a need for strenuous physical activity, a desire for peer approval and increased adventurous behaviour. Orofacial trauma is not uncommon. Children should be taught to play sports in appropriate, safe, supervised areas, with proper equipment and rules, and with safety equipment (such as a bicycle and other safety helmets, knee, elbow, wrist pads/braces, etc.). Safety instruction regarding contact sports, vehicle use, swimming and water sports, matches, fires, lighters and cooking are important to prevent accidents. Continued emphasis upon wearing seat-belts remains the single intervention most capable of preventing major injury or death due to a motor vehicle accident. Children may also be the subjects of abuse.

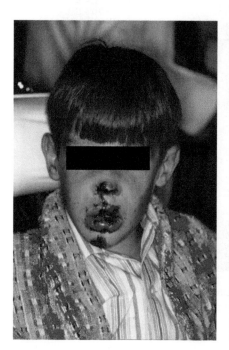

Figure 4.1 Facial contusions caused by accident.

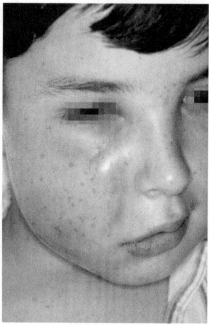

Figure 4.2 Severe facial cellulitis, 24 h postoperatively.

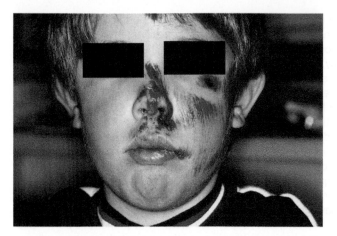

Figure 4.3 Abrasion marks across face.

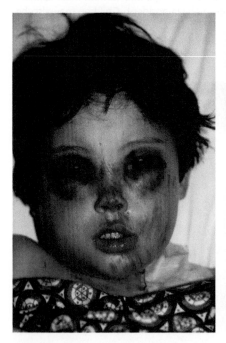

Figure 4.4 Child with Le Fort type II maxillary fracture.

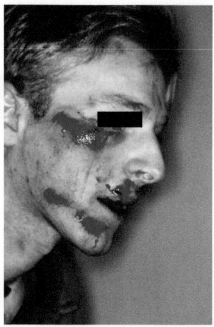

Figure 4.5 Abrasions and lacerations, right side of face.

MEN'S HEALTH

Main dental considerations

Box 4.1 shows diseases more common in males.

There are some conditions that affect only men, and there are gender differences with regard to patterns of many diseases. Men generally also access and use healthcare differently from women (typically less): generally they are less likely to react to health promotion and are more likely to have lifestyle habits that are detrimental to their health (e.g. alcohol or drug abuse). Cancers may lead to metastases that may involve the jaws or mouth; chemotherapy may cause mucositis (see also Section 9).

Box 4.1   Health problems generally more common in men

- Alcoholism
- Balanitis
- Bladder stones
- Cancer
  - Bladder
  - Prostate
  - Testicular
- Drug abuse and addiction
- Hydrocele and varicocele
- Orchitis and epididymitis
- Peyronie disease
- Phimosis and paraphimosis
- Prostate – prostatitis – benign prostatic hyperplasia
- Snoring and obstructive sleep apnoea
- Testicular torsion
- Tinea
- Trauma

Bladder cancer

Definition

The fourth most common cancer in males: 90% are transitional cell and 8% are squamous cell carcinomas.

Aetiopathogenesis

Incidence is increasing. Risk factors may include:

- Older age.
- Male sex (men 2–3 times more than women).
- Family history positive for bladder cancer.
- Race (Caucasians twice as common as Africans, with lowest rates in Asians).
- Carcinogens concentrated in the bladder – from cigarette smoking (raises risk 2–3 times) or occupation (e.g. workers in rubber, chemical, leather, metal, print, textile industries, hairdressing, machinists, painters, or truck drivers), or cyclophosphamide or arsenic.
- Infections – particularly schistosomiasis.

Clinical presentation and classification

Common presentation is painless haematuria but dysuria, urgency, polyuria and/or urinary obstruction may be seen – symptoms also common in benign prostatic hypertrophy (BPH).

Bladder cancer can invade to involve nearby organs such as the prostate (or uterus/vagina) and can metastasize to regional lymph nodes and to lungs, liver or bones.

Diagnosis

Malignant cells may be seen on urine cytology; intravenous urography may show a filling defect, but cystoscopy and biopsy give the definitive diagnosis.

Treatment

Surgery is the common treatment; other treatments include transurethral resection (TUR) for superficial cancer; segmental cystectomy for localized cancer and radical cystectomy for more widespread disease. Radiation, intravesical chemotherapy or immunotherapy using intravesical BCG may also be used.

Prostate cancer

Definition

90% are acinar adenocarcinomas.

Aetiopathogenesis

BPH does *not* seem to raise the chance of prostate cancer. Risk factors include:

- Age (mainly age >55).
- Dietary factors (animal fat may possibly increase the risk, and diets high in fruits and vegetables may lower it).
- Ethnicity (more common in African heritage).
- Family history of prostate cancer.

Clinical presentation

Most prostate cancer is slow-growing initially and may never cause any problems. Later features can mimic BPH or infection and can include:

- Blood in urine or semen.
- Difficulty in erection, painful ejaculation.
- Difficulty starting urination or holding back urine.
- Pain or stiffness in lower back, hips or thighs.
- Inability to urinate; weak or interrupted urine flow.
- Painful or burning urination.
- Urinary frequency, especially at night (nocturia).

Diagnosis

Digital rectal examination (DRE) (Fig. 4.6): all men over 40 should have an annual DRE to screen for cancer.

Blood prostate-specific antigen (PSA), urinalysis for blood or infection and, in some, blood prostatic acid phosphatase or PCA3 (sometimes known as UPM3) is helpful, especially if PSA results are positive. If results are positive, prostate biopsy is needed.

Treatment

Prostate cancer can be managed by watchful waiting, hormone therapy, or surgery, radiation, and chemotherapy:

- Androgen deprivation therapy (ADT) – aims to reduce androgens (testosterone and dihydrotestosterone) by: orchidectomy (removal of the testes – the main androgen source); use of luteinizing hormone-releasing hormone (LHRH) agonists (abiraterone, buserelin, goserelin, leuprolide, triptorelin) which prevent the testicles from producing testosterone; or luteinizing hormone-releasing hormone (LHRH) antagonist (abarelix).
- Androgen suppression therapy with anti-androgens (e.g. flutamide, nilutamide or bicalutamide); or drugs to inhibit adrenal androgen production (e.g. ketoconazole and aminoglutethimide).

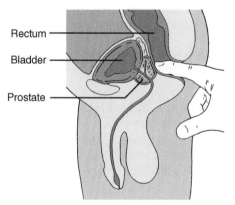

Rectum
Bladder
Prostate

Figure 4.6 Digital rectal examination (DRE) with a gloved hand.

Prostate hypertrophy (benign prostatic hyperplasia or hypertrophy; BPH)

Definition
Prostate enlargement (Fig. 4.7).

Aetiopathogenesis
The prostate almost invariably enlarges with age possibly related to oestrogen or dihydro-testosterone (DHT) production, so that at >50% of men in their sixties and as many as 90% in their seventies have symptoms.

Clinical presentation
As prostate hypertrophies it constricts the urethra causing a hesitant, interrupted or weak urine stream; the bladder then begins to contract even when it contains little urine, causing urgency, frequency, nocturia and leaking or dribbling. The bladder may become distended and atonic leading to overflow incontinence. Urinary infections are also more common. Sustained raised intravesical pressure can cause hydronephrosis and renal damage. Acute urinary retention, an emergency, can be precipitated by alcohol, cold temperatures or immobility.

Diagnosis
Investigations may include prostate-specific antigen (PSA) blood test and digital rectal examination (DRE), mid-stream urine (MSU), urine flow study and blood urea and electrolytes. Cystoscopy should identify the location and degree of any obstruction – and rectal ultrasound with biopsies may be indicated.

PSA level can rise in BPH, infection or prostate cancer, so the result should be interpreted with caution. Urine PCA3 gene level is a more specific cancer marker.

Treatment
BPH symptoms may resolve without treatment in as many as 30% of mild cases. If there are complications or major inconvenience, treatment is recommended.

- Alpha blockers (alfuzosin, doxazosin, indoramin, prazosin, silodosin, tamsulosin or terazosin) act quickly to deal with the 'going' problem – a weak or hesitant stream – by relaxing prostate and urinary tract muscles. PDE5 (phosphodiesterase type 5) inhibitor tadalafil is also approved for BPH.

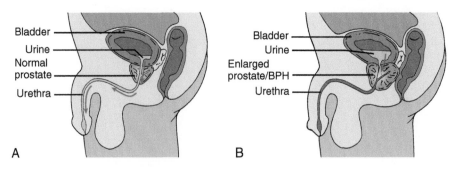

Figure 4.7 Normal and enlarged prostate.

- 5-alpha-reductase inhibitors (dutasteride, finasteride) act slowly over a few months to inhibit BPH growth by inhibiting DHT production and shrinking the prostate; saw palmetto may be as effective as finasteride.
- Surgical treatment includes: transurethral resection of the prostate (TURP); transurethral microwave thermotherapy (TUMT); transurethral needle ablation (TUNA; which delivers low-level radiofrequency energy with fewer side-effects compared with TURP); transurethral laser surgery (Nd:YAG lasers); transurethral incision of the prostate (TUIP); or open excisional surgery (prostatectomy).

Testicular cancer

Definition

Main types are:

- Lymphomas – the most common cancer in the testicles in men >50 (Fig. 4.8).
- Cancer arising in testicular germ cells:
  - Seminomas.
  - Non-seminomas:
    choriocarcinoma;
    embryonal carcinoma;
    teratoma;
    yolk sac tumours.

Aetiopathogenesis risk factors for testicular cancers

- Carcinoma in situ (CIS) of testicle.
- Family history of breast, skin or testicular cancer.
- HIV/AIDS.
- Inguinal hernia.
- Maternal higher androstenedione and oestradiol.
- Men with fertility problems.
- Microlithiasis (calcium in the testes).
- Previous testicular cancer.

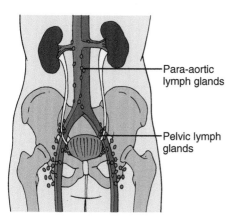

Para-aortic
lymph glands

Pelvic lymph
glands

Figure 4.8 Pelvic and para-aortic lymph nodes.

- Sporting injuries to testes.
- Taller than average height.
- Undescended testicle (cryptorchidism).
- White men – higher risk than other ethnic groups.

Dehydroepiandrosterone sulphate may lower risk of testicular cancer.

Clinical presentation

Features may include;

- Breasts tender or swollen.
- Lump or swelling in part of one testicle.
- Pain in the scrotum, testicle, or lower abdomen (but testicular cancer is not usually painful).
- Symptoms from spread to para-aortic, retro-peritoneal, mediastinal, or pelvic lymph nodes.

Diagnosis

- Blood levels raised of:
  - AFP (alpha feta protein);
  - HCG (human chorionic gonadotrophin);
  - LDH (lactate dehydrogenase).
- Testicular ultrasound.
- MRI.
- Histopathology; removing a testicle – orchidectomy (or sometimes orchiectomy).

Treatment

- Depends on tumour type (seminoma or non-seminoma), and spread orchidectomy, radiotherapy, or chemotherapy. Before treatment starts, semen samples can be stored.
- BEP (bleomycin, etoposide, cisplatin) for non-seminoma or testicular cancer that has metastasized.
- Carboplatin for seminoma.

OLDER PATIENTS

Age does not come alone; diseases are increasingly encountered with aging (Tables 4.1 and 4.2). A growing proportion of the population in many countries, particularly in the resource-rich world, are age >65. In the UK, up to 75% of older people have one or more chronic diseases, 3% are bedridden, 8% walk with difficulty and 11% are house-bound. Gender differences in life expectancy are resulting in a rise in the proportion of older females.

Main dental considerations

Mucosal lesions are more common in older people. Most are fibrous lumps or ulcers, but a minority are potentially or actually malignant lesions. Atypical (idiopathic) facial pain (often related to depressive illness), migraine, trigeminal neuralgia, zoster and oral dysaesthesias are more common as age advances. Many older people with remaining teeth have periodontal disease. Dental caries are usually less acute but root caries are more common. Caries may become active if there is hyposalivation, especially if there is overindulgence in sweet foods. Hyposalivation is even more likely with medications such as neuroleptics or antidepressants. Many older people receive no dental attention whatsoever, despite much evidence of need. Access to care can be a major difficulty for the person who is frail or has limited mobility. Handling of older patients may demand immense patience, but remember always to treat the older patient with sympathy and respect. Domiciliary care may be more appropriate. Older people are often extremely anxious about treatment and should therefore be sympathetically reassured and, if necessary, sedated.

Very many older patients are edentulous and some problems of dental management are thereby greatly reduced. It seems, however, that the proportion of edentulous older patients is gradually falling and, as a consequence, more of them need restorative dentistry or surgery of various types. Many edentulous older people have little alveolar bone to support dentures, and have a dry mouth as well as frail, atrophic mucosa. Implants may be helpful if there is inability to cope with dentures, or a sore mouth for any reason, or to afford appropriate care, readily demoralizes the older patient, and may tip the balance between health and disease.

The major goals of oral healthcare are preventive and conservative treatment for conditions such as hyposalivation, root caries, secondary caries, periodontal disease and gingival recession, and the elimination/avoidance of pain and oral infections. Treatment is often best

Table 4.1 Approximate number of years that older people are likely to remain free from disability

Age group	Men	Women
65–69	9	11
70–74	7	9
75–79	5	7
80–84	3	5
85+	1	3

Table 4.2 Diseases especially affecting older people*

Blood and others	Cardiorespiratory	Genito-urinary	Musculoskeletal	Neuropsychiatric
Accidents	Cardiac failure	Prostatic hypertrophy and cancer	Osteoarthritis	Acute confusional states
Anaemia (especially pernicious anaemia)	Chronic bronchitis and emphysema	Renal failure	Osteoporosis	Alzheimer disease
Cancers	Hypertension	Urinary retention or incontinence	Paget disease	Ataxia
Chronic leukaemia	Ischaemic heart disease			Dependence on hypnotics
Myelodysplasia	Pneumonia			Insomnia
Nutritional deficiencies	Temporal arteritis			Loneliness and depression
				Multi-infarct (cerebrovascular) dementia
				Paranoia
				Parkinson disease or parkinsonism
				Strokes
				Visual impairment

*Multiple conditions are common.

carried out with the patient sitting upright, as few like reclining for treatment, and some may become breathless and/or panic.

Older people tend to be more sensitive to drugs and to trauma. Polypharmacy should be avoided. Older people frequently have difficulties in understanding the medication and in remembering to keep to a regimen. Compliance may therefore be lacking. If there is hepatic or renal disease likely to impair drug metabolism or excretion, drug dosage must be reduced appropriately.

Older people, despite increasing chances of disabilities (Table 4.1), are often reluctant to seek attention, especially if they are ill, apathetic or fear consequent hospitalization and further loss of independence. Many physical disorders affect the older person, particularly a greater incidence and severity of arthritis and cardiovascular disease. Ataxia, fainting and falls are common; may be due to transient cerebral ischaemic attacks, parkinsonism, postural hypotension, cardiac arrhythmias or epilepsy. Mental and emotional disorders are also important and are often also caused by underlying physical disease. Acute confusional states may result from disorders as widely different as minor cerebrovascular accidents, infections, or left ventricular failure. Chronic confusional states may result from such conditions as diabetes, Alzheimer disease, hypothyroidism, carcinomatosis, anaemia, uraemia or drugs and dementia may be seen. Defects of hearing or sight are common.

Disease may present in a less florid and dramatic way in elderly people. Even severe infections, for example, may cause no fever. Atypical symptomatology, polypharmacy and abnormal reactivity towards many drugs further complicate the situation.

Based on the capacity to carry out activities of ordinary life (to dress, to eat, to bathe, etc.), the older patient is classified as functionally independent or dependent. Compliance with treatment can be poor, not least because of forgetfulness or apathy. Inappropriate treatment, poor supervision, excessive dosage, drug interactions and polypharmacy, or impaired drug metabolism, may all contribute.

Drug treatment should be carefully controlled, with the possibility of poor compliance and of adverse reactions always in mind. Drug dosage may need to be reduced when there is hepatic or renal disease. Drugs may precipitate or aggravate physical disorders; antimuscarinic drugs, e.g. atropine or antidepressants, may cause glaucoma, dry mouth or urinary retention. Arrhythmias are common in ambulatory older people, but they are typically benign.

Older patients are often anxious about treatment and should therefore be sympathetically reassured. Handling of older patients may demand immense patience. It can take a long time for a patient in a wheelchair, or using a walking frame, to get into the clinic. Domiciliary care may be more appropriate and avoids the physical and psychological problems of a hospital or clinic visit. Dependent persons often need domiciliary care.

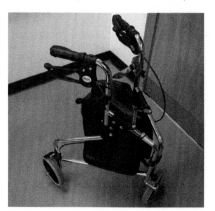

Figure 4.9 Walking frame.

WOMEN'S HEALTH

Box 4.2 shows diseases more common in females. Women generally live longer than men, there are gender differences with regard to patterns of many diseases, and there are some conditions that affect only women. Women generally access and use healthcare differently from men (typically more) and generally react more positively to health promotion.

Box 4.2   Some of the more common problems in women

- Autoimmune disorders
- Bacterial vaginosis
- Cancer
  - Breast
  - Cervical
  - Ovarian
  - Uterine
- Cystitis
- Eating disorders
- Endometriosis

- Female genital cutting
- Fibroids
- Gallstones
- Irritable bowel syndrome
- Menopausal disorders
- Migraine
- Osteoporosis
- Pregnancy-related disorders
- Pyelonephritis
- Sexual abuse

Main dental considerations

Certain diseases that can have orofacial manifestations are especially common in women (e.g. anorexia nervosa/bulimia, atypical facial pain, burning mouth syndrome, facial arthro-myalgia [temporomandibular joint dysfunction], pemphigus and pemphigoid, rheumatoid arthritis and Sjögren syndrome). Cancers may metastasize to jaws or mouth. There has also been discrimination against women across cultures, and subordination and compromised dignity, and women more frequently suffer the consequences of domestic violence and/or sexual abuse than men.

Breast cancer

Definition

The most common cancer, affecting 80% of women over 50 years. It can affect males and younger women.

Classification

There are several types of breast cancer, some quite rare, and a single breast tumour can be a combination of types or a mix of invasive and *in situ* cancer. Ductal carcinoma in situ (DCIS or intraductal carcinoma) is pre-invasive, but there is no good way to know for certain which cases will go on to become invasive cancers. Lobular carcinoma in situ (LCIS) has cells that look like cancer cells, but they are restricted to the milk lobules and this is *not* a cancer or pre-cancer. Most true cancers are invasive (or infiltrating) ductal carcinoma (IDC) which start in a breast milk duct, invades and may metastasize through the lymphatic system and bloodstream. Far less common is invasive lobular carcinoma (ILC) which starts in the milk-producing glands (lobules) and can metastasize.

Aetiopathogenesis

More common in white than in African or Asian women. Risk factors are shown in Box 4.3.

Clinical presentation

Early breast cancer rarely causes pain; more commonly it may be detected on self-examination as a lump or thickening. Later, cancer may result in a change in breast size or shape, nipple discharge, tenderness or inversion, ridging or pitting (the skin looks like orange skin – *peau d'orange*), or a change in the way the skin of breast, areola or nipple looks or feels (e.g. warm, swollen, red or scaly).

Diagnosis

Clinical initially. Current recommendation is 3-yearly screening mammogram from the age of 50, but in cases of increased risk such as a positive family history, screening may start earlier. If an area of the breast looks suspicious on screening, diagnostic mammography is indicated. Ultrasonography can often help. Biopsy is generally needed – by needle or open biopsy.

Treatment

The grade of any tumour, including breast cancer, is given by the histopathologist in order to afford an idea of how quickly the cancer might grow and spread. Tumours are graded between 1 and 3, a higher number indicating the cells are likely to grow and spread more quickly. Grading for ductal carcinoma in situ (DCIS) is different, and is defined as low, medium or high grade. Staging is used to assess the tumour size and extent of any spread. There are two main methods used for defining the stage of a cancer – the TNM (Tumour, Nodes, Metastasis) system and a scale from 0 to 4 (Fig. 4.10).

Invasive breast carcinoma treatment most commonly involves surgery – usually a wide local excision with axillary node sampling or sentinel node biopsy. Histopathology results

---

Box 4.3   Risk factors for breast cancer

- Personal history of breast cancer
- A positive family history: the risk doubles if a woman's mother or sister has had breast cancer, especially at a young age. Genes *BRCA1*, *BRCA2* increase risk
- Having a diagnosis of atypical hyperplasia or lobular carcinoma *in situ* (LCIS)
- Late childbearing (after about age 30)
- Early menarche
- Oestrogen exposure
- Long-term use of combined oral contraceptives or hormone replacement therapy (HRT)
- Radiation therapy
- Breast density
- Alcohol
- Fatty diet
- High body mass index (BMI) and taller stature
- Higher social class.

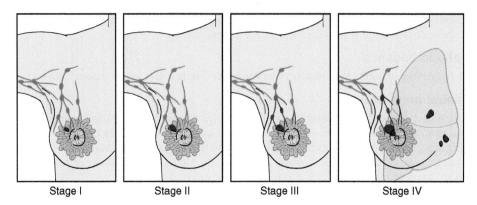

| Stage I | Stage II | Stage III | Stage IV |

Figure 4.10 Stages of breast cancer.

then dictate further treatment, which may be more radical surgery, or adjuvant radiotherapy plus or minus chemotherapy.

Radiation therapy may lead to ischaemic heart disease, and other cardiac conditions, including pericardial disease, peripheral vascular disease, cardiomyopathy, valvular dysfunction, and arrhythmias.

Hormone (oestrogen and progesterone) receptor tests can help determine whether a tumour is hormone-dependent and help predict response to hormone therapy after surgery. Tamoxifen, a hormone receptor blocker, is the most common hormonal treatment used, usually for 5 years following the main treatment, and may cause hot flushes, vaginal discharge or irritation, nausea and irregular periods. Serious adverse effects are rare, but tamoxifen can cause deep vein thrombosis and, in a few women, it can increase the risk of uterine cancer or stroke. Anastrozole is a safer alternative in respect of stroke risk.

Human epidermal growth factor receptor-2 or HER-2 gene may be associated with a higher risk for cancer recurrence. Trastuzumab – a monoclonal antibody that targets breast cancer cells having excess HER-2 – may be given alone or along with chemotherapy such as trastuzumab emtansine – trastuzumab linked to mertansine. HER-2 test results help predict response to trastuzumab and other anti-HER-2 treatments and some types of chemotherapy. Such chemotherapy may include anthracyclines and this and therapies targeting HER-2 can also have a cardiotoxic effect.

Advanced breast cancer may be treated with vinorelbine (a vinca alkaloid); capecitabine (a 5-fluorouracil precursor) may be used for locally advanced or metastatic cancer.

Treatments for DCIS include breast-sparing surgery followed by radiation therapy or mastectomy, with or without breast reconstruction. Tamoxifen may reduce the risk of developing invasive breast cancer.

Tamoxifen is the usual therapy for LCIS, though occasionally women with LCIS may decide to have bilateral mastectomy to try to prevent cancer, but most just have regular screening.

Main dental consideration

(*See also generic guidance under main dental considerations on page 63 top, and also Section 2).

Bisphosphonates used in metastatic disease may cause jaw osteonecrosis (see Section 9).

Cervical cancer

Definition
Cancer of the uterine cervix.

Aetiopathogenesis
The most common genitourinary neoplasm, it is most common in sexually active persons and associated with oncogenic human papillomaviruses (HPV), particularly HPV-16 and HPV-18. Smoking, lower socioeconomic class and HIV disease increase the risk.

Clinical presentation and classification
Most often affects women >40 years. Pre-cancerous changes rarely cause pain. When cancer develops and invades, the most common features are abnormal vaginal bleeding or abnormal vaginal discharge. Consorts and sometimes the patient can have a higher risk of oral cancer.

Diagnosis
Pelvic examination, colposcopy and biopsy. LLETZ (large loop excision of the transformation zone) may be carried out using diathermy, laser ablation or cold coagulation. A cone biopsy removing the entire transformation zone may be carried out. Staging includes cystoscopy, proctosigmoidoscopy, intravenous pyelography (IVP), barium enema, CT scan, ultrasonography and MRI.

Treatment
Surgery, radiotherapy or chemotherapy are employed. Simple local excision may be all required for early cancer. For advanced disease, radical hysterectomy and excision of other involved tissues may be necessary. Radiotherapy may be given alone or with concurrent chemotherapy (e.g. cisplatin).

A vaccine for HPV-16 and HPV-18 is given to girls of 12–13 years of age; there will be a catch-up programme for older girls. Screening for pre-cancerous cells is carried out by a 'cervical smear' test – 3-yearly on women aged 25–50 and then 5-yearly until 64 years of age. Cells from the cervical canal squamocolumnar junction are reported as normal; mild dyskaryosis (CIN 1 – may resolve spontaneously); moderate dyskaryosis (CIN 2); or severe dyskaryosis (CIN 3, sometimes referred to as carcinoma in situ).

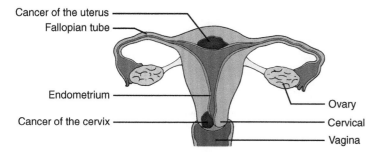

Figure 4.11 Cancer of the uterus and cervix.

Ovarian cancer

Definition
Most ovarian cancer is carcinoma, but there are rare germ-cell tumours and cancers that begin in the stroma.

Aetiopathogenesis
The causes are unclear, but risk factors include:

- Middle age or older.
- Previous breast, uterine or colorectal cancers.
- Family history of ovarian, breast or gastrointestinal cancer.
- BRCA1 or BRCA2 gene mutations.
- Never giving birth.

Factors that reduce the risk include:

- Breastfeeding.
- Use of combined oral contraceptives.
- Low-fat diet.
- Childbearing (the more children a woman has had, the less likely she is to develop ovarian cancer).

Clinical presentation
Ovarian cancer often causes no symptoms or only mild symptoms until the disease is advanced, but may include abdominal discomfort and/or pain; nausea, diarrhoea, constipation or frequent urination; anorexia; weight gain or loss; and abnormal vaginal bleeding. Fluid in the abdomen (ascites) may be seen when it metastasizes to the peritoneum. The BEAT ovarian cancer campaign is the first to engage GPs, women and ovarian cancer charities around the world. It has as its centre piece an easy to remember acronym:
B – bloating that is persistent.
E – eating less and feeling fuller.
A – abdominal pain.
T – telling the GP.

Diagnosis
Pelvic examination together with ultrasound, CA-125 assay, radiography of the lower gastrointestinal tract, or barium enema, CT or MRI and biopsy.

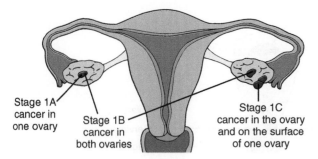

Stage 1A cancer in one ovary

Stage 1B cancer in both ovaries

Stage 1C cancer in the ovary and on the surface of one ovary

Figure 4.12 Stages of ovarian cancer.

Treatment

Surgery (hysterectomy with bilateral salpingo-oophorectomy), chemotherapy or external or intraperitoneal radiation therapy.

Women at high risk due to a positive family history may consider prophylactic oophorectomy.

Uterine cancer (endometrial cancer)

Definition

Cancer of the uterus (womb) is common. Most cancers are endometrial; rare cases are sarcomas.

Aetiopathogenesis

Risk factors may include:

- Older age.
- Hypertension.
- Hormone imbalance (e.g. starting menstruation at an early age – before age 12 – or beginning menopause later; never having been pregnant; HRT that contains oestrogen but not progesterone; tamoxifen; polycystic ovary syndrome; ovarian tumours).
- Obesity.
- Diabetes.
- Hereditary nonpolyposis colorectal cancer (HNPCC) syndrome of colon, which may present with occult radiopaque jaw lesions, and other cancers, including uterine.

Clinical presentation

- Bleeding between periods.
- Pain during intercourse.
- Pelvic pain.
- Vaginal bleeding after menopause.
- Watery or blood-tinged vaginal discharge.

Diagnosis

- CT.
- Endometrial biopsy or dilatation and curettage (D&C).
- Hysteroscopy.
- Pelvic examination.
- Transvaginal ultrasound.

Prophylaxis

Maintaining a healthy weight and the long-term use of some types of contraceptive pills may be preventive.

Treatment

- Surgery:
  - *Hysterectomy* (removal of uterus and cervix):
    through vagina – vaginal hysterectomy;
    through abdominal incision – total abdominal hysterectomy – or via a small incision (laparoscopy) – total laparoscopic hysterectomy.

- *Bilateral salpingo-oophorectomy* – removal of both ovaries and Fallopian tubes
- *Radical hysterectomy* – removal of uterus, cervix, and part of the vagina. The ovaries, Fallopian tubes, or nearby lymph nodes may also be removed.
- Radiotherapy.
- Drugs:
  - Hormones to lower oestrogen levels. Synthetic progestin, a progesterone, stops endometrial cancer growing.
  - Chemotherapy.
  - Monoclonal antibodies and tyrosine kinase inhibitors.

Pregnancy

The normal pregnancy duration is 40 weeks, divided into three trimesters:
- First trimester (weeks 1–12): organs and systems formation.
- Second trimester (weeks 13–28): growth and maturation.
- Third trimester (weeks 29–40): ongoing growth and maturation.

The mother

Pregnancy is associated with changes affecting especially endocrine, cardiovascular and haematological systems, and often attitude, mood or behaviour.

Many hormones increase, especially sex hormones, prolactin and thyroid hormones, but levels of luteinizing hormone (LH) and follicle stimulating hormone (FSH) fall.

Sequelae may include:

- Nausea;
- Vomiting;
- Deepened pigmentation of the nipples and sometimes face (chloasma);
- Glycosuria, impaired glucose tolerance, and sometimes diabetes.
- Tachycardia, and initially often a slight fall in BP with the possibility of syncope or postural hypotension. In later pregnancy, the foetus when mother is supine may press on and occlude the vena cava, causing the 'supine hypotensive syndrome'.

Medical complications in pregnancy

These can include:

- Hypertension – a dangerous complication leading to increased morbidity and mortality in both foetus and mother. Hypertension may be asymptomatic but, when associated with oedema and proteinuria (pre-eclampsia), may culminate in eclampsia (hypertension, oedema, proteinuria and convulsions) which may be fatal. The foetus is also at risk.
- Blood hypercoagulability – can lead to venous thrombosis, particularly postoperatively or occasionally disseminated intravascular coagulopathy.
- Anaemia – expansion of blood volume may cause apparent anaemia but, in about 20%, true anaemia develops, mainly because of foetal demands for iron and folate.
- Supine hypotension syndrome – in up to 10% of patients, there is hypotension if the mother lies supine since the gravid uterus presses on and may occlude the vena cava.

The foetus

Foetal development during the first 3 months of pregnancy is a complex process of organogenesis and the foetus is then especially at risk from developmental defects. The mother may not be aware of pregnancy for 2+ months, when, unfortunately, the foetus is most vulnerable to damage from drugs, radiation and infections. About 10 to 20% of all pregnancies spontaneously abort at this time, often because of foetal defects.

The most critical period is the 3rd to 8th week, when differentiation is occurring. Precautions to avoid foetal damage and developmental defects should, therefore, be adequate if carried out from the time of the first missed menstruation.

Pregnancy causes concern for the parents lest the foetus be damaged, and this is especially the case for the first born of an older mother. Most developmental defects are unexplained; there may be hereditary influences, but drugs (e.g. alcohol and tobacco), infections, materials and radiation, can be implicated in some cases. Some jobs, like farming and working in dry cleaning stores, factories, or healthcare may force the mother to be around or in contact with harmful substances. She may need extra protection at work or a change in job duties to stay safe.

Alcohol can cause serious foetal damage (foetal alcohol syndrome: FAS); even a single exposure to high levels can cause significant brain damage and most will suffer effects ranging from mild learning disabilities to major physical, mental and intellectual impairment.

Tobacco smoking during or after pregnancy can seriously damage the foetus or child. It increases the risks of stillbirth, low birth weight, and impaired mental and physical development.

Infections should be avoided early in pregnancy, especially those that may damage the foetus with consequences ranging from hearing damage to learning disability, cardiac anomalies, or death (TORCH syndrome: acronym of Toxoplasmosis, Rubella, Cytomegalovirus, Herpesviruses). HIV infection of the mother can also be an issue (Section 7), as can influenza in the last trimester.

Concerns about materials in pregnancy revolve mainly around the possible hazards from a wide range of domestic and other materials. Exposure to these should be minimized where possible.

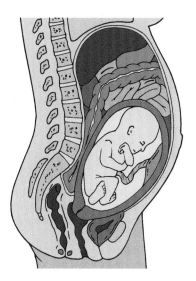

Figure 4.13 Drawing of foetus in the womb (uterus).

Arsenic

Arsenic can enter the environment through natural sources (crumbling rocks and forest fires) and man-made sources (mining and making electronic products). Harmful levels of arsenic may be found in, or near well water near metal smelters (where metal is made) or near harmful waste sites or incinerators. Arsenic should be avoided by pregnant women, and by children.

Lead

Lead was once used in petrol and house paints but is no longer used in many products. Jobs including painting, plumbing, car repair, battery manufacturing and certain kinds of construction may involve lead exposure. Today the most common sources of lead are old house paint, water that comes from wells or through lead pipes, lead crystal glassware and some ceramic dishes, some arts and crafts supplies, including oil paints, ceramic glazes and stained glass materials, old painted toys and some new toys and jewellery, some make-up such as lipstick, that has surma or kohl, canned food from other countries, and sweets from Mexico called Chaca. Lead can especially harm young children and pregnant women.

Pesticides

Contact with large amounts of pesticides may be harmful during pregnancy and may lead to miscarriage, preterm birth, low birthweight, birth defects and learning problems.

Plastics

Plastics may contain phthalates and bisphenol A (BPA) that may be harmful during pregnancy. Phthalates used to be used to make plastic soft and flexible and are found in some dental resins, older toys, medical equipment (such as tubing), shampoos, cosmetics and food packaging. BPA, used to make plastics clear and strong, may be found in baby bottles, metal cans and water bottles.

Solvents

Solvents include alcohols, degreasers, paint thinners and stain and varnish removers. Lacquers, silk-screening inks and paints also contain solvents. Liver, kidney, brain damage and even death can be harmful and in pregnancy may lead to miscarriage, prematurity and birth defects.

Main dental considerations

Oral manifestations in pregnancy may include:
- Pregnancy gingivitis.
- Pyogenic granuloma or 'pregnancy tumour'.
- Strong gag reflex with reflux or possible enamel erosion.
- Halitosis.

Pregnant patients are not medically compromised – and they should not be denied necessary care. Maintain good oral hygiene to minimize the risk for potential problems during later pregnancy and postpartum periods. However, the safest time to treat is during the second trimester.

During the first trimester, defer elective care as this is the period of greatest risk for malformations and miscarriage. Towards the end of pregnancy, there may be potential

Table 4.3 Known risks to foetus of some drugs

Category[a]	A	B	C	D and X
	No risk to foetus in animal model or human studies	Either safe to foetus in animal models without human data, or risk in animal models but safe in human studies	Risk to foetus in animal models but no human studies available, or no human studies support safety	Definitive human data demonstrating risk to foetus
Use	No risk	Where necessary	Only if really essential and after consulting physician	Do not use
Local anaesthetic	–	Lidocaine Prilocaine	Articaine* Bupivacaine Mepivacaine	
Sedative agents	–	Promethazine		Benzodiazepines Nitrous oxide**
Analgesics	–	Meperidine Paracetamol/ acetaminophen	Codeine Diflunisal	Aspirin NSAIDs***
Antimicrobials	–	Azithromycin Cefadroxil Cefuroxime Cephalexin Clindamycin Erythromycin Loracarbef Metronidazole Penciclovir (cream) Penicillins	Aciclovir Ciprofloxacin Clarithromycin Fluconazole	Doxycycline Minocycline Tetracycline
Others	–		Corticosteroids (even topical)	Anti-depressants Carbamazepine Colchicine Danazol Phenytoin Povidone-iodine Retinoids Thalidomide Warfarin

[a]US FDA pregnancy categories.
*Sometimes categorized as B.
**Nitrous oxide, though able to interfere with vitamin B_{12} and folate metabolism, does not appear to be teratogenic in normal use though it is advisable to restrict use to the second or third trimester.
***May be safer in first and second trimesters.
Co-trimoxazole may cause neonatal haemolysis,
Prilocaine at least in theory, can cause methaemoglobinaemia.

patient discomfort, and risk of preterm labour or supine hypotension. Particularly toward the late third trimester use a semi-reclined position and a pillow under the patient's right side, and allow for frequent changes in position. If hypotension occurs, roll the patient to her left side.

Foetal hazards in pregnancy may include drugs, infections, materials, or irradiation.

The decision to administer a drug requires that benefits outweigh potential risks. In general principle, drugs are best avoided where possible (Tables 4.3 and 4.4), particularly in the first trimester. Influenza vaccination is controversial but important (http://www.cdc.gov/flu/protect/vaccine/qa_vacpregnant.htm).

In terms of pain control, the commonly used local anaesthetics (LA) appear safe for use in pregnant women who do not have any specific contraindications, such as allergy. Epinephrine (adrenaline), when used in low concentration as a LA vasoconstrictor, does not cause foetal harm. Paracetamol appears to be the safest analgesic. Anxiolytics, such as benzodiazepines, may cause foetal developmental anomalies and therefore are contraindicated. Exposure to nitrous oxide and cytotoxic drugs is best avoided by pregnant patients or staff.

Most LA and epinephrine are considered safe for pregnant and breastfeeding patients.

Drugs to avoid in pregnancy

Analgesics
- *Bupivacaine hydrochloride and mepivacaine hydrochloride:* may cause foetal bradycardia.
- *Codeine:* in breastfeeding patients, codeine must be avoided owing to rare but fatal effects on the newborn.
- *NSAIDs and high-dose aspirin:* particularly in the third trimester, owing to the risk for maternal bleeding and foetal cardiac malformations.

Antimicrobials
- *Chloramphenicol:* maternal toxicity, grey syndrome and possible death of the infant.
- *Doxycycline:* teeth discolouration, inhibition of bone development in infant.
- *Fluoroquinolones (e.g. ciprofloxacin, nalidixic acid):* risk for abnormal foetal bone growth.
- *Gentamicin:* potential toxicity in foetus.

Sedatives
- *Diazepam and alprazolam:* possible oral cleft in the foetus with prolonged exposure.

Postpartum, especially during the lactation period, the metabolism of many medications remains altered so the potential for transmission of certain drugs and substances through breast milk should be minimized.

Materials

Mercury
Metallic mercury can damage the brain, spinal cord and nerves and can cause hearing and vision problems. Mercury in dental amalgam fillings generally seems not to be a serious issue, but it is best to avoid if possible, placing new or removing old amalgams, or using peroxide – which can increase mercury release.

Plastics
Dental resins may contain phthalates and bisphenol A (BPA).

Table 4.4 Drugs to avoid in pregnant mothers*

Drug	Potential effects on foetus
Aciclovir (systemic)	Teratogenicity?
Alcohol	Foetal alcohol syndrome
Aspirin	Premature closure of ductus arteriosus Persistent pulmonary hypertension Bleeding tendency
Carbamazepine	Neural tube defects Vitamin K impairment and bleeding tendency
Carbimazole	Goitre
Cocaine	Ankyloglossia
Codeine	Respiratory depression
Corticosteroids	Adrenal suppression Growth retardation
Cotrimoxazole	Haemolysis Teratogenicity Methaemoglobinaemia
Diazepam	Cleft lip/palate
Felypressin	Oxytocic
Fluconazole	Congenital anomalies
Gentamicin	Deafness
Lithium	Cardiac abnormalities
Nitrous oxide (repeated)	Congenital anomalies
NSAIDs	Premature closure of ductus arteriosus Persistent pulmonary hypertension Bleeding tendency
Pentazocine	Foetal addiction and withdrawal symptoms
Phenytoin	Foetal phenytoin syndrome
Prilocaine	Methaemoglobinaemia
Retinoids	Neural tube defects
Tetracyclines	Discoloured teeth and bones
Thalidomide	Phocomelia
Valproate	Neural tube defects
Vancomycin	Toxicity (monitor levels)
Warfarin	Long bone and cartilage abnormalities Bleeding tendency

*Most of these are applicable mainly to secondary care. Drugs of abuse may cause neonatal addiction.

Table 4.5 Drug use in pregnancy

Drug	Safe usually	Unsafe/caution
Anxiolytics	None	Alprazolam Diazepam Midazolam
LA	Articaine Lidocaine Prilocaine Adrenaline	Bupivacaine Felypressin
Analgesics	Ibuprofen (1st and 2nd trimester) Paracetamol (all trimesters)	Aspirin Diclofenac Ibuprofen (3rd trimester) Mefenamic acid Naproxen
Antifungals	Fluconazole Miconazole Nystatin	Ketoconazole
Antibacterials	Azithromycin Cephalosporins Clindamycin Erythromycin Penicillins	Aminoglycosides Co-trimoxazole Metronidazole Sulphonamides Tetracyclines

Radiation and radiography

Ionizing radiation can result in harmful effects including cell death and teratogenic effects, carcinogenesis, and genetic effects or mutations in germ cells. It is therefore essential to ensure that the pregnant patient in particular avoids any unnecessary radiation. There may be alternative diagnostic procedures available such as ultrasonography, or magnetic resonance imaging (MRI). Radiographs and radionuclide scans must not be taken unless absolutely necessary and retakes must be avoided. Protective measures in radiography, such as high-speed (E/F speed) films and rectangular collimation should help reduce the dose to the minimum. Modern radiography, carried out following current guidelines, is generally considered safe. 'Undergoing a single diagnostic X-ray procedure does not result in radiation exposure adequate to threaten the well-being of the developing pre-embryo, embryo, or foetus and is not an indication for therapeutic abortion. When multiple diagnostic X-rays are anticipated during pregnancy, imaging procedures not associated with ionizing radiation, such as ultrasonography and MRI, should be considered. Additionally, it may be helpful to consult an expert in dosimetry calculation to determine estimated foetal dose. The use of radioactive isotopes of iodine is contraindicated for therapeutic use during pregnancy (The American Congress of Obstetricians and Gynecologists, 2004).

Menopause

The menopause, the end of a woman's reproductive life – marked by cessation of menstrual periods – can start at any age between 40 and 55 years. Rarely associated with serious physical complications, some women gain weight, lose muscle tone, have hot flushes or develop a few hairs on the chin or upper lip. The menopause is frequently associated with emotional disturbances and stresses, often due to the changes in the pattern of family life around that time. Psychological disorders are not uncommon and are usually mild (e.g. dizziness and insomnia), but depression or paranoia may develop sometimes with complaints of orofacial pain.

Osteoporosis is more common. These changes may sometimes be controlled by hormone replacement therapy (HRT) – replacement of reduced oestrogen secretion after menopause or oophorectomy, with oestrogens taken orally, via a skin patch or implanted; or with oestrogens plus progestogens (progestin).

Consideration of the risks and benefits of HRT has concluded it is beneficial but that combined HRT of oestrogen plus progestogen may cause more harm than good.

Main dental considerations

Bisphosphonates, with calcium and vitamin D can also be used to minimize osteoporosis, but may cause necrotic jaw lesions (Medication Related OsteoNecrosis of the Jaws, MRONJ: Section 9).

References

American Congress of Obstetricians and Gynecologists, 2004. Committee Opinion. Guidelines for Diagnostic Imaging During Pregnancy. Available at: <www.acog.org/Resources-And-Publications/Committee-Opinions/Committee-on-Obstetric-Practice/Guidelines-for-Diagnostic-Imaging-During-Pregnancy> (accessed 14.08.15.).
<https://www.tga.gov.au/prescribing-medicines-pregnancy-database>

5 System synopses

Main dental considerations in most patients

A risk analysis (risk–benefit analysis) is prudent before dental treatment with any patient and medical advice should be obtained if there is any concern about the medical history. Risks are generally greatest when GA or sedation are used and procedures involve haemorrhage and/or are prolonged. Defer elective care until the patient has been medically stabilized. Emergency dental care should be conservative – principally analgesics and antibiotics.

Update the medical history at every appointment. Well-managed medical conditions generally present no or few problems. Ready access to medical help, oxygen and nitroglycerin is vital. Standard infection control measures are necessary. Guidance on oral hygiene and diet are essential.

Valid consent is crucial. All patient information must be kept in a secure location, and discussing a patient's medical status should only occur in a private, closed office to ensure confidentiality.

Short, stress-free appointments are recommended; it is important to avoid anxiety, stress and pain. If local anaesthesia (LA), analgesics, sedative drugs or antibiotics are contraindicated, this is highlighted below. The behaviour, conscious level, pulse, blood pressure and respiratory rate of all patients should be monitored before starting and periodically during treatment, checking with the patient that they feel well. Cardiac monitoring may be indicated. High-risk patients should be offered dental treatment in hospital.

CARDIOVASCULAR

Main dental considerations

(*See also generic guidance under main dental considerations above, and also Section 2). Cardiac monitoring may be indicated.

Anxiety and pain can enhance sympathetic activity and adrenaline release, which increases the load on the heart and the risk of angina or arrhythmias. Appointments should be short. Recent evidence indicates that endogenous epinephrine levels peak during morning hours and adverse cardiac events are most likely in the early morning, so late morning appointments are recommended. Patients with heart disease should take their medications as usual on the day of the dental procedure, and should bring all their medications to the dental office for review at the time of the first appointment. The most important aspect for dentists to consider is how well the patient's heart condition is compensated.

Patients with stable heart disease receiving atraumatic treatment under LA can receive treatment in the dental surgery. The dental team should provide dental care with a stress-reduction protocol and with good analgesia. Pain control is crucial to minimize endogenous adrenaline release. Local anaesthetics must be given with aspiration and it may be prudent to avoid epinephrine-containing LA, since adrenaline/epinephrine in the anaesthetic entering a vessel may theoretically raise the BP or precipitate arrhythmias. If a patient is taking a non-selective beta-blocker (e.g. propanolol), use no more than two carpules of LA with epinephrine (adrenaline) 1:80,000. The use of pulse oximetry and prophylactic sedatives should be considered. Cardiac monitoring is desirable in some instances. Conscious sedation preferably with nitrous oxide can be given with the approval of the physician. General anaesthesia (GA) is a matter for expert anaesthetists in hospital.

The combination of aspirin with other anti-platelet drugs increases the chances for significant postoperative bleeding. Aspirin may cause sodium and fluid retention, which may be contraindicated in severe hypertension or cardiac failure. Indometacin may interfere with antihypertensive agents. Furthermore, drugs such as erythromycin and clarithromycin should be avoided in long QT syndrome (p. 66) and in patients also taking statins (antihyperlipidemics). Macrolides, such as erythromycin, and azoles may cause statins to produce increased muscle damage.

In the case of intraoperative chest pain, medical assistance should be summoned, and emergency management commenced, including the use of sublingual GTN (glyceryl trinitrate) spray, aspirin and oxygen.

An association between periodontal disease and cardiovascular disease has been suggested, but recent evidence-based reviews question this association.

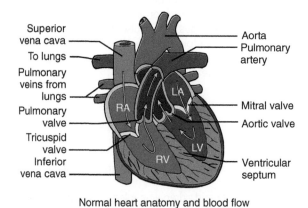

Normal heart anatomy and blood flow

Figure 5.1 Normal heart. Adapted with permission from original artist, Joe Lara III. Available at: http://pediatricheartspecialists.com. RA = right atrium; LA = left atrium; RV = right ventricle; LV = left ventricle.

Aortic valve disease

Aortic stenosis (AS)

Definition
Narrowing of the aortic valve: this generates an increased pressure in the left ventricle.

Aetiopathogenesis
Senile calcification, bicuspid valve (usually asymptomatic, even in athletes – but a high risk for infective endocarditis which may be the first indication of the defect), hypertrophic cardiomyopathy, or Williams syndrome (learning problems, facial dysmorphology, and cardiovascular problems).

Clinical presentation
Angina, dyspnoea, syncope and congestive cardiac failure.

Diagnosis
Echocardiography, ECG and cardiac catheterization.

Treatment
Severe AS necessitates surgical treatment such as percutaneous balloon valvotomy, or commissurotomy, or prosthetic valve replacement. TAVI (Transcatheter Aortic Valve Implantation) is recommended in patients with severe symptomatic AS.

In symptomatic patients, the mean survival is five years. In severe aortic stenosis, sudden death is not uncommon.

Aortic regurgitation (AR)

Definition
The blood propelled to the aorta during systole returns to the left ventricle during diastole.

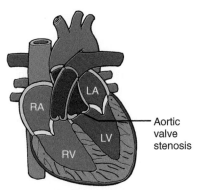

Aortic valve stenosis

Figure 5.2 Aortic valve disease. Adapted with permission from original artist, Joe Lara III. Available at: http://pediatricheartspecialists.com.

Aetiopathogenesis

Congenital defect, rheumatic carditis, infective endocarditis, collagen disorders (Marfan syndrome or Ehlers–Danlos syndrome), hypertension, arthritides, tertiary syphilis, and ankylosing spondylitis.

Clinical presentation

Features may include dyspnoea, palpitations and cardiac failure.

Diagnosis

Echocardiography, ECG, chest radiography and cardiac catheterization.

Treatment

Heart valve replacement/surgical correction by valvotomy, grafts or prosthetic valves. Prosthetic valves are particularly susceptible to infective endocarditis and there is then a high mortality. Infection within the first 6 months usually involving *Staphylococcus aureus*. Replacement of the diseased valve, together with vigorous antimicrobial treatment, frequently eradicates endocarditis.

Main dental considerations

(*See also generic guidance under main dental considerations on page 63 top, and also Section 2); see Endocarditis.

Cardiac arrhythmias (dysrhythmias)

Definition

Alteration in the heartbeat rhythm.

Aetiopathogenesis

Most arrhythmias are because of heart automaticity (impulse formation) or conductivity (block or delay) disorders from cardiac or other disease, or drugs. In some, the cause cannot be determined.

Bradycardia (slow rate)

Intrinsic causes include: myocardial infarction, ischaemia or idiopathic degeneration; infiltrative diseases (sarcoidosis, amyloidosis or haemochromatosis); collagen diseases; myotonic muscular dystrophy; surgical trauma; endocarditis. Extrinsic causes include: autonomically mediated syndromes (vomiting, coughing, micturition, defaecation, etc.); carotid-sinus hypersensitivity from vagal hypertonicity; drugs (beta-adrenergic blockers, calcium-channel blockers, clonidine, digoxin, anti-arrhythmic agents); hypothyroidism; hypothermia; autonomic neurological disorders; or electrolyte imbalances.

Patients with long QT syndrome (LQTS) show on ECG a lengthening of the cardiac cycle repolarization phase. T wave abnormalities may progress to torsades de pointes (TdP) – meaning 'twisting of the spikes', and ventricular fibrillation – and sometimes sudden cardiac death. LQTS clinical presentations range from dizziness to syncope, but for about 10% the condition is not apparent on ECG until after triggering by strenuous physical activity, startling noises or drugs such as LA containing adrenaline or bupivacaine, antimicrobials such as erythromycin and azole antifungals, and GA associated agents

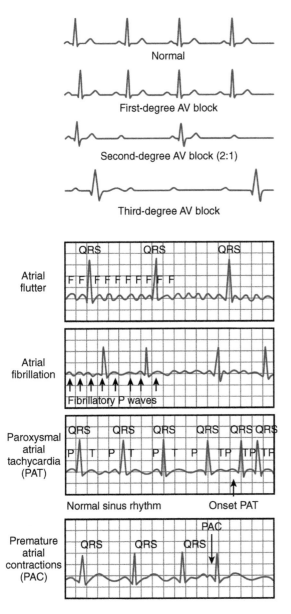

Figure 5.3 Arrhythmia ECGs.

(atropine, succinyl choline or ketamine). LQTS affects about 1–2% of the population and is the second most common cause of sudden cardiac arrest (SCA) in children and young adults. More than half of the people with inherited LQTS die within 10 years.

Tachycardia (fast rate)

May be narrow complex (supraventricular or atrial flutter/fibrillation) or broad complex (ventricular). Causes include: heart disease; congenitally abnormal heart electrical pathways;

anaemia; exercise; stress; hypertension; alcohol, caffeine; smoking; fever; medications; recreational drugs; electrolyte imbalance; and hyperthyroidism.

Clinical presentation and classification

Palpitations are the most frequent symptom, followed by sickness, syncope, dyspnoea and anxiety. Cardiac arrhythmias may cause:

- Ectopic beats (premature atrial, atrioventricular, or ventricular beats)
- Bradycardia (sinus bradycardia, or sinoatrial or atrioventricular heart blocks)
- Tachycardia (sinus, atrial, or ventricular tachycardia)
- Atrial flutter
- Cardiac arrest.

Diagnosis

From electrocardiographic (ECG) findings but electrode catheter technique for intracavitary monitoring may be useful.

Treatment

Arrhythmias are treated by drugs, or pacemaking (using a pacemaker or occasionally implantable cardioverter defibrillator [ICD]), external cardiac defibrillators, cardioversion or catheter ablation (Table 5.1).

Drugs used to control abnormal heart rhythms (or treat related hypertension, coronary artery disease, and heart failure) are mainly:

- Class I drugs (act on *sodium channels;* disopyramide, flecainide, moricizine, procainamide, propafenone, quinidine).
- Class II drugs (*beta-blockers, or beta-adrenoreceptor blocking* drugs; acebutolol, atenolol, bisoprolol, carvedilol, celiprolol, esmolol, labetalol, metoprolol, nadolol, nebivolol, oxyprenolol, pindolol, propranolol, sotalol, timolol).

Table 5.1 Treatment of arrhythmias

Heart rhythm changes	Treatment
Atrial fibrillation (AF)	Cardioversion Digoxin or amiodarone Anticoagulants
Atrial tachycardia	–
Bradycardia (pathological)	Atropine. May need pacemaker
Extrasystoles	–
Paroxysmal supra-ventricular tachycardia (SVT)	Vagal pressure or IV adenosine. Cardiac glycosides or verapamil
Sinus tachycardia	–
Torsades de pointes	Beta-blocker
Ventricular fibrillation (VF)	Defibrillation. Lidocaine, bretyllium, or mexilitine. Acute VF-ICD, flecainide and disopyramide
Ventricular tachycardia	Cardioversion Lidocaine
Wolff-Parkinson-White (pre-excitation) syndrome	Medications or catheter ablation

- Class III drugs (act on *potassium channels;* amiodarone, dofetilide, ibutilide).
- Class IV drugs (*calcium channel blockers* – nifedipine, nicardipine, verapamil).

Anticoagulants may be indicated to reduce stroke risk in some arrhythmias.

Life-threatening cardiac arrhythmias are infrequent but, if it happens, the practitioner should:

- Evaluate vital signs.
- Call for medical assistance.
- Place the patient in the Trendelenburg (legs up) position.
- Administer oxygen.
- Initiate CPR if indicated.
- If there is chest pain, give sublingual GTN.

Main dental considerations

(*See also generic guidance under main dental considerations on page 63 top, and also Section 2).

It is important to avoid stress – it may trigger arrhythmias. Cardiac monitoring may well be indicated. High risk patients and those with severe arrhythmias who should have dental treatment in hospital include those with:

- symptoms;
- resting pulse >100 or <60 associated with any other arrhythmia;
- irregular pulse and bradycardia and wearing a pacemaker.

High frequency, external electromagnetic radiation can interfere with the sensing function of pacemakers and of implantable cardioverter defibrillators (ICDs), and may induce fibrillation. Pacemakers can thus be disrupted by ionizing radiation, ultrasonic, and electromagnetic interference (EMI) from a range of sources. The chief and real hazard to all devices is magnetic resonance imaging (MRI) because of static magnetic, alternating magnetic and radiofrequency (RF) fields produced by MRI. Electrical dental devices (e.g. ultrasonic baths, ultrasonic scalers) induce minor interference with programmers that interrogate implanted cardiac devices but, overall, dental devices do not appear to interfere with pacemakers' and defibrillators' pacing and sensing function. If a pacemaker does shut off, all possible sources of interference should be switched off and the patient given CPR in the supine position.

Use vasoconstrictors with caution. Lidocaine or mepivacaine, which have less of a cardiac affect than some other local anaesthetics, may be preferred for analgesia. LA containing adrenaline or bupivacaine, and antimicrobials such as erythromycin and azole antifungals, and GA associated agents may be contraindicated, particularly if there is any other factor predisposing to TdP. If a LQTS arrhythmia progresses to sudden cardiac arrest, the treatment is prompt shock from an automated external defibrillator (AED).

Arrhythmias can be induced, particularly in older patients and those with ischaemic heart disease (IHD) or aortic stenosis, by:

- Manipulation of the neck, carotid sinus or eyes (vagal reflex).
- LA (rarely).
- Dental extractions or dento-alveolar surgery, which may trigger supraventricular or ventricular ectopics, but these are rarely significant.

- Drugs – GA agents, especially halothane (isoflurane is safer), digitalis, and erythromycin or azole antifungal drugs, especially in patients taking terfenadine, cisapride or astemizole.
- Patients with pacemakers or ICDs do not need antibiotic cover to prevent endocarditis.

Anticoagulants may be given to reduce the stroke risk in some arrhythmias.

Cardiac failure

Definition
The heart functions inefficiently as a pump, and cardiac output and BP fail to meet body needs.

Aetiopathogenesis
Usually cardiac disease (Table 5.2) (e.g. ischaemic heart disease, cardiomyopathy, aortic stenosis, bradycardia), pulmonary disease or overload (e.g. severe anaemia or excess fluid).

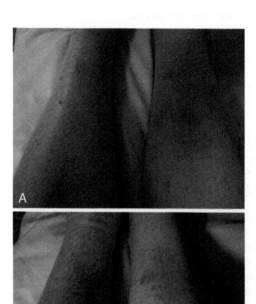

Figure 5.4 (A & B) Pitting oedema in heart failure (**A,** at rest; **B,** after finger pressure over tibia).

Table 5.2 Heart failure; main causes

Left-sided mainly	Right-sided mainly	Bi-ventricular
Aortic valve disease	Chronic obstructive	Aortic valve disease
Hypertension	pulmonary disease	Arrhythmias
Ischaemic heart disease	Pulmonary embolism	Cardiomyopathies
Mitral valve disease		Chronic anaemias
		Hypertension
		Hyperthyroidism
		Ischaemic heart disease
		Mitral valve disease

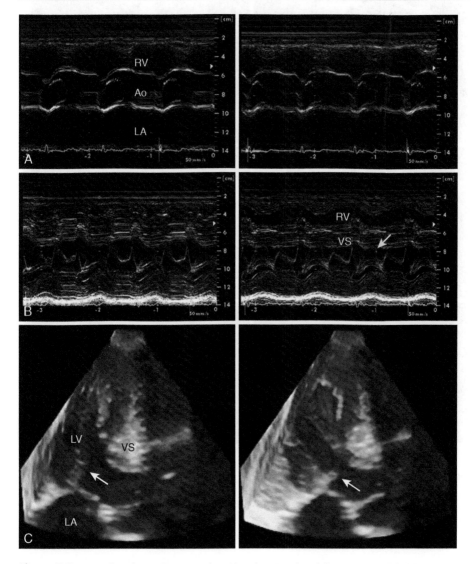

Figure 5.5 M-mode echocardiogram of aortic valve. Reprinted from Bonow RO, Mann DL, Zipes DP (2011) Braunwald's Heart disease: A Textbook of Cardiovascular Medicine, 9e, Elsevier Saunders with permission from Elsevier. *Continued*

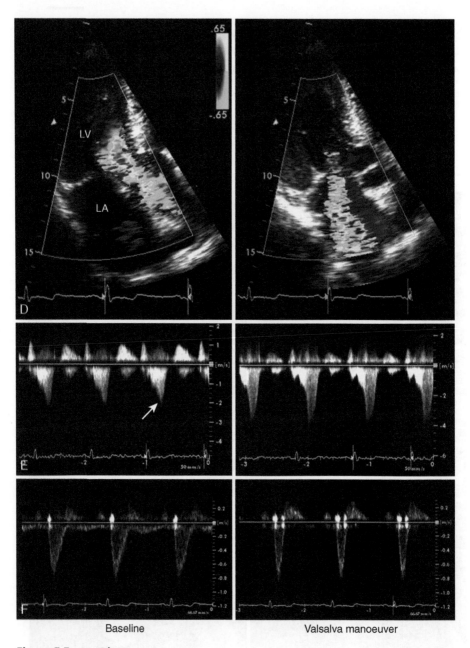

Baseline   Valsalva manoeuver

Figure 5.5, cont'd

Failure can predominantly affect either left or right sides of the heart. Failure of one side usually leads to failure of the other (bi-ventricular).

Clinical presentation

Left-sided heart failure is more common and results in damming back of blood from the left ventricle to the pulmonary circulation causing pulmonary hypertension and pulmonary oedema, with dyspnoea (orthopnoea – dyspnoea on lying), weakness, nocturnal cough, dependent oedema (ankles, sacral area) and cold peripheries. Right-sided failure often follows, particularly if there is mitral stenosis – and causes congestive cardiac failure (CCF).

Right-sided heart failure (cor pulmonale – failure because of respiratory disease leading to increased resistance to blood flow in the pulmonary circulation). Manifests with congestion of both systemic and portal venous systems – affecting mainly the liver, gastrointestinal tract, kidneys and subcutaneous tissues and thus causing peripheral (dependent) oedema, ascites (accumulation of fluid in peritoneal cavity), nausea, anorexia and fatigue.

Heart failure is usually progressive. Arrhythmias and sudden death may result.

Classification

Heart failure is graded (by New York Heart Association; NYHA) as:
- Grade I: Asymptomatic.
- Grade II: Slight limitation of physical activity.
- Grade III: Marked limitation of physical activities.
- Grade IV: Dyspnoea at rest.

Diagnosis

Clinical findings, echocardiography, ECG and chest radiography.

Treatment

Treat cause: low salt diet; diuretic (e.g. furosemide); angiotensin converting enzyme inhibitor (ACEI); angiotensin receptor (AR) blocker eplerenone; AR neprilysin inhibitor (ARNI such as sacubitril valsartan); hydralazine–isosorbide dinitrate; ivabradine; or beta-blocker.

Main dental considerations

(*See also generic guidance under main dental considerations on page 63 top, and also Section 2).

The dental chair should be kept erect or in a partially reclining position since to lay any patient with left-sided heart failure supine may worsen dyspnoea. Discharge patient slowly to avoid orthostatic hypotension.

Use vasoconstrictors with caution. Avoid prolonged use of NSAIDs; limit prescription to 4 days or less. Erythromycin and tetracycline can induce digitalis toxicity by reducing gut breakdown.

Cardiomyopathies

Definition
Heart muscle disease. Uncommon disorders.

Aetiopathogenesis
Intrinsic cardiomyopathy causes may include drug toxicity, infections (including hepatitis C), and various genetic and idiopathic causes. Alcohol is a main cause.

Extrinsic or specific cardiomyopathies include those associated with IHD; nutritional diseases; cardiac valvular disease; hypertension; inflammatory diseases or systemic metabolic disease.

Clinical presentation and classification
Frequently, there are no symptoms until complications develop. Cardiac failure with atrial fibrillation or other serious complications (mitral regurgitation, angina, sudden death or infective endocarditis) can, however, result.

Exercise-induced sudden death is a constant risk.

Cardiomyopathies are divided into three main types (dilated, hypertrophic or restrictive) based on the pathologic features.

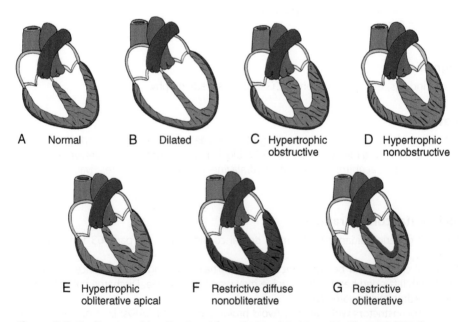

A Normal	B Dilated	C Hypertrophic obstructive	D Hypertrophic nonobstructive
E Hypertrophic obliterative apical	F Restrictive diffuse nonobliterative	G Restrictive obliterative	

Figure 5.6 Cardiomyopathies. Reprinted from Bonow RO, Mann DL, Zipes DP (2011) Braunwald's Heart Disease: A Textbook of Cardiovascular Medicine, 9e, Elsevier Saunders with permission from Elsevier.

Diagnosis

ECG, echocardiography, chest imaging, cardiac MRI.

Treatment

Implanted pacemakers, defibrillators or Ventricular Assist Devices (VADS), or cardiac transplantation often become necessary. Types:

- *Dilated*; diuretics, ACEI, angiotensin II receptor blockers, β-blockers.
- *Hypertrophic*; β-blockers or ablation.
- *Restrictive*; endocardial resection.

Main dental considerations

(*See also generic guidance under main dental considerations on page 63 top, and also Section 2).

Patients with cardiomyopathy are a poor risk for GA because of alcoholism, arrhythmias, cardiac failure or myocardial ischaemia.

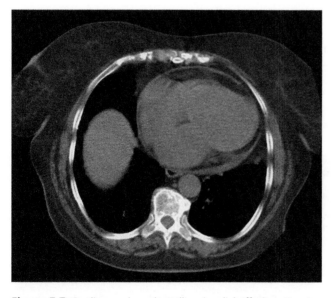

Figure 5.7 Cardiomegaly and small pericardial effusion. Courtesy of Mr A. Kalantzis (Manchester).

Cerebrovascular accidents (CVA); cerebrovascular events (CVE)

Stroke

Definition

A fairly common, sudden, or rapidly progressing, condition with focal CNS signs and symptoms that do not resolve in 24 hours, resulting in impaired motor function, speech and mental damage, and sometimes death.

Aetiopathogenesis and classification

Three types based on aetiology: thrombosis, emboli or haemorrhage. Thrombosis or emboli from heart or great vessels produces focal brain necrosis (infarction). CNS bleeding may follow hypertension, ruptured aneurysm, or trauma (Table 5.3). The risk of stroke is greater in:

- a positive family history of stroke
- cocaine use
- diabetes
- hyperlipidaemia
- hypertension
- ischaemic heart disease
- men
- older people
- smokers
- women on the oral contraceptive pill (OCP).

Table 5.3 Different types of strokes

	Intracerebral haemorrhage	Sub-arachnoid	Thrombosis	Embolism
Underlying diseases	Hypertension Atherosclerosis	Congenital arterial aneurysm (berry aneurysm)	Hypertension Atherosclerosis	Atrial fibrillation Infective endocarditis
Prodromal	None	None	TIAs	None
Onset	Sudden	Sudden	Gradual	Sudden
First symptom	Headache	Headache	Ill-defined	Headache
Hemiplegia and aphasia	Progressive	Progressive	Gradual and intermittent	Almost immediate
Prognosis	Lethal	Lethal	Variable	Recurrence in 80%

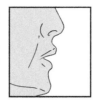 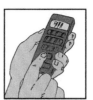

Face	Arm	Speech	Time
Look for an uneven smile	Check if one arm is weak	Listen for slurred speech	Call for help urgently

Figure 5.8 FAST – signs of stroke.

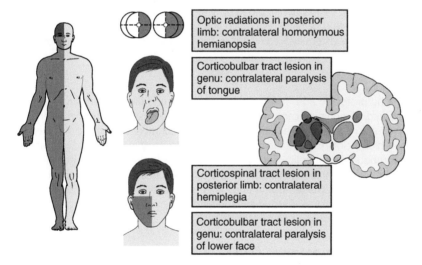

Figure 5.9 Stroke – features.

Table 5.4 CNS complications following stroke

	Right side brain lesion	Left side brain lesion
Side paralysed	Left	Right
Other deficits	Thought, special, perception	Language, speech
Other problems	Memory Problems performing tasks and using mirrors	Memory Problems in organization

Clinical presentations

Acronym FAST:

- **F**ace palsy (paralysis) signifies hemiplegia (loss of voluntary movement of the opposite side of the body to the CNS lesion).
- **A**rm cannot be raised usually on same side (hemiplegia).
- **S**peech loss (aphasia) usually results from a lesion on the left side of the brain.
- **T**ime – rapid deterioration.

There may be vision loss or deterioration. Strokes affecting the brainstem may compromise the gag and swallowing reflexes.

Stroke may cause loss of consciousness, coma or death. About 45% of people with a stroke die within a month.

Diagnosis

Clinical findings and MRI/CT and Doppler blood flow. Tests to determine location and cause of the stroke (e.g. CT or MRI of head; ECG; echocardiogram; carotid duplex ultrasound); cerebral arteriography; brainstem evoked response audiometry; clotting and thrombophilia screens.

Treatment

The airway must be protected and, for most, intensive care and life support, and oxygen are urgently required. Nimodipine can reduce intracranial vasospasm, and neurosurgery to clip an aneurysm in subarachnoid haemorrhage can be curative. In some other cases, removal of brain blood clots may be indicated. Medical care may include anticoagulation if stroke is thrombotic or embolic. Recombinant tissue plasminogen activator (RTPA; alteplase) lyses clots and restores blood flow to the affected area to help prevent further cell death and permanent damage; aspirin and other anti-platelet drugs are also used to prevent non-haemorrhagic strokes. Carotid endarterectomy (removal of plaque from carotid arteries), may help lower the risk of some strokes.

Transient ischaemic attacks (TIA)

Definition

Sudden, or rapidly progressing, focal CNS signs and symptoms that fully resolve in 24 hours.

Aetiopathogenesis

Usually carotid atheroma.

Clinical presentation

Typically embolic, causing focal cerebral deficits (e.g. facial numbness, hemiplegia or dysarthria). About 30% of TIAs progress to strokes.

Reversible Ischaemic Neurological Deficit (RIND) is similar to TIA but persists for >24 hours.

Diagnosis

As for stroke.

Treatment

Aspirin. Treat underlying cause.

Subarachnoid haemorrhage

Definition

Spontaneous arterial haemorrhage into the subarachnoid space from a burst saccular aneurysm (berry aneurysm).

Aetiopathogenesis

Risk factors include:

- Alcohol abuse
- Bleeding disorder
- Genetic tendency (type 3 collagen deficiency, polycystic kidneys, coarctation of aorta, Ehlers–Danlos [hyperflexibility] syndrome)
- Hypertension
- Smoking.

Clinical presentation

- Acute intense headache
- Vomiting
- Collapse
- Neck stiffness or pain
- Coma and death.

Diagnosis

- CT
- ± Lumbar puncture.

Treatment

Neurosurgery (urgent).

Main dental considerations in cerebrovascular events

(*See also generic guidance under main dental considerations on page 63 top, and also Section 2).

In stroke, orofacial features may include:

- Unilateral facial palsy.
- Swallowing problems with an increased risk of aspiration.

Avoid elective dental treatment for 6 months after a stroke or TIA. Arrange stress-free mid-morning appointments with supine positioning and raise the patient slowly to avoid orthostatic hypotension. Monitor BP and heart rate preoperatively and 5 minutes after LA injection. Consider bleeding tendency if patient is anticoagulated. Ensure oral hygiene is maintained.

Congenital heart disease (CHD)

Definition
Any congenital structural defect of the heart or adjacent great vessels.

Aetiopathogenesis
Causes unknown in most cases. The best known acquired causes are maternal infection (e.g. rubella or cytomegalovirus) and drug misuse. The best known genetic cause is Down syndrome.

Classification
Clinical classification is into cyanotic or acyanotic CHD. Anatomically classified as:
- blood outflow obstruction
- intracardiac shunting
- valvular malformation.

Clinical presentation
Affecting about 1% of live births, the most striking feature of some CHD is cyanosis (seen when there is >5 g reduced haemoglobin per dl of blood) caused by shunting deoxygenated blood from the right ventricle directly into left heart and systemic circulation (right to left shunt), leading to chronic hypoxaemia ('blue babies'). Chronic hypoxaemia severely impairs development and causes gross clubbing of fingers (see Fig. 5.12) and toes.

Patients may crouch to increase venous return and, when polycythaemia develops, haemorrhages or thromboses can result. About 20% of patients have cardiovascular or other anomalies elsewhere.

Among the most obvious clinical features of CHD are severe cyanosis, loud cardiac murmurs and effects from chronic hypoxaemia. Paroxysms of cyanosis and breathlessness, which typically cause cerebral hypoxia and syncope, often supervene. In the absence of treatment there is typically heart failure, respiratory infection or infective endocarditis (Table 5.5).

Table 5.5 Possible complications in CHD	
Cardiorespiratory complications	**Liability to infections**
Bleeding tendency	Brain abscess
Cardiac failure	Infective endocarditis
Cyanosis	
Fatigue	
Growth retardation	
Polycythaemia	
Pulmonary oedema	

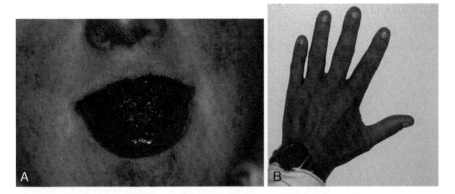

Figure 5.10 Central cyanosis in congenital heart disease showing in **(A)** tongue, lips and **(B)** peripheries.

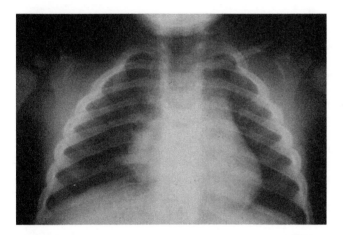

Figure 5.11 Congenital heart disease with cardiomegaly.

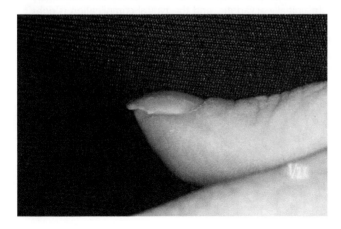

Figure 5.12 Finger clubbing.

Cyanotic CHD

Includes:

- *Eisenmenger syndrome* – cyanosis from reversal of left-to-right shunt, usually through VSD.
- *Fallot tetralogy*:
  - Ventricular septal defect (VSD)
  - Pulmonary stenosis
  - Straddling of the interventricular septum by the aorta
  - Compensatory right ventricular hypertrophy.
- *Pulmonary atresia* – similar to tricuspid atresia – a three-chambered heart but patent tricuspid valve.
- *Transposition of great vessels* – reversal of pulmonary artery and aorta origins.
- *Tricuspid atresia* – includes absence of the tricuspid valve, right ventricle and pulmonary valve. The ductus arteriosus is patent.

Acyanotic CHD

Includes:

- *Aortic stenosis* – see above.
- *Atrial septal defect* (ASD) – often located near the foramen ovale, and termed a secundum defect and, in 10–20%, is associated with mitral valve prolapse. It may have little effect or cause right ventricular failure. An embolus from a vein can pass from the right ventricle into the left and therefore directly to the systemic circulation and can occasionally cause a stroke and be fatal (paradoxical embolism).
- *Coarctation of aorta* – aortic narrowing, beyond the origin of the subclavian arteries, with severe hypertension in the upper body and a low BP below – with strong radial pulses but weak or absent femoral pulses (radio-femoral delay). Secondary enlargement of collateral arteries (such as intercostals) and degenerative changes in the aorta can lead to a fatal aneurysm. Infective endocarditis or left ventricular failure are other possible causes of death.
- *Mitral valve prolapse* (see above).
- *Patent ductus arteriosus* (PDA) – a persistent opening between aorta and pulmonary arteries. Shunt is left to right, initially acyanotic, and the typical complication is right ventricular failure.
- *Pulmonary stenosis* – narrowing of the pulmonary valve. The main symptoms are breathlessness and right ventricular failure, often in childhood.
- *VSD* – one of the most common congenital defects – ranges from pinholes compatible with survival into middle age, to defects so large as to cause death in infancy. There is a left to right shunt with right ventricular hypertrophy, right ventricular failure, reversal of the shunt and late onset cyanosis. 90% have other cardiac defects.

Diagnosis

- Auscultation (heart murmur)
- Chest radiography
- ECG
- Echocardiography
- Arterial blood gases
- Cardiac catheterization
- Angiocardiography.

Treatment

Surgical correction of the anatomic defects is often the treatment of choice. Digitalis, diuretics and anticoagulants to control complications.

Surgery has enormously improved CHD prognosis but residual defects may still predispose to infective endocarditis. Children with CHD receiving modern surgical and medical care now often survive into adult life when they are sometimes called 'Grown-up congenital heart disease'.

Main dental considerations

(*See also generic guidance under main dental considerations on page 63 top, and also Section 2); see Endocarditis.

Endocarditis (infective bacterial endocarditis; IE)

Definition
Infection of heart valves or endocardium.

Aetiopathogenesis
Platelets and fibrin deposit at endothelial sites where there is turbulent blood flow (non-bacterial thrombotic endocarditis) because of valve damage. Such sterile 'vegetations', if there is subsequent bacteraemia, can become infected (IE). Medical, or surgical procedures on genito-urinary or gastrointestinal tract, or dental procedures, can initiate a bacteraemia.

Cardiac valves already damaged by IE or rheumatic carditis, or prosthetic cardiac valves, can readily become infected. Comparable diseases result if there is infection in: arterio-venous shunts for haemodialysis or intravascular access devices such as central intravenous lines, Hickman lines or Uldall catheters. The variables which determine whether microorganisms will infect are unclear. Highly virulent bacteria, e.g. staphylococci, can be introduced into the bloodstream with a drug addict's needle and can cause particularly severe IE – usually on the right side of an apparently previously healthy heart.

Clinical presentation
IE may cause progressive heart damage; infection or embolic damage of many organs, especially the kidneys, brain; immune complex-mediated vasculitis, arthritis, and renal damage; or Osler's nodes – small, tender skin vasculitic lesions. In IE due to viridans streptococci, there is insidious low fever and mild malaise. Skin pallor (anaemia) or light (café-au-lait) pigmentation, joint pains and hepatosplenomegaly are typical. Without treatment, IE may be fatal in about 30%.

Diagnosis
Clinical and
- Changing cardiac murmurs
- ECG

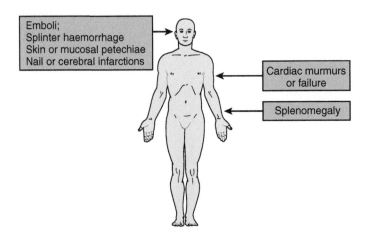

Emboli;
Splinter haemorrhage
Skin or mucosal petechiae
Nail or cerebral infarctions

Cardiac murmurs
or failure

Splenomegaly

Figure 5.13 Endocarditis – features.

- Echo (Doppler and trans-oesophageal)
- Blood culture positive.

Treatment

Antibiotics. In severe cases, early removal of infected valves and insertion of a sterile replacement.

Main dental considerations

(*See also generic guidance under main dental considerations on page 63 top, and also Section 2).

Endocarditis prophylaxis

In the past, patients with nearly every type of congenital and some acquired heart defects were recommended to receive antibiotics one hour before procedures or operations on the teeth, mouth, throat, gastrointestinal genital, or urinary tract. However, the risk: benefit ratio of antimicrobial prophylaxis for endocarditis remains questionable since infective endocarditis:

- only rarely follows dental procedures;
- it has not been proven that antimicrobial prophylaxis effectively prevents endocarditis;
- there is always a risk of adverse reactions to the antimicrobial.

In countries where there are national guidelines on antimicrobial prophylaxis against IE, it may be mandatory for medicolegal reasons to give such prophylaxis to patients at risk. For example, in 2007 the ADA (American Dental Association), endorsed by the Infectious Diseases Society of America and Pediatric Infectious Diseases Society, recommended prophylaxis, but in only high-risk circumstances such as:

- History of IE.
- Artificial heart valves.
- Certain specific, serious congenital heart conditions, namely:
  - Unrepaired cyanotic congenital heart defects, including palliative shunts and conduits.
  - Completely repaired congenital heart defects with prosthetic material or device, whether placed by surgery or by catheter intervention, during the first 6 months after the procedure (prophylaxis is recommended for first 6 months because endothelialization of prosthetic material occurs within 6 months after the procedure).
  - Repaired congenital heart defect with residual defects at the site or adjacent to the site of a prosthetic patch or prosthetic device (which inhibit endothelialization).
  - Cardiac transplantation recipients who develop heart valve dysfunction.

The UK National Institute for Health and Clinical Excellence (NICE) issued recommendations in 2008, completely removing the need for antibiotic prophylaxis in relation to dentistry. *Antibiotic prophylaxis is now not recommended for patients at risk of endocarditis undergoing dental procedures.* Patients at risk of endocarditis should achieve and maintain high standards of oral health. NICE recommended that patients at risk for endocarditis should receive intensive preventive oral healthcare, to try and minimize the need for dental intervention. http://pathways.nice.org.uk/pathways/prophylaxis-against-infectiveendocarditis www.nice.org.uk/guidance/CG64/chapter/introduction. Guidance is being revised.

Hypertension

Definition
Hypertension is when either or both systolic or diastolic BP are persistently raised, with systolic BP over 140 mmHg and diastolic BP over 90 mmHg, and on re-measurement. The ideal BP is <140/80 (systolic/diastolic, at two or three separate readings at rest).

Aetiopathogenesis
Primary (essential) hypertension
BP tends to rise with age but in more than 90% of people with hypertension the cause is unknown and it is then termed essential hypertension. It appears related to genetic influences, obesity and other factors.

Secondary hypertension
About 40% of hypertensive patients have raised levels of catecholamines (epinephrine [adrenaline] and norepinephrine [noradrenaline]) levels and have excess sympathetic activity. Hypertension may also be due to causes such as renal or endocrine disorders, pregnancy or use of oral contraceptive or recreational drugs.

Clinical presentation
About 20% of the population are hypertensive, but about one third are unaware of it. In severe hypertension (≥180/110 mmHg) there may be dizziness and headache. Hypertension increases risk of heart and kidney disease and stroke.

Uncomplicated hypertension causes no symptoms or trivial complications such as epistaxes. Symptoms may include headache, blurred vision, tinnitus, fatiguability and dizziness (Table 5.6).

However, complications related mainly to arteriosclerosis (stroke, myocardial infarct, cardiac and renal failure) may predispose to damage to:
- Heart – mainly IHD (ischaemic heart disease);
- Kidneys;

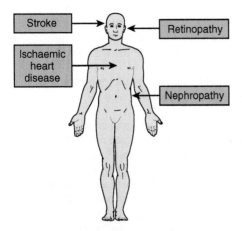

Figure 5.14 Hypertension – features.

Table 5.6 Features of hypertension

Symptoms (advanced hypertension)	Signs
Headaches	Hypertension on testing
Visual problems	Retinal changes
Tinnitus	Left ventricular hypertrophy
Dizziness	Proteinuria
Angina	Haematuria

Table 5.7 ASA (American Society of Anesthesiologists) hypertension grading

BP mmHg (systolic/diastolic)	ASA grade	Hypertension stage
<140/<90	I	–
140–159/90–99	II	1
160–179/95–109	III	2
>180/>110	IV	3

- Brain – particularly stroke;
- Eyes – retinal damage;

and shortened life by 10–20 years.

Malignant hypertension; (BP >200/>130 mmHg) causes retinal haemorrhage and exudates.

Classification

Borderline, mild (stage 1), moderate (stage 2) and severe (stage 3) grades (Table 5.7).

Diagnosis

BP is measured with a sphygmomanometer, in units of millimetres of mercury (mmHg).

Treatment

Acute emotion, particularly anger, fear and anxiety, can raise catecholamine output and increase BP, and should therefore be avoided or minimized. BP control measures are shown in Table 5.8.

Specific antihypertensive therapy is urgently indicated where the systolic BP exceeds 200 mmHg, or the diastolic exceeds 110 mmHg, and it may be indicated at lower levels, particularly if there are vascular or end-organ complications such as renal impairment, or diabetes. Lifelong treatment of hypertension is usually necessary, and typically includes agents shown in Table 5.9; statins and aspirin are prophylaxis of complications.

Table 5.8 Lifestyle risk factors modifying BP

Factors raising BP	Factors lowering BP
Obesity	No obesity
Salt intake high	Salt intake low
Alcohol excess	Alcohol intake low
Smoking	Smoking cessation
Physical inactivity	Physical activity
Stress or anxiety	Peace and relaxation
Drugs such as cocaine	Drugs such as antihypertensives
	Omega-3 fatty acids
	Fruit and vegetables
	Supplemental potassium
	High fibre diet

Table 5.9 Antihypertensive drugs

Antihypertensive agents	Examples
Diuretics	Bendrofluazide
Angiotensin converting enzyme inhibitors (ACEI)	Enalapril
Angiotensinogen II receptor (AR) blockers	Losartan
AR neprilysin inhibitor (ARNI)	LCZ696
Calcium channel blockers	Nifedipine
Alpha-adrenergic blockers (less commonly)	Doxazosin

Main dental considerations

(*See also generic guidance under main dental considerations on page 63 top, and also Section 2).

Defer elective care if BP is ≥180/110. BP should be controlled before elective dental treatment or the opinion of a physician should be sought first. Dental management can be complicated, since the BP often rises even before a visit for dental care; preoperative reassurance is important and sedation using temazepam may be helpful. Use vasoconstrictors with caution. Under most circumstances, the use of adrenaline/epinephrine in combination with LA is not contraindicated in the hypertensive patient unless the systolic pressure is >200 mmHg and/or the diastolic is >115 mmHg. Epinephrine (adrenaline)-containing LA should not be given in large doses to patients taking beta-blockers, since interactions between adrenaline/epinephrine and the beta-blocker may induce hypertension and cardiovascular complications. Lidocaine should be used with caution in patients taking beta-blockers. Continuous BP monitoring is indicated.

Raising the patient suddenly from the supine position may cause postural hypotension and loss of consciousness if the patient is on antihypertensive drugs.

Ischaemic heart disease (IHD)

Also known as coronary heart disease (CHD) or coronary artery disease (CAD).

Definition

Progressive myocardial ischaemia due to reduced coronary artery blood flow. Cardiovascular diseases kill more persons than all other diseases combined.

Aetiopathogenesis

Atherosclerosis (Greek, *athere* [porridge] and *sclerosis* [hardening]) – also termed atheroma or arteriosclerosis (Table 5.10), caused by lipid accumulation in artery walls and now often termed atherosclerotic cardiovascular disease (ACVD). High blood cholesterol is a major risk factor for IHD: very low density lipoproteins (VLDL) are associated with high risk, but high density lipoproteins (HDL) appear to be anti-atherogenic. High blood cholesterol itself causes no symptoms.

   Atherosclerosis is a disease predominantly of males, linked to age, race (high in Africans and Asians), smoking, diabetes mellitus, lack of exercise, hypertension and hyperlipidaemia. Restricted blood flow may cause angina, and rupture of atheromatous plaque may cause myocardial infarction (MI), emboli, coronary arterial spasm or vasculitis.

Clinical presentation

Impaired coronary artery blood flow causes ischaemia which in itself is symptomless and only manifests by its dramatic complications of acute coronary syndromes (ACS) – namely angina pectoris or myocardial infarction which often appear without warning or IHD history. However, a chronically reduced myocardial blood supply progressively damages the heart, which can lead to cardiac failure and/or dysrhythmias. There may be other features of atherosclerosis (Table 5.11).

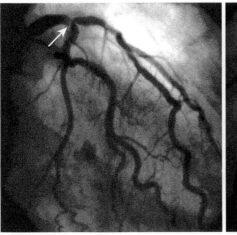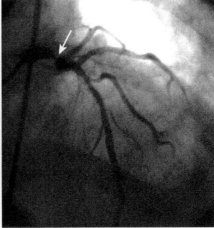

Figure 5.15 Coronary angiography in ischaemic heart disease (IHD). Arrows show stenoses. Reprinted from Bonow RO, Mann DL, Zipes DP (2011) Braunwald's Heart Disease: A Textbook of Cardiovascular Medicine, 9e. Elsevier Saunders, with permission from Elsevier.

Table 5.10 Ischaemic heart disease risk and protective factors

Primary risk factors	Secondary risk factors	Unclear effects	Protective factors
High LDL	Low HDL	Low dietary fibre	Increased HDL: LDL
Hypertension	Diabetes	Hard water	Exercise
Smoking	Obesity	High plasma fibrinogen	Moderate red wine or alcohol
	Family history of CHD	Raised blood factor VII	
	Physical inactivity	Raised lipoprotein levels	
	Type A personality		
	Gout		
	Ethnicity (Asians)		
	Male gender		
	Increasing age		
	Low socioeconomic class		
	High homocysteine levels		
	Chronic renal failure		

Table 5.11 Main sites and results of atherosclerosis

Site	Clinical syndromes
Coronary arteries	Chest pain (angina) or myocardial infarction
Cerebral arteries	Stroke
Peripheral arteries	Impaired oxygenation, and leg pain (intermittent claudication) and sometimes gangrene

Acute coronary syndrome usually occurs as a result of one of three problems: ST elevation myocardial infarction (STEMI), non ST elevation myocardial infarction (NSTEMI), or unstable angina.

- *Stable (classic) angina* – is pain predictably brought on by exercise or emotional upset, relieved by rest, not changed in last 2 months; responds to nitroglycerine.
- *Unstable angina* (pre-infarction) recent increase in severity or frequency; decreased threshold of precipitants; unpredictable response to nitroglycerine.
- *Myocardial infarction* differs from angina in that it:
  - causes severe and persistent pain (>20 min)
  - causes pain not controlled by rest
  - leads to irreversible heart damage or death.

Diagnosis

Clinical, confirmed by ECG which shows the following:

- *In angina,* normal ECG, or shows ST depression, flat or inverted T waves.
- *In MI,* shows hyperacute T waves, ST elevation or Q wave. ST segment elevation MI (STEMI) occurs when a coronary artery is totally occluded.

- Exercise ECG – also usually carried out, reveals the ECG changes in angina.
- Coronary arteriography (angiography) – shows arterial stenosis or occlusion and allows for intervention if necessary (percutaneous coronary intervention; PCI) using angioplasty and placement of stents to correct any stenosis. A radionuclide such as [201]thallium (MIBI or sestamibi, MPS or technetium) scan can enhance sensitivity.
- Cardiac enzymes; increase in serum. In MI, troponin rises within 6 hours and others (creatine kinase, aspartate transaminase, lactic dehydrogenase) – over 12–36 hours.
- Coronary calcium scoring or carotid intima-media thickness test (CIMT). Troponin I test is a fluorescent new rapid immunoassay.

Treatment

The most effective way to prevent, or to treat patients with IHD includes:

Lifestyle changes

- *Reducing*:
  - alcohol
  - animal fats
  - body weight
  - salt
  - smoking
  - stress and tension.
- *Increasing*:
  - exercise 30 minutes on most, if not all, days;
  - fruits and vegetables, which are high in antioxidants, or omega 3 oils (fish such as salmon, tuna, and mackerel).

Drugs

- Anticoagulant/antiplatelet (aspirin, clopidogrel, ticlopidine, warfarin) to inhibit clotting.
- Beta-blockers (atenolol, metoprolol, propranolol) if BP 140/90 or higher.
- Angiotensin converting enzyme inhibitors (ACEI) (captopril, enalapril, fosinopril, lisinopril, ramipril), lower peripheral resistance and cardiac workload.
- Drugs to lower VLDL; statins (pravastatin, simvastatin etc) reduce LDL.

Treatment of angina

During angina attacks, or before anticipated precipitants, nitroglycerine (glyceryl trinitrate; GTN) 0.3 to 0.6 mg sublingually may prevent or treat pain. Long-acting nitrates (isosorbide dinitrate) may prevent attacks.

Surgical management includes angioplasty, stents and coronary artery bypass graft (CABG; 'cabbage').

Treatment of MI

MI (coronary thrombosis or heart attack) is the most severe and lethal form of ACS, in which atherosclerotic plaques rupture, leading to platelet activation, adhesion and aggregation and thus thrombosis impeding filling of the coronary arteries. Under 50% of patients with MI have premonitory symptoms. Sometimes MI is preceded by angina, often felt as indigestion-like pain. The pain is often unmistakable and described as an unbearably severe sense of strangling or choking, or tightness, heaviness, compression or constriction of the chest, and is not relieved by rest or relieved by nitrates. Vomiting, facial pallor, sweating, restlessness and apprehension are common. About 10% have silent (painless) infarctions and the first signs may then be the sudden onset of left ventricular failure, shock, collapse, or death.

Death soon after the onset of chest pain is common, often from ventricular fibrillation or cardiac arrest. Up to 50% of patients die within the first hour of MI and a further 10–20% within the next few days. Cardiac failure and dysrhythmias may develop in survivors.

Diagnosis

Clinical features, supported by ECG (ST segment may be normal or raised, with hyperacute T and acute Q waves) and serum enzyme changes – earliest are troponin T rises; later are raised creatine kinase MB, aspartate transaminase and lactic dehydrogenase.

Treatment

An ambulance should be called: immediate hospital admission and treatment of acute MI, halves the mortality rate. The patient should be:

- kept at rest and reassured as well as possible;
- given oxygen by a face mask or intranasally; nitrous oxide with at least 28% oxygen, to relieve pain and anxiety;
- given 300 mg of soluble aspirin by mouth.

Main dental considerations

(*See also generic guidance under main dental considerations on page 63 top, and also Section 2).

Angina is a rare cause of pain in the mandible, teeth or other oral tissues, neck or pharynx.

For high-risk patients – (unstable) angina or myocardial infarction (MI) within the past 30 days) – defer elective treatment. Delay routine dental treatment for 6 weeks if patient has had a revascularization procedure (i.e., coronary artery bypass graft or stent placement). A physician's opinion is strongly advised.

Patients with stable angina, and those who are at least 3 months post-MI, may be treated in primary care; as a precaution, ask patients to bring their nitroglycerine medication with them. Patients with unstable angina and those with MI <3 months previously, should have dental treatment in a hospital environment. Conscious sedation should be deferred for at least 3 months for patients after MI, recent-onset angina, unstable angina or recent development of bundle branch block and, in any case, should be given in hospital. GA should be avoided wherever possible and at least deferred for 3 months after MI.

Care with NSAIDs which if used for more than 3 weeks, can impair beta-blockers and ACE inhibitors. Macrolide antibiotics such as erythromycin and clarithromycin, and azole antifungals interact with statins to increase muscle damage (rhabdomyolysis).

Mitral valve disease

Mitral stenosis

Definition
Narrowing of the mitral valve which generates an increasing pressure in the left atrium of the heart.

Aetiopathogenesis
Rheumatic fever, CHD and others.

Clinical presentation
Features are related to increased pressure in pulmonary veins:
- Chest pain
- Dyspnoea and fatigue
- Systemic emboli.

Life expectancy of untreated symptomatic patients is about 5 years.

Diagnosis
- Doppler echo
- Echocardiography
- ECG
- Cardiac catheterization.

Treatment
- Anticoagulants
- Digoxin
- Diuretics
- Surgery (balloon valvuloplasty, valvotomy or valve replacement).

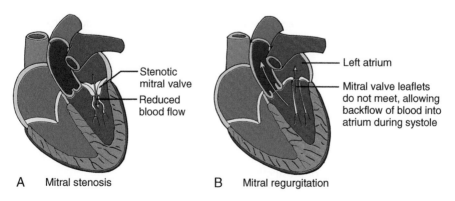

A   Mitral stenosis   B   Mitral regurgitation

Figure 5.16 Mitral valve disease.

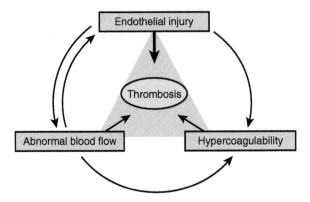

Figure 5.17 Thrombosis – predisposing factors.

Mitral regurgitation

Definition

Blood propulsed to the left ventricle during systolic contraction returns into the left atrium during diastolic dilatation due to defective mitral valve closure.

Aetiopathogenesis

Regurgitation may arise in left ventricular dilatation, valve prolapse, calcification or damage (rheumatic carditis, infective endocarditis), damaged chordae tendinae or muscles, or with some drugs (fenfluramine, phentermine).

Clinical presentation

Features include:

- Dyspnoea
- Fatigue
- Palpitations.

Regurgitation may lead to pulmonary hypertension, cardiac failure, and endocarditis.

Diagnosis

- Echocardiography
- Doppler echo
- Cardiac catheterization
- ECG.

Treatment

- Digoxin
- Surgery (valvotomy, grafts or prosthetic valves).

Functional mitral valve regurgitation (FMR) is considered a disease of the left ventricle, NOT of the mitral valve.

Mitral prolapse

Definition

Protrusion of the valves into the left atrium during systole.

Aetiopathogenesis

There is a strong hereditary tendency and it is a characteristic feature of other conditions (e.g. Ehlers–Danlos syndrome, Marfan syndrome, Down syndrome, Turner syndrome, cardiomyopathies, pseudoxanthoma elasticum, muscular dystrophy, polycystic kidney disease, osteogenesis imperfecta, thyrotoxicosis, ischaemic heart disease, panic disorder and lupus erythematosus).

Clinical presentation

May be no symptoms but some patients develop pain, irregular or racing pulse, or fatigue. Most who exhibit symptoms are actually experiencing dysautonomia from panic disorder (up to 50% of patients with panic disorder have mitral valve prolapse).

Mitral valve prolapse may also be associated with:

- Atrial septal defect
- Mitral regurgitation
- Patent ductus arteriosus.

Usually mitral valve prolapse has a good prognosis, especially in mild cases without regurgitation. Patients may be susceptible to infective endocarditis (see Endocarditis).

Diagnosis

- Echocardiography
- ECG.

Treatment

- Beta-blockers (propanolol).
- Prosthetic valve replacement (particularly susceptible to infective endocarditis).

Main dental considerations

(*See also generic guidance under main dental considerations on page 63 top, and also Section 2); see Endocarditis.

Rheumatic fever (RF)

Definition
Acute fever and arthritis following pharyngitis caused by beta haemolytic bacterium *Streptococcus pyogenes*.

Aetiopathogenesis
Autoimmune reaction to streptococcal cell walls with antibodies that may cause vasculitis and inflammatory lesions of joints, skin, nervous system, and sometimes heart (rheumatic carditis) – mitral valve is often affected.

Clinical presentation
Stenosis and regurgitation of mitral and aortic valves are the most common sequelae of rheumatic heart disease. This leads to atrial fibrillation, cardiac failure and thromboses.

Major features
- Carditis – tachycardia, murmurs.
- Polyarthritis – involving large joints (ankles, knees).
- Skin – subcutaneous nodules or erythema marginatum.
- Sydenham's chorea (St Vitus dance) – involuntary movements.

Minor features
- Arthralgia.
- Blood CRP, ESR, leukocytes, anti-streptolysin O titre (ASOT) increased.
- ECG alterations (PR prolonged).
- Fever.
- Previous rheumatic fever.

Diagnosis
Streptococcal infection (throat swab, raised ASOT and DNase B titre) plus two major manifestations or one major and two minor features.

Treatment
- Bed rest
- Benzyl penicillin
- NSAIDs and possibly corticosteroids.

Prevention
Recurrence rate is high – 50% during the first 5 years. Thus penicillin prophylaxis (once a month) is required, sometimes even until the age of 20 years.

Main dental considerations
(*See also generic guidance under main dental considerations on page 63 top, and also Section 2); see Endocarditis.
Many of these patients take anticoagulants; avoid use of NSAIDs for pain management.

Surgery

Cardiac (heart) surgery can:

- Replace occluded coronary arteries
- Repair or replace heart valves
- Repair abnormal or damaged structures
- Use implant devices to help control the heart beat or support function and blood flow
- Replace a damaged heart.

Traditional heart surgery, called *open-heart surgery*: done by splitting the sternum to open the chest wall for access to the heart. Often, the patient is connected to a heart–lung bypass machine to allow the surgeon to operate on a non-beating heart that has no blood flowing through it. In *off-pump, or beating heart, surgery* such as for *coronary artery bypass grafts* (CABG), however, a heart–lung bypass machine is not used.

Percutaneous transluminal coronary angioplasty (PTCA): aims to open up the coronary blood flow by inserting a balloon-tipped catheter through the groin up via the femoral artery and aorta into the area of arterial blockage. Stents (miniature wire coils) may be inserted to keep arteries open. Cardiac stents are small tubes (typically wire mesh) that are placed in obstructed coronary arteries after angioplasty (balloon dilation of a stenosis) to ensure proper blood flow. Patients after angioplasty are usually given antiplatelets (aspirin forever, plus clopidogrel, prasugrel or ticagrelor for 1 to 12 months; see Section 9).

Coronary artery bypass grafts (CABG): the most common cardiac surgery for adults uses a healthy artery or vein from outwith the heart to graft to and bypass, a blocked coronary artery. Saphenous veins (from the leg) are placed by full sternotomy but minimally invasive surgery uses arteries such as the internal mammary artery without the need for full sternotomy. CABG usually improves or completely relieves angina for 10–15 years and may also reduce MI risk.

Minimally invasive heart surgery (limited access coronary artery surgery): includes port-access coronary artery bypass (PACAB or PortCAB) and minimally invasive coronary artery bypass graft (MIDCAB) involves access via small incisions (termed ports) between the ribs to reach the heart. In PACAB, the heart is stopped and blood is pumped through an oxygenator or 'heart–lung' machine. MIDCAB is used to avoid the heart–lung machine.

Transmyocardial revascularization (TMR): may be used to relieve severe angina in ill patients who are not candidates for bypass or angioplasty. TMR involves an incision on the left breast to expose the heart. Then, a laser is used to drill a series of holes from the outside of the heart into the interior. In some patients TMR is combined with bypass surgery. In those cases an incision through the breastbone is used for the bypass.

Cardiac valve surgery: valve defects may be corrected by valvotomy, grafts or prosthetic valves.

Cardiac transplantation: see Section 9.

Main dental considerations

(*See also generic guidance under main dental considerations on page 63 top, and also Section 2).

Patients scheduled for cardiac surgery should ideally have excellent oral health established before operation, particularly before a valve replacement, major surgery for congenital anomalies or a heart transplant.

For the first 6 months after cardiac surgery elective dental care is best avoided. Emergency dental care should be in a hospital setting. For the first couple of weeks after surgery, the patient may feel severe pain when reclining in the dental chair as a side-effect of the surgery.

The concerns include the risk of post-treatment bleeding and the possibility of interactions with drugs plus the effects of possible bacteraemia on recently stented vessels.

Some patients are on anticoagulants, immunosuppression or other drugs, or may also have a residual lesion. Local anaesthetics with epinephrine may alter BP and PR, although cardiac ischaemic alterations or other cardiovascular complications are rare. Appropriate action is required to deal with any bleeding tendencies but most patients are on aspirin or clopidogrel rather than warfarin. Post-coronary artery bypass graft, patients should not receive an adrenaline/epinephrine-containing LA, since it may possibly precipitate arrhythmias.

Prosthetic valves are particularly susceptible to infective endocarditis and there is then a high mortality rate. Endocarditis within the first 6 months is usually by *Staphylococcus aureus*, rarely of dental origin, and has a mortality rate of around 60%. Patients with vascular stents that are successfully engrafted may warrant antibiotic coverage if emergency dental treatment is required during the first 6 weeks postoperatively.

Thrombosis

(See also Cerebrovascular disease).

Definition
Blood clots that develop, usually in a vein – usually a deep vein thrombosis (DVT).

Aetiopathogenesis
Virchow's triad of predisposing factors is:
- decreased blood flow rate;
- increased tendency to clot (hypercoagulability or thrombophilia); and
- changes to the vessel wall.

Venous thrombosis typically affects calf veins, is more common with advancing age, and risk factors include:
- Hypercoagulability:
  - Autoimmune anti-phospholipid (Hughes) syndrome.
  - Family history of thrombosis.
  - Genetic factors; e.g. thrombophilia due to deficiencies of proteins that normally prevent clotting (antithrombin, protein C and S); blood type non-O (increased factor VIII and vWF); mutations in prothrombin genes and factor V (factor V Leiden makes factor V resistant to inactivation by active protein C).
  - High homocysteine levels (liability to endothelial injury, vessel inflammation and atherogenesis).
  - Medical conditions (e.g. trauma, cancer, heart failure).
  - OCP; oral contraceptive pill.

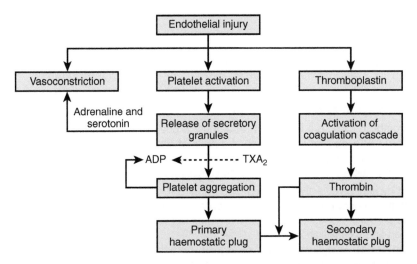

Figure 5.18 Thrombosis aetiopathogenesis. Adapted from Blood as a circulatory fluid and the dynamics of blood and lymph flow. In: Barrett KE, Barman SM, Boitano S, Brooks HL (2012) Ganong's Review of Medical Physiology (24e), McGraw-Hill, Ch. 31, with kind permission from TBC. ADP = adenosine dipjosphate. TXA = thromboxane.

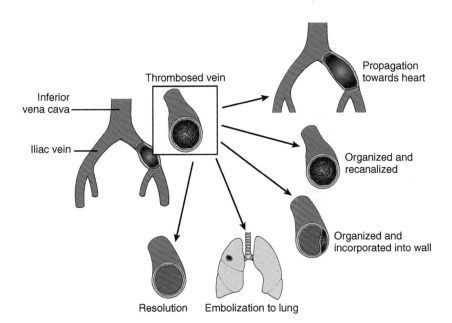

Figure 5.19 Potential outcomes of venous thrombosis. Adapted from Robbins and Cotran Pathologic Basis of Disease (7e) by Kumar V, Abbas, AK, Fausto, N (2007) Philadelphia: Elsevier Saunders.

- Pregnancy.
- Previous venous thromboembolism.
- Inactivity – e.g, postoperatively or long travels.
- Obesity or being overweight.
- Smoking.

Clinical presentation and classification

Deep vein thrombosis (DVT) is a blood clot (thrombus) in one of the deep veins, usually in the leg. This can cause leg pain and swelling. If a piece of clot (embolus) breaks off it may block a lung blood vessel (pulmonary embolism [PE]). Together, DVT and PE are termed venous thrombo-embolism (VTE). Thrombosis outcomes may include death or:

- Dissolution by fibrinolytic activity – when blood flow is re-established.
- Embolization – thrombus may detach and embolize to other sites in the vasculature.
- Organization and recanalization.
- Propagation of clot – may increase and enlarge in size and obstruct blood vessels.

DVT: in some cases may cause no symptoms, but can cause leg pain and swelling. Dorsiflexion at the ankle may aggravate calf pain (Homan sign).

PE: main features include:
- chest pain (sharp, stabbing) worse on inspiration;
- cough – usually dry, but maybe mucus or blood;
- dyspnoea – appearing suddenly or gradually;
- faintness or dizziness.

Diagnosis

DVT: clinical, D-dimer (a blood protein found after a clot has broken down) assay, ultrasound.
PE: clinical, D-dimer, imaging, computerized tomography pulmonary angiography (CTPA), ventilation and perfusion scan.

Prevention

DVT: smoking cessation, weight loss, regularly walking.
PE: methods recommended include:
- anticoagulants, such as aspirin or other antiplatelets, NOACs (Section 9) or warfarin;
- avoiding inactivity;
- calf exercises;
- early and frequent walking;
- graduated compression stockings or devices;
- inferior vena cava filter (e.g. Greenfield filter).

Treatment

DVT: usually involves anticoagulants such as low molecular weight heparin, and compression stockings.
PE: treated with anticoagulants.

Main dental considerations

(*See also generic guidance under main dental considerations on page 63 top, and also Section 2).
Postoperative thrombosis and subsequent bleeding tendency from anticoagulants.

ENDOCRINE AND METABOLIC

Acromegaly

Definition
A chronic, progressive disorder caused by growth hormone (GH) hypersecretion after normal growth cessation. Excess GH production before epiphyseal closure results in gigantism.

Aetiopathogenesis
Usually caused by eosinophilic adenoma of anterior pituitary gland.

Clinical presentation
- broadened nose
- excess tissue growth
- large hands and feet
- macroglossia
- prognathism
- prominent supraorbital ridge
- spaced teeth
- thick skin.

Complications due to organ enlargement
- Cardiomyopathy
- Diabetes
- Hypertension
- Local effects of the pituitary tumour (headache, visual defects).

Diagnosis
- Clinical, laboratory and radiographic findings
- Plasma GH – raised
- Oral glucose tolerance test – fails to suppress GH
- Serum insulin-like growth factor 1 – raised
- CT and MRI.

Treatment
- Neurosurgery and/or radiation.
- Dopamine agonists (bromocriptine).
- Somatostatin analogues (sandostatine).

Main dental considerations
(*See also generic guidance under main dental considerations on page 63 top, and also Section 2).
Skull thickened, paranasal air sinuses enlarged, mandibular enlargement with class III malocclusion and spaced teeth, possible sleep apnoea. Kyphosis and other deformities affecting respiration may make GA hazardous; fatalities have followed orthognathic surgery.

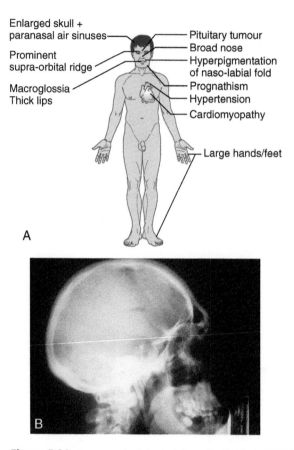

Enlarged skull +
paranasal air sinuses
Prominent
supra-orbital ridge
Macroglossia
Thick lips

Pituitary tumour
Broad nose
Hyperpigmentation
of naso-labial fold
Prognathism
Hypertension
Cardiomyopathy

Large hands/feet

A

B

Figure 5.20 Acromegaly. Adapted from Scully et al. (2007) Special Care in Dentistry: Handbook of Oral Care. Churchill Livingstone Elsevier.

Addison's disease

Definition
Adrenocortical hypofunction with low plasma cortisol.

Aetiopathogenesis
Autoimmune (associated sometimes also with diabetes, Graves' disease, pernicious anaemia, vitiligo or hypoparathyroidism) particularly in women. Rare causes include adrenal tuberculosis, histoplasmosis or tumours.

Secondary hypofunction may follow abrupt systemic corticosteroids withdrawal.

Clinical presentation
Low cortisol leads to raised adrenocorticotrophic hormone (ACTH), weight loss and:
- hypotension (weakness, lethargy, tiredness, collapse);
- hyperpigmentation (skin and mucosae);
- shock and death if the individual is stressed by operation, infection or trauma.

Diagnosis
Postural hypotension and plasma:
- cortisol level – low
- sodium – low
- potassium – high, plus:
  - ACTH stimulation test – impaired
  - adrenal antibodies.

Treatment
Glucocorticoids (cortisone) and mineralocorticoids (fludrocortisone).

Patients undergoing routine surgical procedures rarely need supplemental steroids, but doubling the normal daily dose on the day is often recommended in surgery, extensive procedures and for anxious patients.

During the 2 weeks after cessation of systemic steroid administration, supplemental steroids on the day of the procedure are advised.

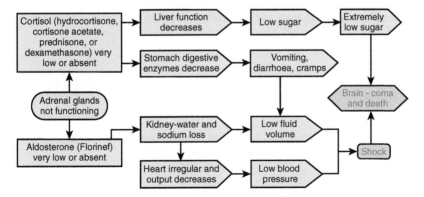

Figure 5.21 Addison's crisis pathway.

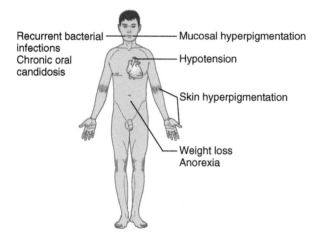

Recurrent bacterial infections
Chronic oral candidosis
Mucosal hyperpigmentation
Hypotension
Skin hyperpigmentation
Weight loss
Anorexia

Figure 5.22 Addison's disease – features. Adapted from Scully et al. (2007) Special Care in Dentistry: Handbook of Oral Care. Churchill Livingstone, Elsevier.

Main dental considerations

(*See also generic guidance under main dental considerations on page 63 top, and also Section 2).
Oral mucous membranes may show brown macular pigmentation. Take caution when prescribing:

- NSAIDs, *or* aspirin simultaneously with steroids – increased risk of peptic ulceration.
- Benzodiazepines – enhance cortisol metabolism.

The concern, especially when undertaking surgery under GA, is of precipitating hypotensive collapse (Addisonian or adrenal crisis). Most patients undergoing routine nonsurgical dental procedures need no supplemental steroids. Best are brief, morning appointments when circulating cortisol levels are highest, with supine positioning and discharge patient slowly to avoid orthostatic hypotension.

However steroid cover is advisable for patients with primary or secondary adrenal insufficiency undergoing surgery, more extensive procedure, or are particularly anxious as they may be at risk for adrenal crisis. The Addison's Clinical Advisory Panel (www.addisons.org.uk/) recommend doubling the steroid dose before significant surgical treatment under LA and continuing this for 24 hours.

Adrenal crisis

Collapse in a patient with Addison disease (or a history of systemic corticosteroid therapy) may be caused by adrenal insufficiency, triggered by GA, trauma, infections or other stress.

Diagnosis

From pallor – rapid, weak or impalpable pulse, rapidly falling BP and loss of consciousness.

Management

- Lay the patient flat with legs raised.
- Give 200 mg hydrocortisone intravenously or orally.
- Give oxygen.
- Summon assistance.

Cushing's syndrome

Definition
The clinical picture resulting from persistently increased adrenal cortex production of hormones, especially cortisol and androgens.

Aetiopathogenesis
Main cause is Cushing's disease – usually caused by a pituitary microadenoma which produces adrenocorticotrophic hormone (ACTH), which then stimulates the adrenals to produce excess corticosteroid hormones.

Other causes include:

• ACTH or corticosteroid administration
• ACTH production by other tumours
• Adrenal tumours.

Clinical presentation
• Amenorrhoea
• Facial swelling ('moon face')
• Fat redistribution with swelling over back of neck ('buffalo hump')
• Hirsutism
• Hyperglycaemia (from gluconeogenesis)
• Hypertension

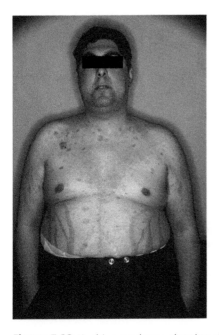

Figure 5.23 Cushing syndrome showing obesity and striae.

- Immunodeficiency and liability to infections
- Protein breakdown (skin striae, bruising, myopathy and osteoporosis)
- Weight gain.

Diagnosis

- Plasma cortisol – raised, and also loss of circadian rhythm of cortisol release.
- Overnight dexamethasone suppression (of cortisol) test – reduced.
- Urinary cortisol excretion – raised.
- CT – to locate any responsible tumour.

Treatment

Trans-sphenoidal surgery, or irradiation of pituitary tumour; resection of any adrenal tumour; steroid antagonists.

Main dental considerations

(*See also generic guidance under main dental considerations on page 63 top, and also Section 2).

Patients show a round plethoric 'moon face'. Patients have an increased susceptibility to infection and poor wound healing and are at risk from an adrenal crisis if subjected to surgery, anaesthesia or trauma. Consult the physician about need for steroid supplementation.

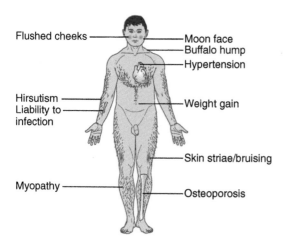

Figure 5.24 Cushing's disease – features. Adapted from Scully et al. (2007) Special Care in Dentistry: Handbook of Oral Care. Churchill Livingstone, Elsevier.

Diabetes insipidus (DI)

Definition

A rare disorder characterized by increased water intake and elimination, due to low posterior pituitary secretion of antidiuretic hormone (ADH) (cranial or central DI), or renal resistance to ADH (nephrogenic DI).

Aetiopathogenesis

Although idiopathic and hereditary types have been recognized, most cases are:
Cranial DI – caused by:

- Autoimmune disease
- Head injury or trauma
- Meningitis
- Sarcoidosis
- Tumours (craniopharyngioma)
- Vascular.

Nephrogenic DI – caused by:

- Drugs (demeclocycline, lithium)
- Hypercalcaemia or hypokalaemia
- Renal disease.

Clinical presentation

Sudden onset polydipsia and polyuria, with normal urine and blood glucose. Weakness, fever and psychiatric disorders are common in cases of dehydration.

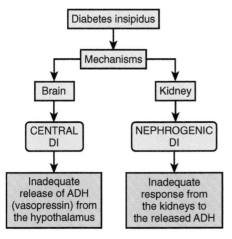

Figure 5.25 Diabetes insipidus. ADH = antidiuretic hormone.

Diagnosis

- Clinical findings
- Plasma osmolality – high
- Urine osmolality – low
- Water deprivation test – fails to significantly alter plasma osmolality.

Treatment

- Treat the cause.
- Desmopressin.

Main dental considerations

(*See also generic guidance under main dental considerations on page 63 top, and also Section 2).

Carbamazepine used to treat trigeminal neuralgia may have an additive effect with other drugs used to treat diabetes insipidus.

Diabetes mellitus

Definition
A relative or absolute lack of insulin. An increasingly common disorder.

Aetiopathogenesis and classification
Primary diabetes
May be:
- Type 1 (insulin-dependent; IDDM) – insulin deficiency with liability to ketosis and weight loss, associated with antibodies to pancreatic islet of Langerhans cells and to Zinc Transporter 8 (ZnT8Ab). Genetic predisposition or infectious agents (e.g. Coxsackie viruses) may be implicated.

Table 5.12 Different types of diabetes mellitus

Type	Also called	Other	Typical onset	Aetiopathogenesis
1	Insulin-dependent	IDDM	Juvenile	Insulin deficiency
2	Non-insulin-dependent	NIDDM	Maturity	Insulin resistance
3	Gestational diabetes	Pregnancy diabetes	2nd or 3rd trimester	Placenta hormones interfere with insulin

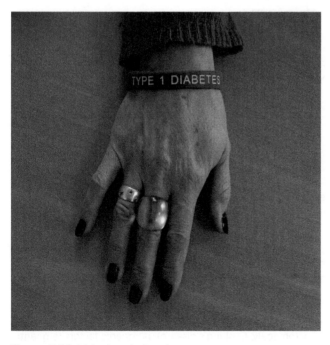

Figure 5.26 Diabetic wrist band.

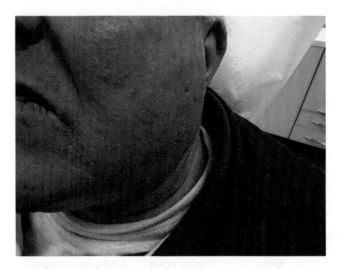

Figure 5.27 Sialosis in diabetes.

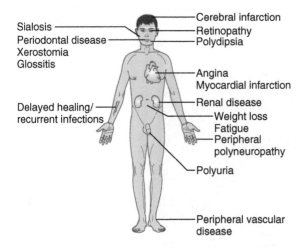

Figure 5.28 Diabetes features. Adapted from Scully et al. (2007) Special Care in Dentistry: Handbook of Oral Care. Churchill Livingstone, Elsevier.

- Type 2 (non-insulin-dependent or NIDDM) – due to lack of insulin, or resistance to it (this is by far the most common type of diabetes).

Secondary diabetes
Caused by: Obesity, lack of exercise, pancreatic islet destruction (e.g. pancreatitis or neoplasm), endocrinopathies (e.g. acromegaly, Cushing's disease), iatrogenic factors (e.g. antipsychotics, corticosteroids, diuretics, beta-blockers, antipsychotics, hormone therapy for

prostate cancer and HIV treatments). Long-term use of the antidepressants SSRIs and TCAs has been linked to an increased risk of developing type 2 diabetes.

Risk factors for diabetes
These include:

- A positive family history of diabetes
- Inactivity
- Older age
- Overweight
- Race: Type 1 diabetes is more common in Caucasians and in Finland and Sweden. Type 2 is more common in people of colour, Asians and Hispanics.

Clinical presentation

Low insulin output, or insulin resistance in peripheral tissues, means glucose cannot enter cells but accumulates in the blood (hyperglycaemia) and spills into the urine (glucosuria), osmotically taking with it, abundant water (polyuria). Since glucose is lost as an energy source, fats must be metabolized to fatty acids and there is over-production of acetoacetate which is converted to the other ketone bodies, hydroxybutyrate and acetone. These all can appear in the blood, causing acidosis (ketosis) and hyperventilation, and in urine (ketonuria) and breath (acetone). Diabetes is also associated with immune deficiencies.

Diabetes may thus present with (Table 5.13):

- Dry mouth;
- Fatigue;
- Macroangiopathy – predisposing to angina pectoris, claudication, myocardial and cerebral infarction;
- Microangiopathy – predisposing to retinopathy, renal disease and peripheral polyneuropathy (Table 5.14);
- Polydipsia, polyphagia, polyuria (increased drinking, appetite, urination);
- Skin infections or oral or vaginal candidosis;
- Weight loss.

Diabetes is a leading cause of death and disability and prevalence is rising, with it affecting at least 2% of the population but recognized in only about 50% of these.

Table 5.13 Possible presenting features of diabetes

Early features	Later features
Confusion and behavioural changes	Abdominal pain
Constipation	Coma
Itching	Dehydration
Polydipsia	Hyperventilation
Polyphagia	Muscle wasting
Polyuria	Nausea
Thirst	Paraesthesiae
Weakness	Renal failure
Weight loss	Shock
	Vomiting

Table 5.14 Complications of diabetes

Microvascular	Macrovascular
Nephropathy	Ischaemic heart disease
Neuropathy	Hypertension
Retinopathy	Peripheral vascular disease

Table 5.15 Glucose assays in diabetes diagnosis*

Plasma glucose test	Confirms diabetes	Excludes diabetes
Fasting (after 8 hour fast)	>7.0 mmol/L	<6 mmol/L
Random (any time of day)	>11.1 mmol/L	< than 8 mmol/L
Oral glucose tolerance test (OGTT) 2 hours after a drink of 75 grams of glucose	> 11.1 mmol/L*	<11.1 mmol/L*

*Persons with equivocal results have 'impaired glucose tolerance'. Some eventually progress to diabetes.

Diagnosis

From clinical features and raised blood glucose. The fasting plasma glucose is preferred (Table 5.16). Diabetes is confirmed when the fasting blood glucose is >7.0 mmol/L (hyperglycaemia), the random blood glucose is >11.1 mmol/L, or the blood glucose is >11.1 mmol/L 2 hours after a glucose tolerance test (GTT) giving 75 g glucose. Glycosuria is usually also present.

Long-term assessment of glucose control is by blood assay of glycosylated (glycated) haemoglobin (HbA1c or HbA1) – a cumulative index of control over the preceding 3 months.

Treatment

The objectives are to avoid acute complications, especially hypoglycaemia; maintain blood glucose levels at near normal; and avoid complications.

Diet

Meals should be regular, with a high fibre and relatively high carbohydrate content – avoiding sugars, and with a caloric intake strictly related to physical activity. The diet efficacy is monitored by checking weight and glucose.

Care in Type 1 diabetes

Insulin or oral hypoglycaemic agents (sulphonylureas, metformin, alpha glucosidase inhibitors or thiazolidinedione). Insulin via injection or a pump is the basic care, the amount being balanced against food intake and daily activities, and blood glucose levels must be monitored. *Inhaled insulin* is as effective, but no better than injected short-acting insulin.

Care in Type 2 diabetes
Controlled eating, physical activity, and blood glucose testing but oral hypoglycaemic drugs – mainly sulphonylureas – may be needed. Urine test for glucose at intervals from daily to once a week and adjust drugs or diet to keep the urine glucose-free.

Diabetes prevention
- Weight reduction and increased physical activity.
- Daily eating less sugar and sweets but more starches such as bread, cereal, and starchy vegetables (5 portions of fruits and vegetables).

Main dental considerations
(*See also generic guidance under main dental considerations on page 63 top, and also Section 2).

Gingivitis and periodontitis are common. Other oral features may include dry mouth, burning mouth sensations, infections such as candidosis and occasionally salivary gland swelling (sialosis). The main hazard during dental treatment is of hypoglycaemia – avoidable by planning. Advise patient to take insulin as always, and eat regularly. Always treat patient on a full stomach; short morning appointments following a regular breakfast; and ensure you do not interfere with patient's usual meals or snacks. Consider giving oral glucose just before treatment, and ensure patients inform the clinician if they feel a hypoglycaemic episode starting. Autonomic neuropathy in diabetes can cause orthostatic hypotension; therefore the supine patient should be slowly raised upright in the dental chair. Otherwise, guidelines for diabetics are similar to those for patients with cardiovascular issues.

Poorly controlled diabetics (whether Type 1 or 2), should be referred for improved control of their blood sugar before non-emergency surgery is performed. If emergency surgery is needed, prophylactic antibiotics are prudent.

Treat even small infections aggressively with appropriate antibiotic therapy and necessary surgical intervention. Severe dentoalveolar abscess with fascial space involvement in a seemingly healthy individual may signify diabetes. Severe diabetics with ketoacidosis are predisposed to fungal infections such as paranasal sinus mucormycosis.

Drugs that can disturb diabetic control – aspirin and steroids – must be avoided. Drugs should be sugar-free. Doxycycline and other tetracyclines may enhance insulin hypoglycaemia.

Hyperaldosteronism

Definition
A rare syndrome consequent upon adrenal aldosterone overproduction.

Aetiopathogenesis
Conn's syndrome (adrenocortical adenoma) is the main cause, but other causes include:
- adrenocortical hyperplasia
- adrenal carcinoma
- glucocorticoid-remediable aldosteronism (abnormal control by ACTH).

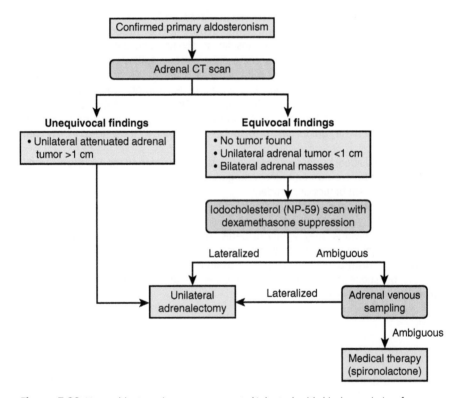

Figure 5.29 Hyperaldosteronism management. (Adapted with kind permission from University of Wisconsin School of Medicine and Public Health. Department of Surgery. Conn's disease. www.surgery.wisc.edu/specialties/endocrine-surgery/conditions/conns-disease).

Clinical presentation

Aldosterone induces in distal renal tubules, sodium retention and potassium secretion, which result in:

- Alkalosis – may produce tetany (muscle twitching)
- Headache
- Hypertension
- Hypokalaemia – responsible for most clinical findings such as muscular weakness and possibly paralysis.

Classification

Primary hyperaldosteronism – increased plasma aldosterone and reduced plasma rennin levels.

Secondary hyperaldosteronism – a consequence of rennin-angiotensin system activation, seen in renal, cardiac and hepatic failure.

Diagnosis

CT/MRI, iodocholesterol scan, and plasma:

- aldosterone – raised
- potassium – reduced
- rennin – reduced
- sodium – often raised.

Treatment

- Spironolactone
- Surgery (adrenalectomy).

Main dental considerations

(*See also generic guidance under main dental considerations on page 63 top, and also Section 2).

If bilateral adrenalectomy has been carried out, the patient is at risk from collapse during dental treatment and therefore requires corticosteroid cover.

Competitive muscle relaxants used in GA should be used with restraint, as they can cause profound paralysis.

Hyperparathyroidism

Definition
Parathyroid hormone (PTH) overproduction.

Aetiopathogenesis
Primary hyperparathyroidism – usually caused by parathyroid adenoma or hyperplasia – with autonomous secretion of PTH.

Secondary hyperparathyroidism – caused by hypocalcaemia in renal failure or vitamin D deficiency – resulting in raised PTH.

Tertiary hyperparathyroidism – parathyroids become autonomous after secondary hyperparathyroidism.

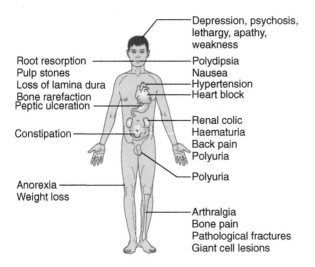

Depression, psychosis, lethargy, apathy, weakness

Root resorption
Pulp stones
Loss of lamina dura
Bone rarefaction
Peptic ulceration

Polydipsia
Nausea
Hypertension
Heart block

Constipation

Renal colic
Haematuria
Back pain
Polyuria

Polyuria

Anorexia
Weight loss

Arthralgia
Bone pain
Pathological fractures
Giant cell lesions

Figure 5.30 Hyperparathyroidism. Adapted from Scully et al. (2007) Special Care in Dentistry: Handbook of Oral Care. Churchill Livingstone, Elsevier.

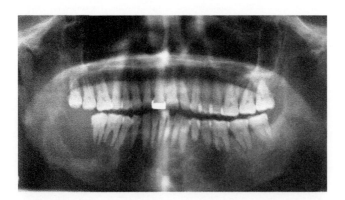

Figure 5.31 Bone radiolucent lesions in hyperparathyroidism.

Clinical presentation

Increased gastrointestinal calcium absorption, renal calcium resorption, and mobilization of calcium from bones (osteoclastic resorption) leads to hypercalcaemia which may, if severe, result in arrhythmia, bronchospasm, convulsions, lethargy, stupor, and finally coma and death. Other features ('stones, bones and abdominal groan') include:

- Anorexia and constipation
- Arthralgias
- Band keratopathy in the cornea
- Dehydration
- Mental confusion and lethargy
- Myopathy
- Osteopenia, bone radioluciencies and rarely giant-cell lesions
- Polyuria
- Renal calculi
- Thirst.

Diagnosis

Radioisotope scan.
CT
Blood plasma analysis:
- alkaline phosphatase – raised
- calcium – raised
- phosphate – reduced
- PTH – raised.

Treatment

- Diuresis – lowers the plasma calcium level
- Mithramycin
- Calcitonin
- Surgery.

Main dental considerations

(*See also generic guidance under main dental considerations on page 63 top, and also Section 2).
Primary hyperthyroidism: oral findings are late and uncommon, and include teeth sensitive to mastication, root resorption and pulp stones. Jaw bone pain, loss of the lamina dura and cortical bone of the inferior mandibular border and mandibular canal, generalized rarefaction (ground-glass appearance) or giant cell lesions (brown tumours) are possible. Brown tumours need not necessarily always be removed, particularly where the risk of fracture is high.

Hyperthyroidism

Definition
Raised thyroid hormone (T3 and T4) levels.

Aetiopathogenesis
Thyroid overactivity (leading to low thyroid stimulating hormone [TSH]) because of:
- Graves' disease (autoimmunity against TSH receptors)
- Toxic goitre
- Toxic thyroid adenoma.

Clinical presentation
Mimics epinephrine (adrenaline) excess, with thyrotoxicosis i.e.:
- dislike of heat
- hypertension
- irritability and anxiety
- raised pulse rate
- tremor.

May also be associated with:
- Appetite increase
- Diarrhoea
- Exophthalmos or proptosis
- Eyelid lag
- Thyroid swelling/lump
- Warm, moist and erythematous skin.

Thyrotoxic crisis (thyroid storm) is severe starting with extreme anxiety, nausea, vomiting and abdominal pain; then fever, sweating, tachycardia, and pulmonary oedema; finally stupor, coma and occasionally death.

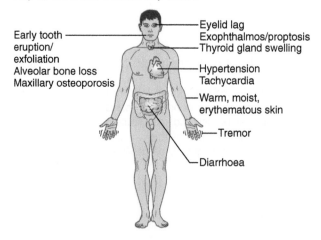

Figure 5.32 Hyperthyroidism features. Adapted from Scully et al. (2007) Special Care in Dentistry: Handbook of Oral Care. Churchill Livingstone, Elsevier.

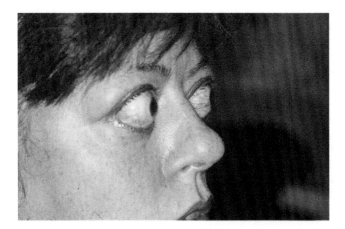

Figure 5.33 Exophthalmos.

Diagnosis

Thyroid function tests (TFT) include serum:

- T3, T4, levels – raised.
- TSH – reduced.
- Antibodies.

Treatment

Control symptoms with beta-blockers (e.g. propranolol or nadolol). Treat hyperthyroidism with: antithyroid drugs (carbimazole or propylthiouracil, and methimazole), radioiodine (^{131}I), or surgery.

Main dental considerations

(*See also generic guidance under main dental considerations on page 63 top, and also Section 2).

Medical treatment of hyperthyroidism with carbimazole occasionally leads to agranulocytosis – with oral ulceration. Use vasoconstrictors with caution though risks of giving epinephrine/epinephrine-containing LA are more theoretical than real. If concerned, prilocaine with felypressin can be given, but not known to be safer. An increased risk of cardiovascular complications in patients taking nonselective beta-blockers and antithyroid agents (e.g. propylthiouracil, tapazole, or methimazole). Radio-iodine can cause salivary damage and hyposalivation.

Behavioural control and techniques to allay anxiety are essential. These patients may be difficult to manage as a result of heightened anxiety and irritability. The sympathetic overactivity may lead to fainting. A thyroid storm (crisis) may be provoked during dental treatment by the stress, or by epinephrine, infection or traumatic surgery. Short, stress-free appointments, as anxiety and stress can trigger a thyrotoxic crisis. Treat acute oral infections with antibiotics to prevent the development of thyrotoxic crisis. Patients in crisis must immediately be admitted to hospital.

The hyperthyroid patient is especially at risk from GA because of the risk of precipitating dangerous arrhythmias. After hyperthyroidism treatment, the risk is from hypothyroidism.

Hypoparathyroidism

Definition

Parathyroid hormone (PTH) underproduction.

Aetiopathogenesis

The most common cause is thyroidectomy (but this resolves when the remaining parathyroid undergoes compensatory hyperplasia).

Rare cases of idiopathic hypoparathyroidism may be associated with CATCH 22, (other endocrine defects – especially hypoadrenocorticism – associated with multiple autoantibodies and cataracts, calcification of the basal ganglia, defects of the teeth and, occasionally, chronic mucocutaneous candidosis).

Clinical presentation

Hypocalcaemia and hyper-phosphataemia lead to muscle irritability and tetany – with facial twitching (Chvostek sign; contracture of the facial muscles upon tapping over the facial nerve), carpopedal spasms (Trousseau sign; contracture of the hand and fingers [main d'accoucheur – obstetrician's hand] on occluding the arm with a cuff), numbness and tingling of arms and legs, and even laryngeal stridor.

Severe complications include seizures, cardiac arrhythmia and bronchospasm.

Pseudo-hypoparathyroidism, characterized by normal or raised PTH secretion but unresponsive tissue receptors, has features similar to idiopathic hypoparathyroidism also with short stature, small fingers and toes, liability to cataracts, but no dental defects. A similar appearance in patients with normal biochemistry is termed *pseudo-pseudohypoparathyroidism*.

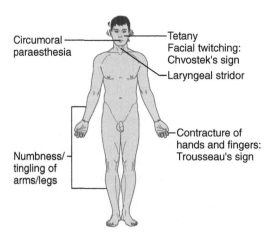

Figure 5.34 Hypoparathyroidism features. Adapted from Scully et al. (2007) Special Care in Dentistry: Handbook of Oral Care. Churchill Livingstone, Elsevier.

Diagnosis

Blood plasma

- calcium-reduced
- phosphate-raised.

PTH stimulation test – reduced response

Treatment

Replacement therapy includes vitamin D and calcium. A low phosphate diet is recommended.

Main dental considerations

(*See also generic guidance under main dental considerations on page 63 top, and also Section 2).
Oral manifestations in congenital hypoparathyroidism may include: enamel hypoplasia and shortened roots. Chronic mucocutaneous candidosis may be seen in Catch 22, candida–endocrinopathy syndrome. Candidosis and hypoparathyroidism are seen in autoimmune polyendocrinopathy–candidosis–ectodermal dystrophy (APECED); this is an autosomal recessive disease which presents with chronic mucocutaneous candidosis and dental abnormalities. Adrenocortical and gonadal failure are common.

In postpubertal hypoparathyroidism there may be circumoral paraesthesia and facial twitching (Chvostek's sign). Dental management may be complicated by: tetany (twitching), seizures, arrhythmias or other endocrinopathies. Patients with calcium levels below 8 mg/100 mL should be treated in a hospital environment and receive only emergency dental care. Conscious sedation or GA should be undertaken with caution in view of the systemic complications of hypoparathyroidism, particularly laryngeal stridor.

Hypopituitarism (dwarfism)

Definition
Complete or partial loss of anterior pituitary hormones (adrenocorticotrophic; follicle-stimulating growth; luteinizing; prolactin and/or thyroid-stimulating).

Aetiopathogenesis
Main causes – pituitary surgery or irradiation.
Rarer causes are disease in/around pituitary gland:
- Haemorrhage
- Infections
- Trauma
- Tumours (craniopharyngioma).

Clinical presentation
- Constipation, mood change (low thyroid stimulating hormone; TSH).
- Obesity, weakness (low growth hormone; GH).
- Oligomenorrhoea, libido loss, infertility, and hypogonadism (low follicle stimulating hormone; FSH: luteinizing hormone; LH: prolactin).
- Weakness, weight loss, hypotension (low ACTH).

Diagnosis
- Hormone assays and stimulation tests.
- CT/MRI.

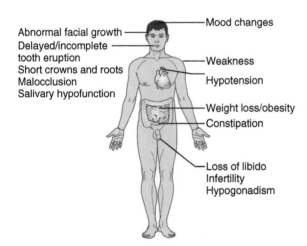

Figure 5.35 Hypopituitarism features. Adapted from Scully et al. (2007) Special Care in Dentistry: Handbook of Oral Care. Churchill Livingstone, Elsevier.

Treatment

Hormone replacement.

Main dental considerations

Abnormal facial size (small), delayed and incomplete tooth eruption, short crowns and roots, crowding and malocclusion are common. Patients are at risk from adrenal crisis and hypopituitary coma. If possible, conscious sedation and GA should be avoided in view of multiple systemic complications, and risk of drug-induced hypopituitary coma.

The patient is at risk of postural hypotension, and thus the patient is best not treated supine.

Hypothyroidism

Definition
Thyroid hormone deficiency.

Aetiopathogenesis
The most common causes include:

- autoimmunity
- drugs (e.g. amiodarone, lithium, radio-iodine)
- thyroid surgery or radiotherapy.

Clinical presentation
Usual findings in children include:

- delayed physical and mental development
- feeding problems
- hypothermia
- somnolence.

Usual findings in adults include:

- bradycardia
- constipation
- depression/dementia
- dislike of cold
- hoarse voice
- myxoedema
- tiredness/lethargy
- weight gain.

Diagnosis
- Thyroid function tests (TFT) include serum; T3, T4, levels – low.
- TSH – raised.
- Thyroid autoantibodies (Table 5.16).

Table 5.16 Thyroid autoantibodies		
Antibody	**Acronym**	**Present in**
Thyroid peroxidase antibody	TPOAb	Autoimmune thyroid disease: Hashimoto's thyroiditis (95%); primary myxoedema (90%); Graves' disease (18%)
Thyroglobulin antibody	TgAb	Autoimmune thyroid disease
TSH receptor antibody	TRAb	Hyperthyroidism; Graves' disease

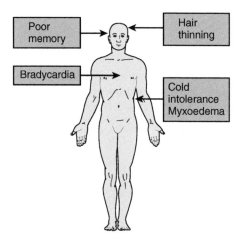

Figure 5.36 Hypothyroidism – features.

Treatment

Thyroxine (thyroid hormone replacement).

Main dental considerations

(*See also generic guidance under main dental considerations on page 63 top, and also Section 2).
Macroglossia is a common finding.

The main danger is of precipitating myxoedematous coma by the use of CNS depressants such as sedatives (including diazepam), opioid analgesics (including codeine), other tranquillizers or general anaesthetics. These should therefore either be avoided or given in low dose. Myxoedema coma may also be precipitated by stress, infection or traumatic surgery, especially in older people.

Obesity

Definition
'Obesity' means to be overweight. However, 'overweight' is sometimes defined as an excess amount of body weight that includes muscle, bone, fat and water, while 'obesity' specifically refers to excessive body fat. Men with >25% body fat and women with >30% body fat are obese. Obesity is increasingly common.

Aetiopathogenesis
Obesity results from eating more than the body needs.
Environmental factors include lifestyle behaviours, such as what a person eats and their level of physical activity.
Psychological factors may play a role; many eat in response to boredom, sadness or anger. Antidepressants or steroids may cause weight gain.
Genetic factors: hypothalamic disease (Frohlich, Laurence–Moon–Biedl or Prader–Willi syndromes), endocrinopathies (hypothyroidism, Cushing disease or insulinoma).

Clinical presentation
Obese patients have a threefold increase in premature deaths from heart disease, hypertension, diabetes, stroke and cancer. Accident risks are increased. Obese men are more likely than non-obese men to die from colorectal or prostate cancer. Obese women are more likely to die from gallbladder, breast, uterus, cervix or ovarian cancer.

Diagnosis
A simple method to measure subcutaneous fat thickness is with skin calipers. The most accurate methods are to weigh the person under water or to use Dual-Energy X-ray Absorptiometry (DEXA or DXA). Body Mass Index (BMI), equals weight in kilograms divided by height in metres squared ($BMI = kg/m^2$). Weight-for-height tables do not distinguish between muscle and excess fat.

Treatment
Bariatric medicine (from Greek *baros* [weight] and – *iatros* [doctor]) is the specialty of caring for obese patients. Weight loss is recommended, particularly if there are two or more of the following:

- family history of heart disease or diabetes
- hypertension, hyperglycaemia or hyper-cholesterolaemia
- 'apple' body shape.

Treatment may include a combination of diet, exercise, behaviour modification and sometimes drugs or surgery. People with a BMI exceeding 30 can improve health by weight loss. Sympathomimetic appetite suppressants are used only in short-term treatment since their effect decreases after a few weeks. Tesofensine is of possible benefit.

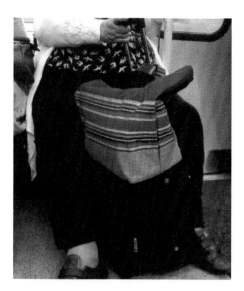

Figure 5.37 Obesity.

In severe obesity, bariatric surgery aims at:

- *Reducing stomach size by*:
  - sleeve gastrectomy
  - transoral gastroplasty
  - vertical banded gastroplasty (Mason procedure, stomach stapling)
  - Laparoscopic adjustable gastric band (LAGB; REALIZE band – lap band).
- *Reducing food absorption by*:
  - biliopancreatic diversion (Scopinaro procedure – rare)
  - mixed procedures (gastric bypass; sleeve gastrectomy with duodenal switch; implantable gastric stimulation).

Obese people often meet healthcare access problems.

Main dental considerations

(*See also generic guidance under main dental considerations on page 63 top, and also Section 2).

Appetite suppressants, including sibutramine and phentermine, and herbal supplements containing ephedrine alkaloids/caffeine (ma huang, kola nut), can cause dry mouth.

Jaw wiring of obese patients appears to be an effective and safe way of substantially reducing weight, but relapse is common. Bariatric surgeries may increase gastro-oesophageal reflux.

Dental treatment may be complicated mainly by the sheer size and weight of the patient and difficulties in accessing dental care. Bariatric dental chairs suitable for all patient groups up to 1000 lb (454 kg; 71 st) are available for large, overweight, obese and bariatric patients to be safely treated (e.g. Diaco, Barico). Respiration is impaired if the patient is supine. Some 10% have hypoventilation, cor pulmonale and episodic somnolence (Pickwickian syndrome). Sleep apnoea is more common.

GASTROINTESTINAL

Coeliac disease (CD)

(Gluten-sensitive enteropathy; coeliac sprue, non-tropical sprue.)

Definition

Small intestine mucosal hypersensitivity to the gliadin component of gluten (prolamine), a group of proteins in all wheats (including durum, semolina, spelt, kamut, einkorn and faro), and related grains (rye, barley, triticale).

Aetiopathogenesis

CD is the most common genetic disease in Europe, but rare in Africans, Chinese or Japanese. Strongly associated with a background of HLA-DQw2 or DRw3 and may have a familial tendency. CD4+ T cells specific for dietary gluten and interleukin 15 (IL-15) contribute to the pathogenesis. Gluten ingestion causes jejunal villous destruction (villous atrophy) and inflammation, leading to malabsorption.

Clinical presentation

Many affected people are asymptomatic and undiagnosed. One of the great mimics in medicine, CD may present at any age and can result in malabsorption (leading to growth retardation, vitamin and mineral deficiencies, which may result in anaemia, osteomalacia, bleeding tendencies and neurological disorders), abdominal pain, steatorrhoea and behavioural changes. Intestinal lymphomas arise in ~6%.

Diagnosis

Often misdiagnosed as lactose intolerance or irritable bowel. Clinical, and malabsorption tests such as low blood folate and carotene levels (the screening method of choice), and assays for serum antibodies to substances such as transglutaminase, endomysium (the connective tissue stroma covering individual muscle fibres or cells), or gliadin (see Fig. 5.39). To confirm the diagnosis, a jejunal biopsy is needed, and if positive with villous atrophy and a Marsh histopathological score above 2, is repeated after a 3 month gluten-free diet.

Treatment

Rectify nutritional deficiencies, and take a gluten-free diet for life. Instead of wheat flour, potato, rice, soy or bean flour and gluten-free bread, and pasta are used. Follow-up because of lymphoma risk.

Main dental considerations

(*See also generic guidance under main dental considerations on page 63 top, and also Section 2).
Oral features may include enamel defects, recurrent aphthous-like ulcers, cheilosis and/or atrophic glossitis.

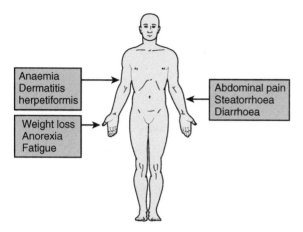

Figure 5.38 Coeliac disease – features.

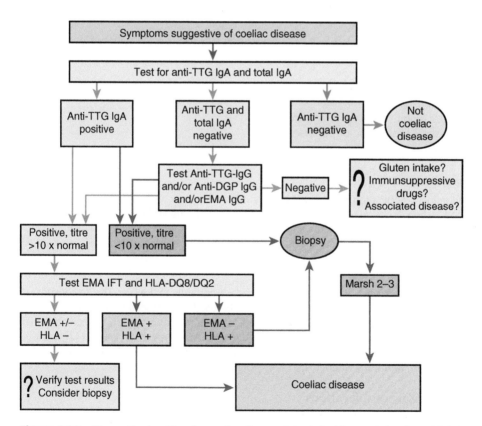

Figure 5.39 Diagnostic algorithm for coeliac disease. Adapted with permission from ORGEN-TEC www.autoimmunityblog.wordpress.com. TTG = tissue transglutaminase; EMA = endomysial antibody; HLA = human leucocyte antigen; Marsh = histopathology score; DGP = deamidated gliadin peptide.

Colorectal cancer

Definition
Carcinoma of the colon; a common cancer.

Aetiopathogenesis
Peak incidence is in the sixth or seventh decades, mainly in males. Risk factors include:
- Crohn's disease.
- Diabetes.
- Family history of colon cancer.
- Lynch syndrome (hereditary nonpolyposis colorectal cancer; HNPCC) and familial adenomatous polyposis (FAP).
- Obesity.
- Smoking.
- Ulcerative colitis.

Clinical presentation
The tumour is usually in the rectum or pelvic (sigmoid) colon, often symptomless, but may cause:
- abdominal pain
- anaemia
- bowel habit change
- faecal blood or melaena (tarry stools)
- intestinal obstruction or perforation
- weight loss.

Diagnosis
Abdominal examination may reveal a mass. Sigmoidoscopy and sometimes faecal occult blood testing (stool guaiac), MRI, ultrasound, barium enema and colonoscopy. Methylated Septin 9 (SEPT9) a plasma screening test has a sensitivity and specificity similar to stool guaiac or faecal immune tests (immunochemical faecal occult blood test).

Treatment
Surgical resection is the usual treatment. Spread is frequently to the liver. The 5-year survival rate is overall about 30%. Chemotherapy may be used in advanced cancer: 5-flurouracil, oxaliplatin, capecitabine, irinotecan, raltitrexed, bevacizumab and possibly cetuximab. Serial monitoring for serum carcino-embryonic antigen (CEA) or serum or faecal M2-pyruvate kinase (M2-PK) antigen may help detect recurrences. Radiotherapy may be useful for dealing with pain from recurrences.

Main dental considerations
(*See also generic guidance under main dental considerations on page 63 top, and also Section 2).
Familial adenomatous polyposis with the extra-colonic manifestations of desmoids, osteomas (sometimes in jaws) and epidermoid cysts is termed Gardner's syndrome. Peutz–Jeghers

syndrome, an autosomal dominant disorder characterized by mucosal pigmentation with multiple intestinal hamartomatous polyps is associated with an increased risk of malignancies, especially gastro-oesophageal, small bowel, colorectal, pancreatic, ductal breast cancer, thyroid, lung, uterine, Sertoli cell testicular tumours or ovarian sex cord tumours.

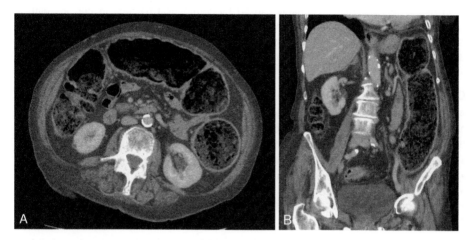

Figure 5.40 (A) Distended colon due to distal carcinoma; **(B)** coronal view of obstructed colon. Courtesy of Mr A. Kalantzis (Manchester).

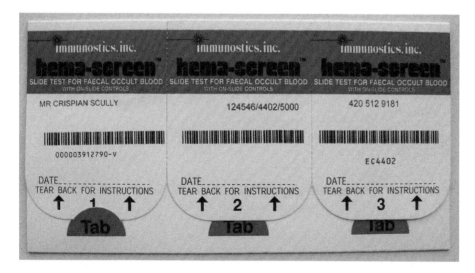

Figure 5.41 Faecal occult blood screening kit.

Crohn's disease (CD)

Definition

A heterogeneous group of disorders with chronic granulomatous inflammation, grouped with ulcerative colitis as inflammatory bowel disease.

Aetiopathogenesis

Seen mainly in Caucasians, probably caused by commensal bacteria in persons with a genetically determined dysregulation of mucosal T-lymphocytes. The inflammatory response is probably mediated by factors such as tumour necrosis factor alpha. Microscopically, there is submucosal chronic inflammation with many mononuclear, interleukin-1 producing cells and non-caseating granulomas.

Clinical presentation

Affects the ileocaecal region mainly, with ulceration, fissuring and fibrosis and may cause abdominal pain that often mimics appendicitis, with malabsorption or abnormal bowel habits. Alternating diarrhoea and constipation are typical. May also cause:

- Mouth – ulcers, lip or oral mucosal swellings ("cobbllestoning"), or cheilitis.
- Skin – pyoderma, erythema nodosum.
- Joints – arthritis, sacroiliitis.
- Eyes – conjunctivitis, episcleritis, iritis.
- Liver – various.

Complications may include weight loss, gastrointestinal obstruction, internal or external fistulas, perianal fissures, abscesses, sclerosing cholangiitis or renal damage (renal stones or infections).

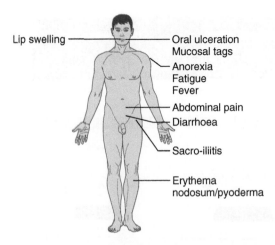

Figure 5.42 Crohn's disease features. Adapted from Scully et al. (2007) Special Care in Dentistry: Handbook of Oral Care. Churchill Livingstone, Elsevier.

Diagnosis

There is no specific diagnostic test for CD. There may be anaemia, raised faecal calprotectin, ESR and acute phase proteins such as C-reactive protein (CRP) and seromucoid, and depressed serum potassium, zinc and albumin. Sigmoidoscopy, colonoscopy, MRI enterography, barium enemas of large and small bowel, or barium meal and follow-through may help diagnosis which is confirmed by mucosal biopsy showing the typical granulomas. Isotope leukocyte intestinal scans may help to diagnose active disease.

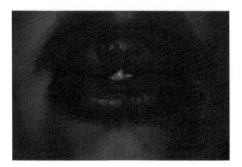

Figure 5.43 Lip swelling and splitting in Crohn's disease.

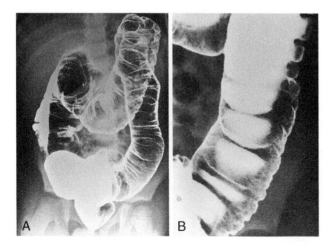

Figure 5.44 Crohn's disease. This figure was published in Marcdante KJ, Kleigman RM. Inflammatory bowel disease. In: Nelson's Textbook of Pediatrics, 19e © Elsevier (2014).

Table 5.17 Comparison of Crohn's disease and ulcerative colitis

	Crohn's disease	Ulcerative colitis
Main site affected	Ileum	Colo-rectum
Sites occasionally affected	Any part of gastrointestinal tract, including mouth	Terminal ileum
Pathology	Transmural inflammation	Superficial inflammation
Abdominal pain	Prominent	Not prominent
Bloody diarrhoea	Not prominent	Prominent
Fistulae and abscesses	Possible	Rare
Colonic carcinoma	Low risk	High risk
Iron deficiency	Common	Common
Folate deficiency	Common	Common
Other deficiencies	Vitamin B_{12}	–

Treatment

Early recognition of lesions and initiation of treatment may improve the prognosis:

- Elemental diets.
- Anti-inflammatory drugs:
  - metronidazole;
  - sulfasalazine or newer 5-amino-salicylates (balsalazide, mesalazine or olsalazine).
- Immunosuppressive drugs:
  - corticosteroids;
  - azathioprine and 6-mercaptopurine;
  - biologic agents such as Adalimumab, Certolizumab pegol, Infliximab, Golimumab, Natalizumab or Vedolizumab.
- ± Surgery: over a 20-year period: about 80% of patients need surgical intervention.

No treatment is curative, but periods of spontaneous remission may occur. An increased prevalence of intestinal cancer has been described in Crohn's disease.

Main dental considerations

(*See also generic guidance under main dental considerations on page 63 top, and also Section 2).

Oral features may include recurrent ulcers, cheilosis and/or atrophic glossitis, or granulomatous swellings.

Cystic fibrosis (CF)

Definition
A defect in chloride and sodium transport, causing viscous mucus, especially in pancreas and lungs.

Aetiopathogenesis
An autosomal recessive condition.

Clinical presentation
Change in composition of exocrine secretions causes:
- Gastrointestinal – pancreatic insufficiency.
- Lungs – cough, wheeze, recurrent infection, and possibly bronchiectasis (permanent enlargement of parts of the airways with liability to infection).
- Mouth – dryness.
- Nose – polyps.
- Sinuses – sinusitis.
- Testes – infertility.

Diagnosis
- Sweat or salivary sodium and chloride – increased.
- Faecal elastase – increased.

Treatment
- Physiotherapy and postural drainage.
- Bronchodilators.
- Antimicrobials.
- High-protein, high-calorie and low-fat diet, plus fat-soluble vitamins and pancreatic enzymes.

CF is progressive and finally fatal, mostly as a consequence of pulmonary complications and cor pulmonale (right ventricular failure from respiratory disease). Lung transplant may be indicated.

Main dental considerations
(*See also generic guidance under main dental considerations on page 63 top, and also Section 2).
Oral manifestations may include delayed dental development and eruption, dry mouth, salivary gland swelling, and recurrent sinusitis.

Semi-supine or upright patient positioning may be necessary. Conscious sedation and GA may be contraindicated due to poor respiratory function. Liver disease or diabetes may be complicating factors to treatment.

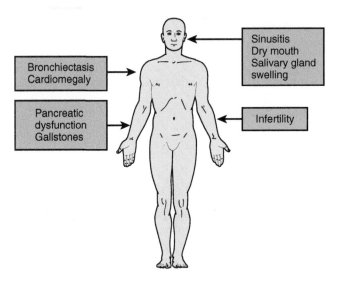

Figure 5.45 Cystic fibrosis – features.

Diverticular disease

Definition

Diverticulosis (small colonic pouches – diverticula – that bulge out through weak spots of the large intestine wall) and diverticulitis (inflammation of these diverticula).

Aetiopathogenesis

Most common in developed or industrialized countries, where it affects >50% of those >60 years. It may result from a low-fibre diet.

Clinical presentation

Left-sided diverticular disease (involving the sigmoid colon) is most common in the West. *Right-sided diverticular disease* is more prevalent in Africans and Asians.
Diverticular disease may be asymptomatic, but is often accompanied by abdominal pain, constipation, dyspepsia, and flatulence. Complications include pericolic abscess, perforation and peritonitis, or fistula.

Diagnosis

Conditions to be excluded include IBD (irritable bowel disease), IBS, cancer, and urological and gynaecological disorders. Abdominal imaging is indicated.

Treatment

Management includes a high-fibre diet and reassurance. Antibiotics and surgery may be needed.

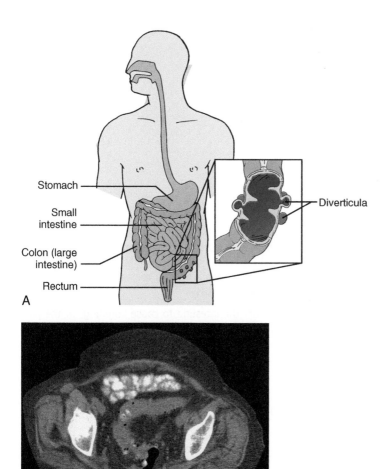

Figure 5.46 (A) Diverticulitis – features. **(B)** Diverticular disease, sigmoid colon. Courtesy of Mr A. Kalantzis (Manchester).

Gastric cancer

Definition
Usually adenocarcinoma, a common cancer.

Aetiopathogenesis
- Age 55 or older.
- Diet of salted and pickled foods.
- Infection due to bacterium *Helicobacter pylori*.
- Men affected nearly twice as often as women.
- Smoking.

Clinical presentation
- Early symptoms – can mimic peptic ulcer, with indigestion, heartburn, burping or vague upper abdominal pain.
- Later features – may be anorexia, bloating, haematemesis or melaena (stools black and tarry with blood), nausea, vomiting, weight loss.

The tumour spreads locally, and may obstruct the intestine to cause vomiting, or the bile duct to cause jaundice. Metastases are mainly to liver, peritoneum (causing ascites), lungs, bones or brain, occasionally to a lower cervical (supraclavicular, or Virchow) lymph node, usually on the left side (Troisier sign).

Diagnosis
Gastroscopy and biopsy. Barium imaging may help, but diagnosis is often delayed by lack of symptoms.

Treatment
Surgery, but it is frequently only palliative. The prognosis is poor, with about a 7% 5-year survival rate. Chemotherapy with trastuzumab may help.

Gastro-oesophageal reflux disease (GORD; GERD)

Definition
The return of stomach contents into the oesophagus.

Aetiopathogenesis
The lower oesophageal sphincter (LES) becomes dysfunctional; normally it opens to allow food to pass into the stomach and closes to prevent food and acidic stomach juices from returning back into the oesophagus. Risk factors include:

- Alcohol.
- Fried or fatty foods, chocolate, peppermint, coffee.
- Hiatal hernia (the upper part of the stomach moves up into the chest through an opening in the diaphragm (diaphragmatic hiatus). This may arise from coughing, stooping, straining, vomiting, by any change in position or sudden physical exertion causing increased intra-abdominal pressure.
- Obesity.
- Pregnancy.
- Smoking.

Clinical presentation
Features depend on the type and amount of fluid regurgitated, and the neutralizing effect of saliva. Common symptoms include:

- acid reflux – an unpleasant taste in the mouth.
- dysphagia and heartburn – burning retrosternal pain or discomfort after eating (heartburn that occurs more than twice a week may be considered GORD).
- odynophagia (pain when swallowing).

GORD may lead to oesophagitis and rarely, oesophageal cancer.

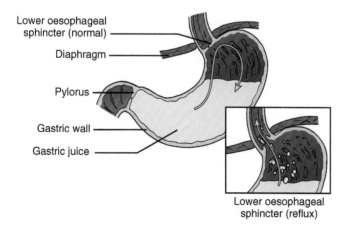

Figure 5.47 Gastro-oesophageal reflux disease.

Diagnosis

- Clinical.
- Endoscopy.

Treatment

Heartburn can usually be relieved through diet and lifestyle changes, but some people may require the bed propped up at the head end at night, and:

- Drugs; proton pump inhibitors (PPIs) and histamine type 2 receptor antagonists (H2Ras) to reduce acid production with antacids to neutralize stomach acid effects.
- Surgery if medication fails to control symptoms.

Main dental considerations

(*See also generic guidance under main dental considerations on page 63 top, and also Section 2).

Oral manifestations may include dental erosion, sweet, saline, sour, and bitter taste sensations and/or halitosis. Although it is safe to place most patients in a supine position for dental care, some need to be at 45°: asking patients in what position they sleep best can help decide what should be done. NSAIDs are contraindicated because of gastric irritating effect.

Head and neck cancer

Definition

Head and neck cancer is usually squamous cell carcinoma (HNSCC) and mainly oral (OSCC).

Aetiopathogenesis

Commoner in males and with increasing age. High rates seen particularly in India, Sri Lanka, Brazil, northern France and Eastern Europe.

The risk factors include:

- Alcohol.
- Betel (areca) nut.
- Diet (i.e. Plummer–Vinson syndrome of iron deficiency and candidosis; low fruit/ vegetables).
- Genetic factors.
- Immunosuppression.
- Infectious agents (i.e. chronic candidosis, syphilis and human papillomaviruses [HPV]).
- Marijuana.
- Poor oral health status.
- Potentially malignant disorders – mainly erythroplasia (erythroplakia), speckled or nodular leukoplakias, submucous fibrosis, lichen planus.
- Sun-exposure.
- Tobacco.

Clinical presentation

The clinical appearance of oral cancer is highly variable, including any single **R**ed or white area, **U**lcer, **L**ump, or fissure **E**xceeding 3 weeks (the 'RULE'). Common sites are the lip, lateral border of tongue and floor of mouth. There may be widespread dysplastic mucosa ('field change') or even a second primary tumour (SPT) anywhere in the oral cavity, oropharynx or upper aerodigestive tract.

Features which suggest malignancy include:

- abnormal blood vessels supplying a lump;
- cervical lymph node enlargement (Fig. 5.50);
- dysphagia or dysarthria;
- erythroplasia;
- fixation of the lesion (or lymph node);
- granular appearance;
- induration;
- non-healing ulcer or extraction socket.

Diagnosis

History, physical examination and lesional biopsy are essential. SPTs are excluded by chest radiography and panendoscopy. Grading is by histological findings and staging by the international Tumour Node Metastases (TNM) system (see Table 5.22).

Treatment

Many early carcinomas can be treated by either surgery or radiotherapy. In later stages, surgery is often the first option. Feeding may need to be via a nasogastric (NG) tube (Figure 5.51) or per-endoscopic gastrostomy (PEG). Targetted biologic therapies (e.g. against epidermal growth factor receptor [EGFR]) are being introduced.

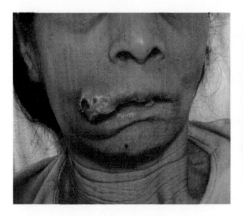

Figure 5.48 Lip cancer. Courtesy of N Kalavrezos and L Newman, London.

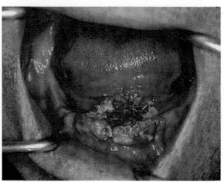

Figure 5.49 Cancer in floor of mouth.

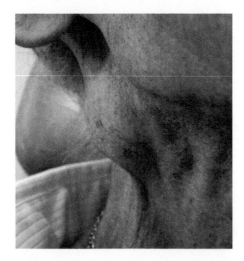

Figure 5.50 Cervical lymph node enlargement.

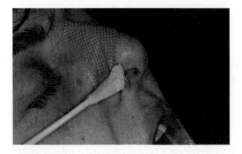

Figure 5.51 Nasogastric (NG) feeding.

Table 5.18 TNM staging of malignant neoplasms

Primary tumour size (T)	
Tx	No available information
T0	No evidence of primary tumour
Tis	Only carcinoma in situ
T1, T2, T3, T4	Increasing size of tumour
Regional lymph node involvement (N)	
Nx	Nodes could not or were not assessed
N0	No clinically positive nodes
N1	Single ipsilateral node less than 3 cm in diameter
N2a	Single ipsilateral nodes 3–6 cm
N2b	Multiple ipsilateral nodes less than 6 cm
N2c	Bilateral or contralateral nodes less than 6 cm
N3	Any node greater than 6 cm
Involvement by distant metastases (M)	
Mx	Distant metastasis was not assessed
M0	No evidence of distant metastasis
M1	Distant metastasis is present

Several other classifications are available, e.g. STNM (S = site).
T1 maximum diameter 2 cm; T2 maximum diameter of 4 cm; T3 maximum diameter over 4 cm. T4 massive tumour greater than 4 cm diameter, with involvement of adjacent anatomical structures

Prognosis

Survival rate 5 years after diagnosis is about 50%.
  Major complications and death are often related to:

- Infiltration into major vessels (e.g. carotid artery).
- Local obstruction of breathing and swallowing.
- Metastases with impaired function of organs.
- Secondary infection.
- Treatment complications.
- Wasting syndrome.

Main dental considerations

(*See also generic guidance under main dental considerations on page 63 top, and also Section 2).
Some cancer patients may have poor oral hygiene, poorly maintained dentitions, periodontal disease, and effects of tobacco/alcohol/betel use. The main risk factors for oral complications of cancer therapy are pre-existent oral or dental disease and poor subsequent oral care. Planning and timely oral healthcare before, during and after cancer therapy can reduce complications. Pre-cancer treatment, the aim is to eliminate or stabilize oral disease to

minimize local and systemic infection. Elective dental treatment should be avoided during radiotherapy: dental management is best limited to treating acute dental infections and symptoms must be managed. After surgery, patients will often require rehabilitation to restore mastication, speech, swallowing and appearance. Radiotherapy may induce mucositis, hyposalivation and infections, and endarteritis obliterans, and hence predispose to osteoradionecrosis (ORN) (Section 9). Detail on dental care advised is available in the UK guidelines *'The Oral Management of Oncology Patients Requiring Radiotherapy, Chemotherapy and/or Bone Marrow Transplantation. Clinical Guidelines.* Updated 2012, The Royal College of Surgeons of England/The British Society for Disability and Oral Health'. See www.rcseng.ac.uk/fds/publications-clinical-guidelines/clinical_guidelines/documents/clinical-guidelines-for-the-oral-management-of-oncology-patients-requiring-radiotherapy-chemotherapy-and-or-bone-marrow-transplantation), accessed 29.8.15.

Irritable bowel syndrome (IBS)

(Spastic colon; mucous colitis, irritable bowel disease)

Definition

IBS is recurrent abdominal pain together with colon increased tone and activity, and abnormal bowel habits, often with urgency. May affect ~30% of the population.

Aetiopathogenesis

Unclear: may occur at any age and has a slight female predominance and may begin after an infection or stressful life event; often a positive family history, anxious personality type and history of migraine or psychogenic symptoms. FODMAPs (fermentable oligo-, di-, and monosaccharides and polyols), and cytokines (IL-1, IL-6 and TNF) and serotonin have been implicated.

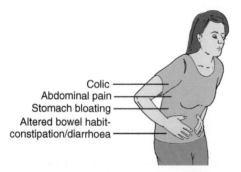

Colic
Abdominal pain
Stomach bloating
Altered bowel habit-
constipation/diarrhoea

Figure 5.52 Irritable bowel syndrome (IBS or spastic colon).

Clinical presentation and classification

Most common cause of referrals to gastroenterologists. IBS causes recurrent abdominal pain together with increased tone and activity of the colon, and abnormal bowel habits, often with urgency (tenesmus) and other symptoms.

Diagnosis

Exclude coeliac disease, inflammatory bowel disease and colon cancer (full blood count and haematinics; inflammatory markers (ESR); contrast radiography; endoscopy and mucosal biopsy).

Treatment

Stress reduction and high-fibre diet. Anti-spasmodics (mebeverine, loperamide or an anti-muscarinic such as dicyclomine, or peppermint oil) may help. Cognitive behavioural therapy or antidepressants may be of benefit. Cilansetron is a selective 5HT3-antagonist in clinical trials for IBS. Probiotics may have a role.

Oesophageal carcinoma

Definition

Usually squamous carcinoma in the upper and middle oesophagus, or adenocarcinoma in the lower third.

Aetiopathogenesis

More frequent in people from China, Asia and Africa. Risk factors include:

- Achalasia (lower oesophageal sphincter does not relax properly).
- Age over 50.
- Alcohol.
- Dry cleaning solvents.
- Gastro-oesophageal reflux disease (GORD) and resultant Barrett's oesophagus (metaplasia).
- Hot foods/drinks or caustics.
- Male gender.
- Obesity.
- Plummer–Vinson syndrome (Paterson–Kelly syndrome; webs in upper oesophagus, anaemia, glossitis, brittle fingernails, and sometimes an enlarged thyroid gland or spleen).
- Tobacco.
- Tylosis (inherited palmar-plantar hyperkeratosis and oesophageal papillomas).

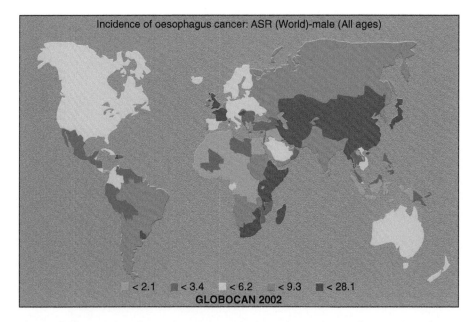

Figure 5.53 Incidence of oesophagus cancer in the male population of the world. Adapted from www.startoncology.net/en/professional-area/esophageal-cancer/

Clinical presentation

Early oesophageal cancer usually causes few or no symptoms but later features may include:

- Chronic cough.
- Dysphagia.
- Hoarseness.
- Pain (in throat or back, behind sternum or between the shoulder blades).
- Vomiting or haematemesis (coughing up blood).
- Weight loss.

Metastases are typically to the lymph nodes, liver, lungs, brain and bones.

Diagnosis

Chest radiography, barium swallow, oesophagoscopy (endoscopy), CT, MRI and biopsy. Bone scan and bronchoscopy may be needed.

Treatment

Surgery (oesophagectomy) is the common treatment. Laser therapy or photodynamic therapy are sometimes used. Sometimes, a stent is used for palliation or a plastic tube or part of the intestine is used to re-connect with the stomach. Radio- or chemoradiotherapy may be used, and cetuximab may help.

Patients who have had oesophageal cancer have a greater chance of developing a second primary cancer in the head and neck.

Peptic ulcer (PUD: Peptic ulcer disease)

Definition
Ulceration in or close to acid-secreting areas in stomach (gastric ulcer) or proximal duodenum (duodenal ulcer).

Aetiopathogenesis
- *Helicobacter pylori*, a spiral bacterium, is found in 70–90% of ulcers. In the developed world, some 20–50% of normal adults are infected, higher in poor socioeconomic circumstances, though most carriers have no disease. *H. pylori* resists gastric acid via urease, an enzyme which converts urea, abundant in the stomach (from saliva and gastric juices), into bicarbonate and ammonia – both strong bases. This reaction is important for diagnosis by the 'breath test'.
- Alcohol.
- Corticosteroids.
- Gastrin levels raised (e.g. Zollinger–Ellison syndrome [gastrin-producing tumour], hyperparathyroidism and chronic kidney disease).
- NSAIDs.
- Smoking.
- Stress.

Clinical presentation
PUD affects up to 3% of the population, mostly men >45 years. Many patients are symptomless or suffer mild dyspepsia. The main feature is epigastric pain, often relieved by antacids. Complications include bleeding, perforation, or pyloric obstruction (stenosis) with vomiting.

Diagnosis
Endoscopy. Studies of gastric acid or serum gastrin levels may help. Patients <45 years old who have ulcer symptoms should be screened for *H. pylori* by breath test, biopsy, serologically, lesional culture or stool test.

Treatment
- Triple therapy (amoxicillin, clarithromycin, metronidazole plus proton pump inhibitors (e.g. omeprazole) to treat *H. pylori* – usually a 7-day course (effective in 90% with few relapses). An additional reason to treat *H. pylori* is that it may lead to gastric cancer or mucosa-associated lymphoid tissue (MALT) lymphomas.
- *H. pylori*-negative PUD is usually associated with NSAID use. Histamine (H2) receptor blockers, such as cimetidine and ranitidine or proton pump inhibitors (PPIs) such as omeprazole or lansoprazole, are therefore used to reduce gastric acid. Prostaglandin analogues such as misoprostol promote healing in PUD and are indicated in patients from whom NSAIDs cannot be withdrawn.
- Diet (milk, antacids and frequent small meals with no fried foods).
- Stopping smoking.
- Limiting alcohol intake.
- Surgery is usually reserved for those with complications. Gastric ulcers may be managed by antrectomy with gastroduodenal anastomosis or partial gastrectomy. Duodenal ulcers are sometimes managed with vagotomy and pyloroplasty or antrectomy.

Main dental considerations

(*See also generic guidance under main dental considerations on page 63 top, and also Section 2).

Oral manifestations may include dry mouth or altered taste perceptions (from proton pump inhibitors). Consider semisupine chair position for patient comfort. NSAIDs are contraindicated because of the gastric irritating effect. Benzodiazepines may interact with cimetidine (and other H2 receptor agonists): sedation is increased and prolonged. Take antibiotics 2 hours before or 2 hours after antacids which will otherwise impair their absorption.

Pancreatitis

Definition
Inflammation of pancreas.

Aetiopathogenesis and classification

Acute pancreatitis – mainly caused by gallstones, with acinar damage and activation
of enzymes leading to local fat necrosis. It may be precipitated by alcoholism, drugs
(e.g. azathioprine, OCP, corticosteroids, furosemide or phenothiazines), endoscopic
retrograde cholangio-pancreatography, hypercalcaemia, hyperlipidaemia, mumps or
other viral infections, or trauma.

Chronic pancreatitis – mainly caused by gallstones and alcoholism particularly, results in
acinar atrophy and deterioration in both exocrine and endocrine function. Exocrine
dysfunction causes a decline in pancreatic secretion volume, bicarbonate and enzyme
content. Endocrine dysfunction often includes abnormal glucose tolerance or frank
diabetes. Sometimes implicated are carcinoma, cystic fibrosis, malnutrition,
haemochromatosis, hyperlipidaemia or hyperparathyroidism.

Clinical presentation

Mainly seen in adult younger males.
Acute pancreatitis effects include severe abdominal pain, and shock, and may include:

- Abdomen distended
- Anxious
- Bowel sounds reduced
- Distressed
- Epigastric tenderness with voluntary and involuntary guarding +/– rigidity
- Fever
- Hypotension

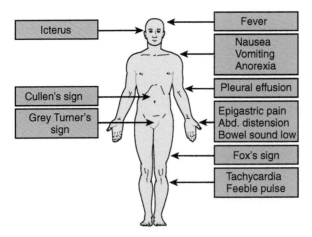

Figure 5.54 Pancreatitis – features. Adapted from Medchrome Magazine. Available at: http://
medchrome.com/major/medicine/review-acute-pancreatitis/ (see p. 151 for signs).

- Jaundice
- Nausea and vomiting
- Pleural effusion – usually left sided (sometimes)
- Tachycardia
- Tachypnoea.

Uncommon signs associated with severe necrotizing pancreatitis may be:

- Cullen's sign (periumbilical discolouration due to peritoneal haemorrhage).
- Fox's sign (discolouration below inguinal ligament or at the base of penis).
- Grey–Turner's sign (flank discolouration due to retroperitoneal haemorrhage).
- Red skin nodules (subcutaneous fat necrosis).

Chronic pancreatitis causes chronic dull abdominal pain and is punctuated by episodes of acute pancreatitis. Weight loss is common, as are nausea, steatorrhoea (floating faeces), vomiting and pruritus (from bile salt accumulation).

Diagnosis

Suggested clinically and by high faecal fat, low chymotrypsin and undigested meat fibres. Raised serum alkaline phosphatase, transaminases, amylase and lipase. CT may demonstrate pancreatic calcification. Barium meal, duodenography, cholangiography and endoscopy (endoscopic retrograde cholangiopancreatography; ERCP), MRI, and ultrasonography aid diagnosis. Pancrealauryl and para-aminobenzoic acid testing assess exocrine function.

Treatment

Acute pancreatitis if mild usually resolves in a few days, but in fulminating pancreatitis, the patient is severely ill with retroperitoneal haemorrhage, pleural effusion and paralytic ileus. Shock, metabolic complications and pain must be urgently treated.
Chronic pancreatitis treatment includes analgesics, treatment of diabetes and oral administration of pancreatic enzymes to aid digestion.

Pancreatic cancer

Definition
Adenocarcinomas, usually involving head of pancreas, in the exocrine duct (acinar cells). Tumours of islet cells (endocrine tumours) are rare but may release hormones.

Aetiopathogenesis
Usually unclear but 10% of pancreatic cancers result from inherited tendency in:
- familial adenomatous polyposis
- familial breast cancer associated with the BRCA2 gene
- non-polyposis colonic cancer.

Clinical presentation
Pancreatic carcinoma frequently invades to cause biliary obstruction (jaundice), pancreatitis and diabetes mellitus. Extra-pancreatic complications, such as peripheral vein thrombosis (thrombophlebitis migrans), pruritus, nausea and vomiting, are common.

Diagnosis
Plain radiography, CT, MRI, ultrasound, endoscopy retrograde cholangiopancreatography (ERCP) or percutaneous transhepatic cholangiography.

Treatment
Pancreatic carcinoma has the worst prognosis of any cancer, with a 1-year survival of 10% and a 5-year survival of 3%. It is usually treated surgically, often with a bypass sometimes with stenting to relieve obstructive jaundice. Gemcitabine may help.

Main dental considerations
(*See also generic guidance under main dental considerations on page 63 top, and also Section 2).
Peutz–Jegher syndrome may rarely be associated. As association with periodontal disease has been muted. Patients with pancreatic cancer may have higher levels of the oral bacteria, *Leptotrichia* and *Campylobacter*, compared to any other healthy or diseased states.

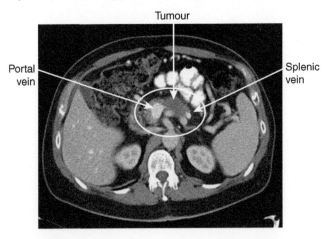

Figure 5.55 Pancreatic cancer. Reprinted from Palliative therapy for pancreatic cancer, Conrad C, Lillemoe KD. In: Current Surgical Therapy, 10e, Cameron JL, Cameron AM, eds. ©Elsevier (2011).

Ulcerative colitis (UC)

Definition

An inflammatory bowel disease affecting most frequently the lower colon (colitis) and rectum (proctitis).

Aetiopathogenesis

Although allergy, infective agents, stress and immunologic factors have been suggested to play a role, the aetiology remains unknown.

Clinical presentation

Most often affecting people aged 15–40 years, UC can affect the whole or any part of the large intestine. Ulcers and inflammation are followed by pseudopolyp formation.

Typical features are diarrhoea with stools containing intermixed mucus, blood and pus and, in severe cases, abdominal pain, fever, anorexia and weight loss.

Complications can include iron deficiency anaemia, arthralgia, iritis and uveitis, finger clubbing, or skin lesions (e.g. pyoderma, erythema nodosum). Disease extension through the muscular layers may result in toxic megacolon (the colon dilates and can perforate) but the most serious complication is colon cancer which is 30 times more frequent than in the general population.

Diagnosis

Differentiate ulcerative colitis from Crohn's disease, Behcet's and Sweet's (acute febrile neutrophilic dermatosis) syndromes. Abdominal radiography and barium enema, full blood count, haemoglobin and haematocrit (iron deficiency anaemia) can help. Sigmoidoscopy and rectal biopsy establish the diagnosis.

Treatment

Treatment includes aminosalicylates (sulphasalazine or olsalazine) and local corticosteroids. Systemic steroids or azathioprine may be required in acute exacerbations. Anti-tumor necrosis factor (TNF) agents increasingly used for treating inflammatory bowel disease, include infliximab, adalimumab, golimumab, and an anti-adhesion therapy (etrolizumab or vedolizumab), or a Janus kinase inhibitor – tofacitinib. Regular colonoscopy is indicated. Colectomy may be indicated if symptoms are severe, drug response is poor, there are complications, or to eliminate the risk of malignant change.

Proctocolectomy and ileostomy is most common.

Main dental considerations

(*See also generic guidance under main dental considerations on page 63 top, and also Section 2).

Oral manifestations may include ulcers, glossitis, cheilitis or pyostomatitis vegetans (multiple, friable pustules, erosions, and ulcerations). NSAIDs are contraindicated in patients treated with methotrexate or steroids.

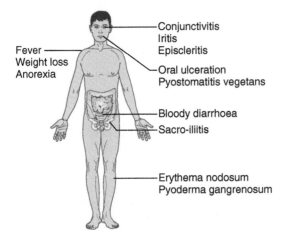

Conjunctivitis
Iritis
Episcleritis

Fever
Weight loss
Anorexia

Oral ulceration
Pyostomatitis vegetans

Bloody diarrhoea

Sacro-iliitis

Erythema nodosum
Pyoderma gangrenosum

Figure 5.56 Ulcerative colitis – features.

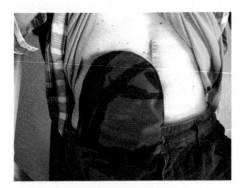

Figure 5.57 Ileostomy bag.

GENITO-URINARY

Chronic kidney disease (CKD); or chronic renal failure (CRF)

Definition
A low *estimated glomerular filtration rate* (volume of blood filtered by kidneys over a given time – eGFR; calculated from age, sex and blood creatinine level) persisting for >3 months.

Aetiopathogenesis
Increasingly common with advancing age, mainly males, people of Caribbean or South Asian origins, with a family history of CKD, and as a sequel to many disorders, particularly (alphabetically):

- Amyloidosis
- Chronic glomerulonephritis
- Chronic kidney diseases such as in:
  - Diabetes mellitus
  - Hypertension
  - Myeloma
  - Nephrotoxic drugs (e.g. 'analgesic nephropathy' – NSAIDs, acetaminophen/paracetamol), aminoglycosides, or amphotericin
  - Poisoning (e.g. lead poisoning)
  - Polycystic renal disease
  - Renal artery stenosis
  - Systemic lupus erythematosus
  - Urinary obstruction (calculi; stones).

Clinical presentation
Raised urea levels are usually asymptomatic until kidney function has fallen to <25%. Then nocturia and anorexia, raised creatinine (azotaemia) and electrolytes (potassium and hydrogen ions) appear. Advanced CKD affects most body systems. Hypertension is common. Renal osteodystrophy is common; phosphate retention depresses calcium and subsequently raises parathyroid activity (secondary hyperparathyroidism) and deficient renal production of 1,25 dihydroxycholecalciferol (vitamin D3) reduces calcium absorption. Purpura, a bleeding tendency and anaemia are common. Defective phagocyte function causes liability to infection.

End-stage renal disease (ESRD; uraemia) – is when >90% renal function is lost.

The A's of CKD are:

- anaemia
- atherosclerosis
- anti-angiotensin therapy
- albumin
- anions and cations
- arterial BP
- arterial calcifications
- access
- avoid nephrotoxic drugs
- allograft.

Table 5.19 Stages of chronic kidney disease			
Renal health	GFR mL/min/1.73 m²	Stage	Manage, control BP and
Normal	>130	–	
Normal but other evidence of CKD	>90	I	
Mild or early CRF with other evidence of CKD	60–89	II	CVS risk factors
Moderate CRF (azotaemia)	45–59	IIIa	
	30–44	IIIb	
Severe CRF	15–29	IV	Plan for ESRF
Established, very severe or end-stage renal failure (ESRF)	<15	V	Dialysis or transplant

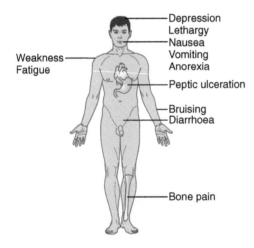

Figure 5.58 Chronic kidney disease – features.

Diagnosis

Mainly by rising plasma urea and creatinine levels and a falling eGFR. Urine: albuminuria/proteinuria.

Treatment

- Underlying causes should be treated if possible.
- Nephrotoxic drugs should be avoided.
- Initial management aims to lower the:
  - BP – using angiotensin converting enzymes inhibitor (ACEIs) and angiotensin-II blockers, which also minimize proteinuria.

- Blood urea, electrolytes, etc. by:
  - Normal diet (low protein diets are rarely advocated now);
  - Potassium restriction;
  - Salt or water control.
- Recombinant erythropoietin or darbepoietin, as treatment for anaemia.
- Calcium carbonate, vitamin D3 or its synthetic analogue, a low phosphate diet, or intravenous clodronate aid bone resorption inhibition. Parathyroidectomy may be necessary in resistant cases.
- Dialysis to remove metabolites becomes essential if renal function deteriorates to ESRD and may be by continuous ambulatory peritoneal dialysis (CAPD), or continuous cyclic peritoneal dialysis (CCPD) or extra-corporeal haemodialysis. Renal transplantation may become necessary (see Section 9).

Main dental considerations

(*See also generic guidance under main dental considerations on page 63 top, and also Section 2).

Oral manifestations may include xerostomia, candidiasis, salivary infections, dysgeusia (taste anomalies), petechiae and ecchymoses, osteodystrophy (radiolucent jaw lesions) or uraemic stomatitis.

For patients being treated for hypertension, use vasoconstrictors with caution. May need to alter the dosage of other drugs according to kidney functioning. Avoid high doses of NSAIDs, paracetamol and tetracycline. Monitor the patient on benzodiazepines for resulting excessive sedation. Defer dental treatment if there is electrolyte imbalance, advanced renal failure or another systemic disease (e.g. diabetes mellitus, hypertension, and systemic lupus erythematosus) until a physician can be consulted and treatment can be provided in a hospital-like setting, or postpone until after haemodialysis. Aggressively manage orofacial infections and consider hospitalization for severe infection or major procedures. Increased risk of bleeding. A patient with ESRD who has been taking large doses of corticosteroids (i.e., 10 mg daily of prednisone or equivalent) may have adrenal hypofunction.

Infection control is of paramount importance, as infection with hepatitis viruses, HIV or other blood-borne agents, and tuberculosis, was common in the past. Consider other comorbid diseases. Patients on haemodialysis are severely compromised, and many are on anticoagulation (see Section 9).

Defer elective dental treatment on day of dialysis. Appointments should be scheduled on day after dialysis. Lidocaine is the safest LA to use, followed by articaine and prilocaine. Midazolam is preferable to diazepam because of its lower associated risk of thrombophlebitis. Diazepam should be safe, except that it is long acting, requires renal dosing and has a risk of propylene glycol toxicity if given via IV (at high/prolonged dosage). It is not dialyzable. Never put a cannula (IV) into the arm with the shunt.

Antimicrobial use may be:

- *Usually safe (no dosage change required):* azithromycin, cloxacillin, doxycycline, flucloxacillin, fucidin, minocycline, rifampicin.
- *Fairly safe (change dosage only in severe CKD):* ampicillin, amoxicillin, benzylpenicillin, clindamycin, co-trimoxazole, erythromycin, ketoconazole, lincomycin, metronidazole, phenoxymethyl penicillin.
- *Less safe (dosage reduction in all patients):* aciclovir, cephalosporin, ciprofloxacin, fluconazole, levofloxacin, ofloxacin, sitafloxacin, and vancomycin.

Avoid *(do not use in any patients):* aminoglycosides, carbenicillin, cefadroxil, cefixime, cephalexin, cephalothin, gentamicin, imipenem, itraconazole sulfonamides, tetracyclines, and valacyclovir.

Analgesic may be:

- *Usually safe (no dosage change required):* acetaminophen/paracetamol.
- *Fairly safe (dosage change only in patients with severe CKD):* codeine.
- *Less safe (dosage reduction in all patients):* NSAIDs.

Avoid *(do not use in any patients):* dextropropoxyphene, meperidine, morphine, opioids, pethidine, and tramadol.

Other drugs:

- Diazepam and midazolam are usually safe *(no dosage change required):* but dosage reduction is needed in all patients given carbamazepine, gabapentin or lamotrigine.

Kidney cancer

Definition
Kidney cancer is the eighth most common cancer in adults. Renal cell carcinoma (RCC – also known as hypernephroma, Grawitz tumour, adenocarcinoma) accounts for most. Rarer cancer types include transitional cell cancer (usually affects men over 50) and Wilms' tumour (affects children).

Aetiopathogenesis
Although the cause is unknown, risk factors include:
- Age
- Dialysis
- Exposure to asbestos, cadmium, lead, or trichloroethylene
- Family history of kidney cancer
- Genetic conditions:
  - Birt–Hogg–Dube syndrome (BHD; with benign skin growths, lung collapse);
  - Hereditary papillary renal cell carcinoma (HPRCC);
  - von Hippel-Lindau disease (VHL; benign and malignant tumours, in retina, CNS and viscera, renal cysts, haemangioblastoma, phaeochromocytoma).
- Hypertension
- Obesity
- Renal failure
- Smoking.

Clinical presentations
Kidney cancer most frequently affects men over 50 years of age. In around half of cases there are no symptoms and the cancer is detected during tests for other unrelated conditions. Signs and symptoms can include:
- abdominal lump
- abdominal or loin pain
- haematuria.

Diagnosis
Renal function tests, imaging (US, MRI, CT, IVP), biopsy.

Treatment
- Surgery (partial, simple or radical nephrectomies); radiofrequency ablation (RFA), cryotherapy, high-intensity focused ultrasound (HIFU).
- Radiotherapy or targeted drug therapies are available.
- Chemotherapy (aldesleukin, axitinib, bevacizumab, everolimus, interferon, pazopanib, sorafenib, sunitinib, temsirolimus) is less effective.

Main dental considerations
(*See also generic guidance under main dental considerations on page 63 top, and also Section 2).
Oral sequelae of chemotherapy (Section 9) are common. Renal metastases to the mouth are rare.

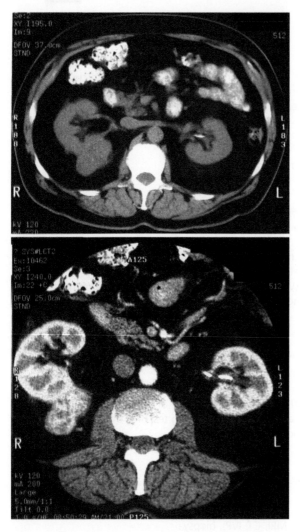

Figure 5.59 Kidney cancer. Reprinted from Wein AJ et al. (2012) Campbell-Walsh Urology, 10e. Elsevier with permission.

Kidney stones (nephrolithiasis)

Definition
Stone-like lumps that develop in one or both kidneys.

Aetiopathogenesis
Kidney stones are quite common and usually affect people aged 30–60 years, men more than women. The waste products in urine can occasionally form crystals in the kidneys which, over time, may build up to form a hard stone-like lump. This is more likely if inadequate amounts of fluids are ingested. The substances implicated can include:

- Calcium (in high levels of vitamin D, hyperparathyroidism, renal disease, sarcoidosis).
- Cystine (cystinuria).
- Magnesium ammonium phosphate (struvite) – often caused by ammonia-producing urinary infections.
- Uric acid (chemotherapy, gout, high protein diets, hyperuricaemia).

Stones are most likely if the person has:

- a high-protein, low-fibre diet or low fluid intake
- too little activity or is bed-bound
- a family history of kidney stones
- had several kidney or urinary infections
- only one functional kidney
- had an intestinal bypass or Crohn's disease.

Drugs that may increase risk of stones include:

- Antacids
- Antibiotics
- Anticonvulsants
- Antiretrovirals
- Aspirin
- Calcium
- Diuretics
- Vitamin D.

Clinical presentation
Small stones may pass painlessly in the urine and may even go undetected. However, it is fairly common for a stone to block the ureter or the urethra when it can cause severe pain in the abdomen or groin and sometimes causes urinary tract infection.

Diagnosis
Clinical, plus ultrasound and radiography of kidneys, ureters, and bladder (KUB).

Treatment
Many kidney stones are small enough to pass in urine. Larger stones may need to be fragmented with ultrasound, or to be surgically removed using:

- extracorporeal shock wave lithotripsy (ESWL);
- open surgery;
- percutaneous nephrolithotomy (PCNL); or
- ureteroendoscopy.

Nephrotic syndrome

Definition
Constellation of proteinuria, hypoalbuminaemia and oedema.

Aetiopathogenesis
Renal glomerular damage from:
- *Renal immune diseases*:
  - Minimal change disease (glomeruli look normal but minor changes allow protein leakage);
  - Membranous nephropathy (glomeruli thickened but 'leaky').
- *Renal other disorders*: membranoproliferative and mesangial proliferative glomerulo-nephritis, fibrillary glomerulo-sclerosis, diffuse mesangial sclerosis, IgM mesangial nephropathy.
- *General conditions*: e.g. amyloidosis, diabetes, Henoch–Schönlein purpura, infections, lupus, polyarteritis nodosa, rheumatoid arthritis and some cancers.
- *Drugs, poisons or toxins*.

Clinical presentation
Proteinuria leads to low blood protein levels (especially albumin), fluid retention and oedema, plus high blood cholesterol and other fats (lipids). Initially kidney function is normal. Then appear:
- Oedematous swelling – usually painless and, in children, affects the face first but, in adults, the ankles swell. As oedema worsens, the calves, then thighs may swell. In severe cases, oedema accumulates in the lower back, the arms, abdominal cavity (ascites – causing abdominal pain and discomfort) or the chest (pleural effusion – causing chest pain and dyspnoea).
- Other symptoms may include:
  - Diarrhoea and/or vomiting;
  - Fatigue, lethargy and anorexia;
  - Muscle wasting;
  - Nails turn white (leukonychia);

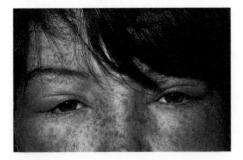

Figure 5.60 Nephrotic syndrome.

- Possible complications from underlying cause of nephrotic syndrome (e.g. diabetes, rheumatoid arthritis) or kidney disease – hypertension or renal failure;
- Protein loss complications:
  - anaemia
  - bone disease from loss of vitamin D-binding protein
  - heart disease
  - infections
  - venous thrombosis.

Diagnosis

- Protein in the urine by 'dipstick'
- 24-hour urine
- Low blood albumin
- Tests to identify the cause of nephrotic syndrome
- Kidney biopsy
- U&Es
- eGFR.

Treatment

- Limit dietary salt
- Diuretics to limit oedema
- Treatment of hypertension
- Treatment of the underlying cause.

Main dental considerations

(*See also generic guidance under main dental considerations on page 63 top, and also Section 2).
Nephrotic syndrome may manifest with swelling of the face, lips, mouth, tongue or throat. Some viruses that cause mouth ulceration, including certain enteroviruses, can cause nephrotic syndrome.

Pyelonephritis

Definition
Infection in the kidney pelvis, usually accompanied by infection within the renal parenchyma (Greek *pyelum*, 'renal pelvis', and *nephros*, 'kidney').

Aetiopathogenesis
Usually arises from lower urinary tract infection (UTI), occasionally from haematogenous spread. Organisms include *Escherichia coli*, *Klebsiella* spp., *Proteus* spp., *Enterococcus* spp. Risk factors may include:

- Calculi (stones)
- Diabetes
- Immunocompromised patients
- Neuropathic bladder
- Pregnancy
- Primary biliary cirrhosis
- Renal structural abnormalities
- Stents or drainage procedures
- Urinary tract catheterization.

Clinical presentation and classification
Acute pyelonephritis can arise at any age. In neonates it is more common in boys and associated with renal tract abnormalities. Beyond infancy, girls have higher incidence. In younger adults it is more common in women but, over 65, the incidence in men rises to match. Onset is usually over a day or so with unilateral or bilateral loin, suprapubic or back pain. Fever is variable. Malaise, nausea, vomiting, anorexia and occasionally diarrhoea occur. There may be accompanying lower UTI symptoms (frequency, dysuria, haematuria or hesitancy). Often pain on kidney(s) palpation and suprapubic tenderness.

Chronic pyelonephritis may ensue after repeated acute pyelonephritis, and then features may include:
- Dysuria
- Fever
- Hypertension.
- Loin pain
- Malaise
- Nausea and vomiting.

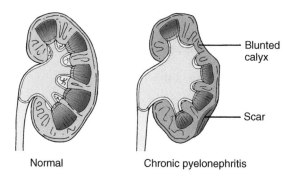

Normal   Chronic pyelonephritis

Figure 5.61 Cross section of normal kidney and kidney with chronic pyelonephritis.

Diagnosis

Clinical and:

- *Urine*:
  - Dipstick urinalysis for blood, protein, leukocyte esterase and nitrite.
  - Mid-stream specimen (MSU) for microscopy, and culture and sensitivity.
- *Blood*:
  - Cultures: positive in >10%.
  - CRP, ESR, and PV (plasma viscosity) may be raised. Procalcitonin may be a marker in children under 2 years.
  - Raised white cell count, with neutrophilia.
- *Imaging*:
  - Ultrasound.
  - Kidneys, ureters, and bladder (KUB) radiography.
  - Intravenous pyelography (IVP) may show small kidneys, ureteric and caliceal dilatation/blunting.
  - Voiding cystourethrography (VCUG) may identify reflux.
  - In children – ultrasound or CT scanning.
  - In adults – contrast-enhanced helical/spiral CT (CECT).
  - MRI is useful in children or adults.
  - Tc-DMSA (Technetium-99m-labelled Di-Mercapto-Succinic Acid) scan.
  - Renal biopsy is rarely used – usually to exclude papillary necrosis.

Treatment

Acute pyelonephritis

Support: rest, adequate fluid intake and analgesia. Antibiotics: empirical treatment while awaiting culture and sensitivity results.

Surgery: may be required to drain abscesses, or relieve obstructions causing the infection.

Indications for hospital admission include:

- Anuria or oliguria
- Co-morbidity, e.g. diabetes
- Complications
- Dehydration
- Inadequate access to follow-up
- Relapse as soon as antibiotics have stopped
- Sepsis (e.g. tachypnoea, tachycardia, hypotension)
- Severe pain, debility or vomiting
- Social issues
- Treatment non-compliance
- Unclear diagnosis
- Urinary tract obstruction.

Chronic pyelonephritis

- Monitor BP, blood lipids, renal function and glucose.
- BP should be controlled with ACEI to slow renal failure – which may eventually require renal transplantation.
- Supervening UTI may require long courses of antibiotics.
- Ureteric surgical re-implantation may be needed in severe cases.

Prevention

Prevention is based on preventing UTI. In children antibiotic prophylaxis is used for those at highest risk of complications (e.g. demonstrable vesicoureteric reflux, recurrent infections or renal scarring on imaging), with consideration of correction of renal structural abnormalities. Women should be encouraged to void after sexual intercourse. Cranberry juice may be helpful and, in women with at least three symptomatic infections a year, prophylactic trimethoprim is widely used. Antibiotics are also used in asymptomatic bacteriuria of pregnancy and in those with severe vesicoureteric reflux.

HAEMATOLOGICAL

Anaemia

A haemoglobin level below the normal for the age and sex (in adult females, below 11.5 g/dl and adult males below 13.5 g/dl), anaemia may be a feature of many diseases (Box 5.1) and is classified on the basis of erythrocyte (red cell) size as:

- *Microcytic* (small red cells – mean corpuscular cell volume [MCV] is reduced below 78 fl) anaemia is most common – usually due to iron deficiency, occasionally to thalassaemia or chronic diseases.
- *Macrocytic* anaemia (large – MCV more than 99 fl) is usually caused by vitamin B_{12} or folate deficiency (e.g. in alcoholics or pregnancy), and sometimes by chronic haemolysis, drugs (methotrexate, azathioprine, cytosine or hydroxycarbamide), liver disease, or aplastic anaemia.
- *Normocytic* anaemia (normal size – MCV between 79 and 98 fl) may result from various chronic diseases, e.g. chronic inflammatory disease, infection, leukaemia, liver disorders, malignancy, renal failure, and sickle cell disease.

Box 5.1   Causes of anaemia

- Blood loss (most common cause)
- Poor dietary intake of haematinics
- Impaired absorption of haematinics (small intestine diseases particularly)
- Increased demands for haematinics (pregnancy and haemolysis)
- Impaired erythropoiesis
- Haemolytic anaemias (sickle cell disease and thalassaemia)

Table 5.20   Main causes and classification of anaemias

Type	Examples	Comments
Microcytic hypochromic	Iron deficiency Thalassaemia	Blood loss from menstruation or occult sources (gastrointestinal or genito-urinary) Dietary deficiency Malabsorption (post-gastrectomy)
Macrocytic	Vitamin B_{12} deficiency Folate deficiency Haemolysis Hypothyroidism Liver disease Aplastic anaemia	
Normocytic anaemia	Chronic diseases Renal failure Haemolysis Hypothyroidism	

Anaemia in the early stages is commonly symptomless but, as blood O_2-carrying capacity falls, dyspnoea and raised cardiac output (palpitations, murmurs, cardiac failure) result. Anaemia is diagnosed from the haemoglobin level, but the precise nature must be established by a full (or complete) blood count/picture (FBC/FBP/CBC).

Haemoglobin levels can be replenished by haematinics (e.g. iron, folic acid or vitamin B_{12}), blood transfusions, or perhaps erythropoietin to stimulate natural haemopoiesis.

Anaemia – deficiency

Aetiopathogenesis

Decrease in circulating erythrocytes due to decreased production. The most common cause in resource-rich countries is chronic blood loss and consequent iron deficiency anaemia, usually in women from heavy menstruation. Folate and vitamin B_{12} (cobalamin) deficiency (pernicious anaemia) are the next most common causes.

Clinical presentations

Consequences of cardiovascular and ventilatory efforts to compensate for oxygen deficiency, include:

- General: tiredness, anorexia and dyspnoea.
- Skin and mucosa: pallor of mucosa, conjunctiva or palmar creases. Splitting and spooning of the nails (koilonychia) may be detected.
- Cardiovascular: tachycardia and palpitations. Anaemia exacerbates, or can cause, heart failure, angina, and effects of pulmonary disease.
- Nervous system: headache, behaviour changes, and in children there can be learning impairment. Paraesthesia of fingers and toes and CNS damage (sub-acute combined degeneration of spinal cord causing loss of joint position and vibration sense and possibly paraplegia) are associated with pernicious anaemia.

Diagnosis

Clinical findings plus:

- Haemoglobin (Hb) assay.
- Complete blood count (CBC or FBC), plus *mean corpuscular* volume (MCV), haemoglobin (MCH) and haemoglobin concentration (MCHC).
- Serum iron and ferritin (iron deficiency anaemia).
- Serum vitamin B_{12} and autoantibodies (pernicious anaemia).
- Red cell folate assays.

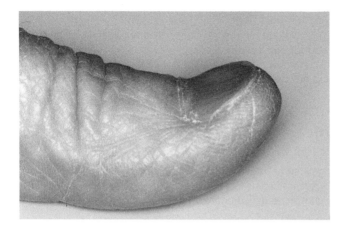

Figure 5.62 Koilonychia (spoon-shaped nail).

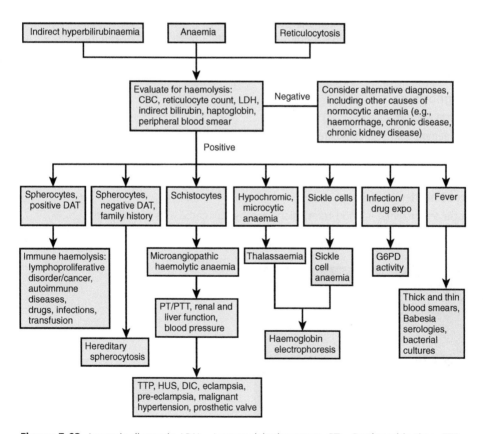

Figure 5.63 Anaemia diagnosis. LDH = Lactate dehydrogenase. PT = Prothrombin time. TTP = Thrombotic Thrmbocytopenic Purpura. HUS = Haemolytic Uraemic Syndrome. DIC = Disseminated Intravascular Coagulopathy.

Treatment

Treat causes and give oral ferrous sulphate for iron deficiency anaemia: vitamin B_{12} by injection for life and/or oral folic acid for macrocytic anaemia.

The main danger in anaemias is when a GA is given, as it is vital to ensure full oxygenation: elective operations should not usually be carried out when the haemoglobin is less than 10 g/dl (male).

Anaemia – haemolytic

Aetiopathogenesis

Erythrocyte damage – usually related to infection (malaria), inherited haemoglobin abnormality (haemoglobinopathy) – such as sickle cell disease or thalassaemia, or an enzyme defect (e.g. G6PD [glucose 6 phosphate dehydrogenase] deficiency).

Clinical presentation

Most symptoms are the consequence of cardiovascular and ventilatory efforts to compensate for oxygen deficiency, and include:

- General: tiredness, anorexia and dyspnoea.
- Thrombosis, jaundice, pain, neuropathy and osteomyelitis may be seen in sickle cell disorders.
- Bone marrow hyperplasia in haemoglobinopathies.

Diagnosis

Clinical findings plus:

- Haemoglobin and complete blood count.
- Haemoglobin electrophoresis (sickle cell anaemia and thalassemia).
- Radiography.

Treatment

Sickle cell anaemia – blood transfusions and hydroxycarbamide (hydroxyurea).
Thalassemias – blood transfusions and folate supplements; chelate excess iron with desferioxamine and ascorbic acid; splenectomy.

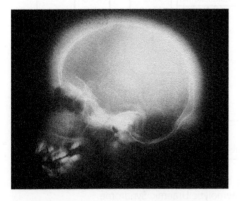

Figure 5.64 Hair-on-end radiographic appearance in haemoglobinopathy.

Main dental considerations

(*See also generic guidance under main dental considerations on page 63 top, and also Section 2).

Oral manifestations in deficiency anaemias may include ulcers, angular cheilitis, or glossitis. In haemolytic anaemias, bone marrow hyperplasia with enlarged bones may be seen, as may pain or infections. Pain/analgesic therapies offered may need to be adjusted if a tolerance has developed. There is a possible risk of medication dependence. Splenectomy causes immune defect. If infection occurs, treat aggressively. It may be prudent to offer prophylactic antibiotics for major surgical procedures. GA is a particular hazard in sickle cell anaemia.

Table 5.21 The sickling disorders

Disorder	Hb	Predominant ethnic groups	Clinical features
Sickle cell anaemia	SS	African, Caribbean, Mediterranean, Indian	Severe anaemia
Sickle cell trait	SA	African, Caribbean, Mediterranean, Indian	Usually asymptomatic
Sickle cell – HbC disease	SC	West African, South-East Asian	Variable anaemia
Sickle cell – HbD disease	SD	African, Indian, Pakistani	Moderately severe anaemia
Sickle cell – HbE disease	SE	South-East Asian	Moderately severe anaemia
Sickle cell – thalassaemia	SAF	Mediterranean, African, Caribbean	Moderately severe anaemia

Haemophilias

Definition and aetiopathogenesis

Inherited deficiencies of a blood coagulation (clotting) factor.

Clinical presentation and classification

Characteristic is excessive bleeding particularly after trauma, and sometimes spontaneously. Haemorrhage appears to stop normally after injury (as a result of normal vascular and platelet haemostatic responses) but, after an hour or more, intractable oozing or rapid blood loss starts and persists. Haemorrhage is dangerous either because of loss of blood or because of bleeding causing damage compressing the brain, larynx and pharynx, or the joints or muscles.

Haemophilia A

An X-linked disorder, affects males and is 10 times as common as haemophilia B, except in Asians, where frequencies are equal. Bleeding severity depends on blood clotting Factor VIII coagulant (VIIIC) activity, and degree of trauma. Factor VIII activity of less than 1% results in spontaneous bleeding typically evident from childhood with bleeding into muscles or joints (haemarthroses), easy bruising and prolonged bleeding from wounds (severe haemophilia). Factor VIII activity of 1 to 5% causes moderate haemophilia, and above 5% is mild haemophilia when comparatively minor trauma can lead to persistent bleeding. A factor VIII level above 25% causes very mild disease and the patient can often lead a relatively normal life and may remain undiagnosed.

Diagnosis

Laboratory findings needed are as follows:

- Activated partial thromboplastin time (APTT) – prolonged.
- Factor VIII assay is required as APTT may be normal in mild haemophilia. Factor VIIIC is low but VIIIR:Ag (von Willebrand factor) and R:RCo (ristocetin cofactor) are normal.
- Prothrombin time (PT) – normal.

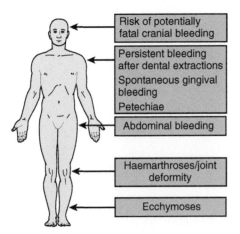

Figure 5.65 Haemophilia – features.

Treatment

Haemophiliacs should be under the care of a recognized Haemophilia Reference Centre. If bleeding starts, or is expected (e.g. perioperatively), Factor VIII must be replaced to a level adequate to ensure haemostasis. Factor VIII replacement is achieved with genetically engineered (recombinant) Factor VIII preparations (eloctate, ruriococtocog, or simoctocog; or porcine Factor VIII. Previously, fresh plasma, or fresh frozen plasma cryoprecipitate or fractionated human factor concentrates obtained from pooled blood sources were used, but these had potential to carry blood-borne pathogens such as hepatitis viruses, HIV and various herpesviruses. Desmopressin (deamino-8-D arginine vasopressin: DDAVP) – a synthetic vasopressin analogue which induces release of Factor VIII, von Willebrand's factor (vWF) and tissue plasminogen activator (tPA) from storage sites in endothelium may help in mild haemophilia mainly. Tranexamic acid, a synthetic derivative of lysine with antifibrinolytic effect by blocking lysine binding sites on plasminogen, can significantly reduce blood losses. Haemophiliacs who develop inhibitors are treated with factor eight inhibitor bypass activity (FEIBA) (activates Factor X directly, by-passing the intrinsic pathway of blood clotting).

Haemophilia B (Christmas disease)

Christmas disease – after the surname of the person first described with the disease – is a sex-linked defect in Factor IX. Males are affected but female carriers (unlike those of haemophilia A) often have a mild bleeding tendency. Christmas disease is clinically identical to haemophilia A, the severity of clinical findings depending on the degree of Factor IX deficiency.

Diagnosis

Prolonged APTT, with normal PT and a Factor IX deficit.

Treatment

Recombinant Factor IX (trenonocog) or synthetic factor VIII are used for replacement. Prothrombin complex (Factor II, VII, IX and X) may be used. Desmopressin however, is not useful.

Haemophilia C (Von Willebrand's disease; vWD; pseudohaemophilia)

A deficiency in von Willebrand factor (vWF), synthesized in endothelium and megakaryocytes, which binds collagen and platelet glycoprotein (Gp) receptors, mediating platelet adhesion and aggregation and, as a carrier for Factor VIII, protects it from degradation.

Clinical presentation

vWD affects females and males, and bleeding is more like that in platelet dysfunction than in haemophilia A or B – with bleeding from mucosae with menorrhagia, epistaxis, gastrointestinal bleeding and purpura of mucosae and skin.

There are various types of vWD, – the most common inherited bleeding disorder (Table 5.22) and the severity in each varies from patient to patient, and from time to time.

Diagnosis

- APTT – usually prolonged.
- Factor VIIIC – low.
- vWF (Factor VIIIR:Ag and VIIIR:RCo [ristocetin cofactor]) levels – low.

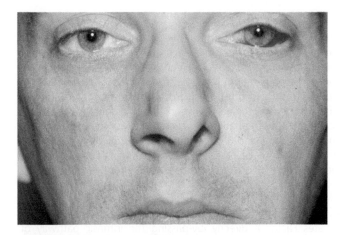

Figure 5.66 Haemophilia subconjunctival bleeding.

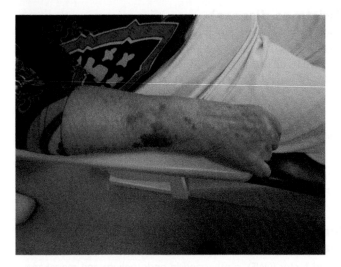

Figure 5.67 Bruising in a haemophilia.

Table 5.22	von Willebrand disease types		
Type	**% vWD**	**vWF defect**	**Factor VIIIc**
1	80	Partial lack	May be normal
2	15	Partial lack but reduced function	Reduced
2B	Rare	Partial lack but reduced function	Reduced
2M	Rare	Partial lack but reduced function	Reduced
2N	Rare	Partial lack but reduced function	Reduced
3	5	Complete lack	Reduced

Treatment

Desmopressin given via a nasal spray is used in type 1 vWD, but contraindicated in types 2B and 3, which require clotting factor replacement. Intermediate purity Factor VIII, cryoprecipitate and fresh frozen plasma are used, though pure Factor VIII may be ineffective. Recombinant vWF is now available.

Main dental considerations

(*See also generic guidance under main dental considerations on page 63 top, and also Section 2).

Spontaneous gingival bleeding may be seen in the haemophilias. General dental procedures and simple restorative procedures are generally not associated with bleeding. Proceed with caution for dental extractions and other dental surgeries. Extractions and surgery, gingival surgery/deep root planing and implant placement all pose a bleeding risk, even in mild haemophilia. For patients with moderate to severe Factor VIII deficiency, proceed with caution until the appropriate replacement factors have been given in consultation with the patient's haematologist. Desmopressin, or antifibrinolytic agents (epsilon-aminocaproic acid [EACA], and tranexamic acid) may help. Avoid NSAIDs – known to aggravate bleeding. Use paracetamol/acetaminophen with or without codeine. Older patients may have blood-borne infections.

Leukaemias

Definition
Malignant haematopoietic proliferation.

Aetiopathogenesis
Predisposing factors may include:

- autoimmune disorders
- blood disorders (e.g. myelodysplasia)
- chemicals (e.g. benzene)
- chemotherapy in the past
- genetic (e.g. Down syndrome, Fanconi anaemia)
- ionizing radiation, or radon
- maternal alcohol use in pregnancy
- smoking
- viruses.

Clinical presentation
Lymphadenopathy is common (especially in lymphatic leukaemias), and the crowding out of normal blood cells from the bone marrow by leukaemic cells, leads to:

- anaemia – fatigue, pallor, etc.
- defective leukocytes – liability to infections.
- thrombocytopenia – purpura and bleeding.

When disease progresses, leukaemic tissue may infiltrate gingivae, testes, liver, spleen, lymph nodes, and CNS.

Classification
Classification is essential because of the implications for treatment and is according to predominant cell types (lymphoid and myeloid cells) and the degree of cell maturity. Leukaemias are also classified by the clinical course (acute or chronic).

Acute leukaemias are most common in children, in whom they account for nearly 50% of malignant disease and are characterized by primitive blast cells in the blood and bone marrow. The onset is sudden, if untreated they are rapidly fatal, but treated have a good prognosis.

Chronic leukaemias are mainly diseases of adult life and are characterized by an excess of mature leukocytes in blood and bone marrow (Table 5.23). The onset is insidious, and untreated patients may survive longer than one year.

Diagnosis
Haematological examination (white blood cells count with differential), supplemented by bone marrow biopsy, chest radiography, CT and MRI scans, and lumbar puncture. Cytochemistry, analysis of membrane markers and immunophenotyping are required for categorization of the cell type.

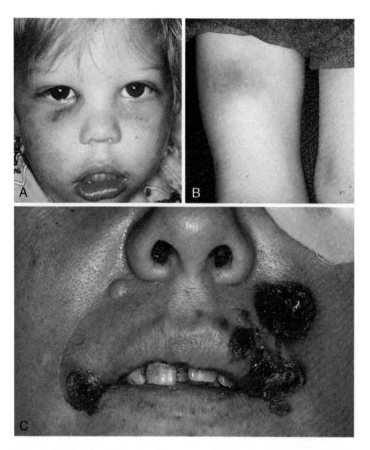

Figure 5.68 (A & B) Leukaemia bruising; **(C)** leukaemic deposits.

Table 5.23	Classification of leukaemias	
Acute	Lymphoblastic	Homogeneous small blast type
	Non-lymphoblastic	Heterogeneous blast type
		Homogeneous large blast type
		Myeloblastic without differentiation
		Myeloblastic with differentiation
		Hypergranular promyelocytic
		Acute myelomonocytic
		Monocytic
		Erythroleukaemia
		Megakaryoblastic
Chronic	Lymphoid	Lymphocytic
	Myeloid	Sezary syndrome (T cell cutaneous lymphoma)
		Hairy cell
		Prolymphocytic
		T-cell
		Granulocytic
		Atypical granulocytic
		Juvenile
		Myelomonocytic
		Eosinophilic

Treatment

Chemotherapeutic cytotoxic agent combinations include:

- Remission induction with cytotoxics and, increasingly, bone marrow transplantation.
- Post-remission treatment (consolidation).
- Maintenance therapy in some instances.

Busulfan, cyclophosphamide, cytarabine, daunorubicin, doxorubicin, mitomycin, hydroxy-urea (hydroxycarbamide), mercaptopurine, methotrexate, or thioguanine are the main agents, used along with:

- Alpha interferon.
- Haemopoietic stem cell transplant (HSCT: Section 9).
- Treatments such as cytokines, colony stimulating factors, monoclonal antibodies (mainly tyrosine kinase inhibitors), peptide vaccines, retinoids and T-cell infusions.

Cytotoxic drugs damage leukaemic cells but also all proliferating cells including epithelium, bone marrow, growth centres and gonads and therefore are often toxic, causing nausea and vomiting, impaired immunity, alopecia and mucositis.

Main dental considerations

(*See also generic guidance under main dental considerations on page 63 top, and also Section 2).

Spontaneous gingival bleeding, ulcers and infections may be seen. Herpetic, varicella-zoster infections and candidosis are particularly common. In severely ill patients, over 50% of systemic infections result from oropharyngeal microorganisms. Other oral findings include tonsillar swelling, paraesthesiae, extrusion of teeth, and painful swellings over the mandible and of the parotid (Mikulicz syndrome). Bone changes may include destruction of the crypts of developing teeth, thinning of the lamina dura, and loss of the alveolar crestal bone. Many of the cytotoxic drugs can precipitate mucositis, with oral ulceration.

Dental treatment should only be carried out after consultation with the physician. Preventive oral healthcare is essential and, where indicated, conservative dental treatment may be possible. General dental procedures and simple restorative procedures are generally not associated with bleeding. Proceed with caution for dental extractions and other dental surgeries. Regional LA injections, extractions and surgery, gingival surgery/deep root planing and implant placement all pose a bleeding risk. Surgery should be deferred (except for emergencies such as fractures, haemorrhage, potential airways obstruction or dangerous sepsis) until a remission phase. Conscious sedation is usually possible. Anaemia may be a contraindication to GA.

Because of the dangers of haemorrhage and infections such as osteomyelitis or septicaemia, desmopressin or platelet infusions or blood may be needed preoperatively, and antibiotics given until the wound has healed; intramuscular injections should be avoided as a haematoma may result. Operative procedures must be performed with strict asepsis and with the least trauma. Sockets should not be packed, as this appears to predispose to infection.

Aspirin and other NSAIDs should not be given, since they can aggravate bleeding.

Lymphomas

Definition and classification

Solid lymphoid cell neoplasms

Hodgkin's lymphoma (HL) – proliferation of multinucleated reticulum cells sometimes with mirror-image nuclei (Reed–Sternberg cells) – histologic types include:
- lymphocyte predominant
- lymphocyte depletion
- mixed cellularity
- nodular sclerosis.

Non-Hodgkin's lymphoma (NHL; the most common lymphoma) histologic types – those without Reed–Sternberg cells, commonly of B-cell origin, arising from lymph nodes or mucosa-associated lymphoid tissue (MALT), include:
- lymphocytic
- mixed lymphocytic-histiocytic
- histiocytic
- undifferentiated.

Other lymphomas include Burkitt's lymphoma, mycosis fungoides and Sézary syndrome.

Aetiopathogenesis

Possibly autoimmune responses to infection.
HL risk factors may include:

- Caucasians
- Family history of HL, NHL or leukaemia, sarcoid or ulcerative colitis
- Immune defects
- Infections (EBV, HCV)
- Obesity
- Previous NHL
- Smoking.

NHL risk factors may include:

- Age; most occur in people >69.
- Autoimmune disorders
- Coeliac disease
- Family history of NHL
- Immune defects
- Infections (e.g. EBV, HIV/AIDS, HTLV-1). NHL in stomach may be caused by *Helicobacter pylori*.
- Previous cancers (e.g. breast, melanoma)
- Previous HL or leukaemia
- Sjögren syndrome.

Clinical presentation of lymphomas

Arise in and spread to distant lymphoid organs (e.g. lymph nodes, spleen, liver or bone marrow), presenting with lymph node swelling and/or hepatosplenomegaly; systemic issues e.g. fever, sweats, or weight loss; or symptoms from compression of nerve roots, vessels or lymphatics.

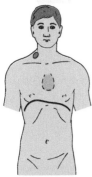
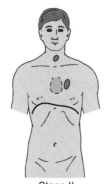
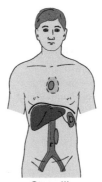
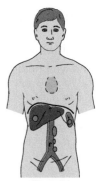

Stage I	Stage II	Stage III	Stage IV
Single lymph node region or single extralymphatic site (Ie)	Two or more sites, same side of diaphragm or c̄ continuous extralymphatic site (IIe)	Both sides of diaphragm or c̄ spleen (IIIs) or continuous extralymphatic site (IIIe)	Diffuse involvement of extralymphatic sites ± nodal disease

Stage subdivision: A-asymptomatic B-unexplained weight loss > 10% and/or fever and/or night sweats

Extralymphatic: =tissue other than lymph nodes, thymus, spleen, Waldeyer's ring, appendix and Peyer's patches

Figure 5.69 Ann Arbor lymphoma staging.

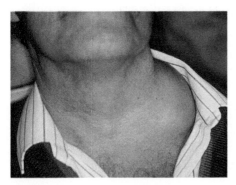

Figure 5.70 Lymphoma causing neck swelling.

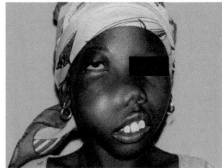

Figure 5.71 Burkitt lymphoma.

About 90% of patients with early HL survive 5 years, but only 50% survive advanced stages. Most patients with high grade diffuse NHL will, after treatment, be disease free for only 3–5 years but 75% of patients with nodular NHL survive 10 years.

Diagnosis

Diagnostic methods, also for staging disease, include chest/abdomen CT/MRI, ultrasonography, lymph node and bone marrow biopsy.

Treatment

- *HL* early stages – radiotherapy – later stages – chemotherapy (Section 9).
- *NHL* – radiotherapy or chemotherapy (Section 9). Biologics (blinatumomab, bortezomib, ibritumomab, rituximab, tositumomab) are increasingly used.

Main dental considerations

(*See also generic guidance under main dental considerations on page 63 top, and also Section 2).

Lymphomas often involve cervical lymph nodes and occasionally are seen in the mouth usually as a lump or ulcer. Dental treatment may be complicated by corticosteroid or cytotoxic therapy, liability to infection, radiation, or anaemia. Respiratory function may be impaired (pulmonary fibrosis due to irradiation) and contraindicate GA.

Myeloma (Myelomatosis: Kahler disease)

Definition
A disseminated plasma cell neoplasm.

Aetiopathogenesis
A disease mainly of the middle-aged and older people with a slight predilection for males. Occasionally related to exposure to ionizing radiation or petroleum products.

Clinical presentation
Neoplastic proliferation of plasma cells in the bone marrow and their release of osteoclastactivating factors, such as interleukin-1 and other cytokines, causes bone resorption (osteolysis), hypercalcaemia, suppression of haemopoiesis, and bone pain. Circumscribed areas of bone destruction are typical, especially in the skull vault. Defective immunoglobulins (Igs) cause liability to infections, plasma hyperviscosity with a clotting or bleeding tendency, renal failure, and neurological sequelae.

Diagnosis
Abnormal serum Igs form early and are occasionally detectable by chance during routine haematological examination, by a raised ESR, rouleaux formation or high plasma viscosity, or by serum protein investigations.

A growing number of asymptomatic patients are found to have myelomatosis by electrophoretic evidence of hypergammaglobulinaemia. Ig light chains (Bence–Jones proteins) may appear in urine.

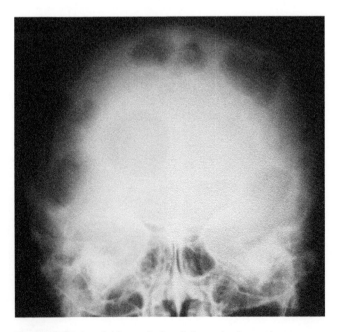

Figure 5.72 Punched out skull radiolucencies in myeloma.

Treatment

Many years may elapse before symptoms appear: such patients must be followed up and treatment started when appropriate.

Symptomatic patients, or those with progressive disease, are treated by chemotherapy (melphalan, cyclophosphamide or chlorambucil plus corticosteroids). Relapses are probably best treated with vincristine, adriamycin (doxorubicin) and dexamethasone (VAD). Newer treatments include bortezomib, daratumumab, ixazomib, bone marrow or stem cell transplantation, interferon, lenalidomide, revlimid, thalidomide) and haemopoietic growth factors.

Main dental considerations

(*See also generic guidance under main dental considerations on page 63 top, and also Section 2).

The skull, especially the calvarium and jaws, may show rounded, discrete (punched-out) osteolytic lesions. Root resorption, loosening of teeth, mental anaesthesia and, rarely, pathological fractures are other effects. Melphalan can cause severe mucositis. Bisphosphonates, such as pamidronate, help prevent pathological fractures but predispose to osteonecrosis (see Section 9).

Neutrophil defects

Definitions
- *Agranulocytosis* – the clinical syndrome resulting from leukopenia or neutropenia.
- *Leukopenia* – low level of functional leukocytes, either in absolute numbers or as effective cells.
- *Neutropenia* – low level of circulating functional polymorphonuclear leukocytes (PMNL), either in numbers ($<2000 \times 10^6$/litre) or as effective phagocytes – leukocyte adhesion defects (LAD); chemotaxis defects; opsonization defects; killing defects (granule alterations, oxidative activity deficiency).

Aetiopathogenesis
Congenital or acquired (Table 5.24).

Clinical presentation
Abnormal susceptibility to infection and oropharyngeal ulceration, periodontitis, sore throat, fever, weakness or prostration. Septicaemia may arise with complications that may include adult respiratory distress syndrome (ARDS), pneumonia, shock or endocarditis, and mortality rates have been as high as 30%. Patients should be in laminar-airflow rooms, with any surgery done under antibiotic cover.

Diagnosis
- Full blood picture. Based on the absolute neutrophil count in peripheral blood, neutropenia is classified as:
  - Mild: $1000–2000$ neutrophils $\times 10^6$/litre
  - Moderate: $500–1000$ neutrophils $\times 10^6$/litre
  - Severe: <500 neutrophils $\times 10^6$/litre.
- Bone marrow biopsy.

Treatment
Treat the underlying cause. Colony Stimulating Factors (CSF) may help. Control infections; if neutropenic patients develop fever, sample blood, urine, sputum and faeces for culture and start empirical systemic antibiotics, usually initially gentamicin plus piperacillin/tazobactam or, if penicillin-allergic, ceftazidime. Gram-positive infections are usually sensitive to penicillin, beta-lactams, vancomycin, roxithromycin, rifampicin, macrolides, teicoplanin, lincosamides and aminoglycosides but co-trimoxazole is not effective. Gram-negative

infections should be treated with ticarcillin, mecillinam or a third generation cephalosporin such as ceftazidime or cefotaxime.

Granulocyte colony stimulating factors (G-CSF) may be of benefit.

Main dental considerations

(*See also generic guidance under main dental considerations on page 63 top, and also Section 2).

The main oral manifestations include infections, ulcers and periodontal disease and even minor infections may result in gangrenous stomatitis, metastatic infections or septicaemia, sometimes fatal. Dental surgical procedures should be covered with antibiotics and particular attention should be paid to the possibility of thrombocytopenia with haemorrhagic tendencies and to the risks associated with corticosteroid treatment.

Table 5.24 Causes of neutropenia

Intrinsic neutropenia

Congenital severe neutropenia (Kostmann's syndrome)
Congenital benign neutropenia
Reticular dysgenesis
Cyclic neutropenia
Schwachman–Diamond syndrome (inherited condition affecting particularly the bone marrow, pancreas, and skeletal system)
Severe chronic neutropenias, related to immunoglobulinopathies, phenotypic abnormalities, metabolic alterations

Acquired neutropenia

Caused by drugs.
Predictable: cytostatics and immunodepressants
Idiosyncratic: penicillins, NSAIDs, phenothiazine, procainamide, quinidine, sulphonamides
Post-infectious
Bone marrow transplantation
Radiotherapy
Nutritional deficiencies:
    vitamin B_{12}
    folate
    copper

Thrombocytopenia

Definition
A platelet count below 100×10^9 per litre.

Aetiopathogenesis
The main causes are platelet:
- altered production (i.e. chemotherapy, radiation, leukaemia, viruses [HIV, EBV, rubella, viral haemorrhagic fevers such as Ebola]);
- disturbed distribution (i.e. splenomegaly);
- increased destruction (i.e. idiopathic [autoimmune] thrombocytopenic purpura [ITP]).

Clinical presentation and classification
Thrombocytopenia can cause petechiae, ecchymoses, postoperative haemorrhage and spontaneous bleeding in/from inflamed tissues. Classified as mild, moderate, severe or life-threatening. Where platelet counts do not fall below 50×10^9 per litre, thrombocytopenia is usually asymptomatic.

Diagnosis
Clinical, FBC and reduced platelet count.

Treatment
Platelets may be needed to cover operative procedures. Avoid drugs that impair platelets (aspirin and other NSAIDs). Therefore, acetaminophen/paracetamol and codeine are recommended analgesics. Other drugs which may affect platelet function include beta lactam antibiotics (amoxicillin, ampicillin, cephalosporins) and diazepam. Thrombocytopenia is treated with corticosteroids or other immunosuppressive agents or sometimes recombinant thrombopoietin or analogues such as romiplostin or eltrombopag, or splenectomy.

Main dental considerations
(*See also generic guidance under main dental considerations on page 63 top, and also Section 2).
Spontaneous gingival bleeding may be seen. General dental procedures and simple restorative procedures are generally not associated with bleeding. Proceed with caution for dental extractions and other dental surgeries. Regional LA injections, extractions and surgery, gingival surgery/deep root planing and implant placement all pose a bleeding risk but this is rarely as severe as in clotting disorders. Platelets can be replaced or supplemented by platelet transfusions, given half just before surgery to control capillary bleeding, and half at the end of the operation to facilitate suture placement. The need for platelets can be reduced by local haemostatic measures and use of desmopressin or tranexamic acid or topical administration of platelet concentrates. Splenectomy predisposes to infections, typically with pneumococci, and especially within the first 2 years but infection involving oral streptococci is rare and antimicrobial prophylaxis is not therefore generally recommended before invasive dental procedures. Drugs such as NSAIDs which damage platelets should be avoided.

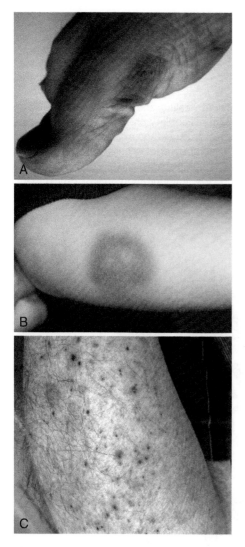

Figure 5.73 (A–C) Examples of purpura in thrombocytopenia.

HEPATIC

Main dental considerations

(*See also generic guidance under main dental considerations on page 63 top, and also Section 2).

Oral manifestations may include bleeding, impaired healing and salivary swelling. Defer elective dental care in patients with active hepatitis. People with hepatitis may have an increased bleeding tendency and metabolize some drugs slowly. Analgesics and/or sedatives should be prescribed with caution. Liver-metabolized anaesthetics, such as lidocaine and mepivacaine, should be used cautiously. Hepatitis viruses transmitted through blood and blood products include HBV, HCV and HDV. Immunization against HBV is mandatory for healthcare staff and students.

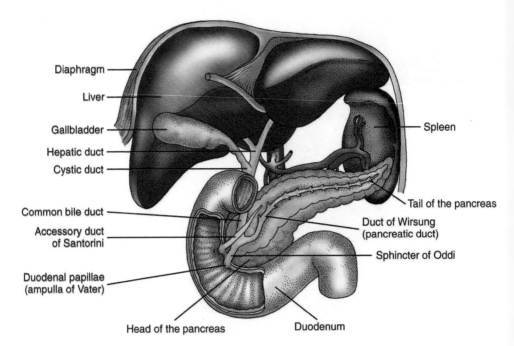

Figure 5.74 Liver and associated structures. This Figure was published in Linton A. Introduction to medical-surgical nursing, 5e. Elsevier Saunders. Copyright Elsevier (2012).

Cholecystitis

Definition
Inflammation of the gallbladder.

Aetiopathogenesis
Chronic cholecystitis leads to gallstones. Acute cholecystitis may result if a stone blocks a bile duct.

Clinical presentation and classification
10–15% of the adult population have gallstones which, in most cases, cause no symptoms.

- *Acute cholecystitis* – is uncommon and features include: a severe, sharp and constant pain in the right hypochondrium (upper abdomen) which may be worse when breathing deeply or touching the abdomen, and fever around 38°C. Around two-thirds of cases affect obese older females ("fair, fat and forty").
- *Chronic cholecystitis* may cause pain and complications:
  - *Pancreatitis* (acute or chronic) since pancreatic enzymes are obstructed.
  - *Jaundice* – if gallstones block the common bile duct.
  - *Cancer of the gallbladder* in 80% is associated with gallstones.

Diagnosis
Abdominal imaging including US; liver function tests (LFTs).

Treatment
Often first treated with antibiotics. Cholecystectomy (open or laparoscopic) is then often needed.

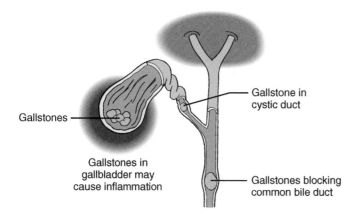

Figure 5.75 Cholecystitis: complication and prognosis.

Hepatitis

Definition
Liver inflammation. The term usually refers to viral or alcoholic hepatitis.

Aetiopathogenesis
Can result from:
- autoimmune disorders
- drugs (e.g. halothane)
- infections (e.g. viral)
- poisons (e.g. alcohol).

Clinical presentation of viral hepatitis
- Jaundice (yellowing of skin and sclerae) is the major feature although anicteric hepatitis (i.e. no jaundice) is more common.
- Malaise, fatigue, fever, arthralgia and urticaria are other findings.
- Hepatitis A (HAV) rarely has serious consequences.
- HBV, HCV and HDV have a small early mortality, and can also cause chronic hepatitis (prolonged infection – sometimes lifelong) and cirrhosis (scarring). HCV especially, can lead to liver cancer.

Diagnosis
LFTs show serum markers of viruses and raised bilirubin, aspartate transaminase (AST), alanine transaminase (ALT) and alkaline phosphatase (Alk Pase) – if there is any biliary obstruction. Patients are sometime co-infected with other hepatitis viruses, or other microorganisms.

Treatment
Bed rest, high carbohydrate diet and avoid hepatotoxins such as alcohol.

Prevention
Cross-infection risk can be minimized by:
- Avoiding tattoo, body piercing or other risks.
- Drug users never sharing needles, syringes, water, or 'works', but being vaccinated against hepatitis A and B.

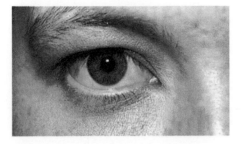

Figure 5.76 Icteric (jaundiced) sclerae.

- General hygiene.
- Healthcare workers always following standard (universal) precautions against infection transmission, safely handling needles and other sharps, and being vaccinated against hepatitis B. All clinical personnel wearing protective clothing, gloves, eye protection and mask.
- Immunizing infants born to HBV-infected mothers – hepatitis B immune globulin (HBIG) and vaccine.
- Never sharing personal care items (razors, toothbrushes).
- Using condoms.

HBV and HCV are present in blood, serum and saliva from infected persons. HBV and HCV infection have followed human bites. HBV, HCV and HDV have been transmitted to patients and staff in healthcare facilities. Needlestick injuries in unvaccinated individuals involving HBV should have hepatitis B immune globulin within 24 hours of contact. The injured person should also receive the first of three shots of the hepatitis B vaccine.

Hepatitis A ('Infectious hepatitis')

Caused by hepatitis A virus (HAV), endemic throughout the world, particularly where living and socioeconomic conditions are poor. In those areas, infection (and consequent immunity) is common in childhood. In resource-rich countries, many people reach adulthood without infection, therefore have no immunity, and are at risk from infection if travelling to endemic areas.

HAV spread is largely faeco-orally via contaminated water or food, particularly shellfish. HAV can also be transmitted sexually and by close person-to-person contact, and in body fluids including saliva. Persons in the armed forces, food handlers, healthcare workers, sewage workers, travellers to areas of high endemicity, children and employees at day care centres, promiscuous individuals who do not practise safe sex, and injecting drug users are at greatest risk.

HAV incubation period is 2–6 weeks. The disease is frequently subclinical or anicteric, but clinical features are similar to those of other forms of viral hepatitis. Blood and faeces become non-infective during or shortly after the acute illness. Recovery is usually uneventful with no evidence of a carrier state or progression to chronic liver disease though about 15% relapse over a 6–9-month period. Hepatitis A can be lethal however, if the patient is also HBV/HCV infected.

The diagnosis can be confirmed if necessary by serum antibodies (HAAb).

No specific treatment is usually needed; normal human immunoglobulin may prevent or attenuate the clinical illness and is used mainly in sporadic outbreaks. Hepatitis A infection gives long-lasting immunity. HAV vaccine is available especially for prophylaxis in travellers to high-risk endemic areas such as Asia, South America and Africa.

A combined HAV/HBV vaccine is also available.

Hepatitis B (HBV: Serum hepatitis: homologous serum jaundice)

HBV infection is endemic throughout the world, especially in poor socioeconomic and resource-poor conditions (Africa, South-East Asia and South America). Spread is mainly parenteral (via unscreened blood or blood product transfusions, particularly by intravenous drug abuse, and by tattooing/ear-piercing), sexually (especially among promiscuous individuals who do not practise safe sex) and perinatally. HBV has been transmitted to patients and staff in healthcare facilities.

Table 5.25 Comparative features of more common forms of viral hepatitis

	A (infectious)	B (serum)	C (Non-A non-B)*	D (delta agent)	E	G
Prevalence in resource-rich countries	Common; 40% urban populations	Uncommon; about 5–10% of general populations	Uncommon; about 1–5% of general populations	In countries with low prevalence of chronic HBV infection, HDV prevalence is low among both HBV carriers (<10%) and patients with chronic hepatitis (<25%).	Rare except in endemic areas in far East	Uncommon; about 1–2% of general populations
Type of virus	Picornaviridae (RNA)	Hepadnaviridae (DNA)	Flaviviridae (RNA)	Delta virus (RNA)	RNA	Flaviviridae (RNA)
Incubation	2–6 weeks	2–6 months	2–22 weeks	3 weeks–2 months	2–9 weeks	?
Main route of transmission	Faecal–oral	Parenteral	Parenteral	Parenteral	Faecal–oral	Parenteral
Vaccine available	+	+	–	–	–	–
Severity	Mild	May be severe	Moderate	Severe	May be severe	No consequences
Complications	Rare. Acute mortality 0.1%	Relatively few. Chronic liver disease in 10–20% Hepatoma, polyarteritis nodosa, chronic glomerulonephritis. Acute mortality 1–2%	Many. Chronic liver disease in >70% Hepatoma	Can cause fulminant hepatitis	Rare except in pregnancy	–

HBV is a DNA virus. Electron microscopy shows three types of particle in serum: the Dane particle probably represents intact HBV, and consists of an inner core containing DNA and core antigens (HBcAg), and an outer envelope of surface antigen (HBsAg); smaller spherical and tubular forms represent excess HBsAg. The other HBV antigen is the e antigen (HBeAg) (Table 5.26).

HBV incubation period is 2–6 months. About 30% of persons have no signs or symptoms. Common findings include jaundice, malaise, fatigue, fever, arthralgia and urticaria.

Most patients with clinical hepatitis recover completely with no untoward effect, apart perhaps from some persistent malaise. There is a small acute mortality rate. Complications may include a carrier state, chronic infection, cirrhosis, carcinoma or death.

Prevention is by avoiding contact with HBV, and having the hepatitis B vaccine. Combined HAV/HBV vaccine is available for some travellers and users of injectable drugs, promiscuous individuals who do not practise safe sex, and persons with clotting disorders who receive therapeutic blood products.

Drugs for HBV treatment include:

- adefovir
- dipivoxil
- interferon
- lamivudine.

Hepatitis C (HCV; non-A, non-B hepatitis; NANB)

The percentage of people who are seropositive for anti-HCV antibodies worldwide is estimated to have increased to almost 3%. Central and east Asia, north Africa, and the Middle East have the highest prevalence, with a moderate prevalence in eastern and western Europe. HCV infection spreads especially via intravenous drug abuse. Transmission in an epidemic in HIV-positive men who have sex with men (MSM), seems to be permucosal rather than parenteral, and is associated with sexual practices (fisting and group sex) and intranasal and intrarectal drug use. HCV now ranks second only to alcoholism as a cause of liver disease and is responsible for much chronic liver disease.

Table 5.26 HBV infection serum markers in relation to disease progress

	HbsAg	Anti-HBs	HBeAg*	Anti-HBe	HbcAg	Anti-HBc	DNA polymerase*
Late incubation	+	−	+	−	Liver only	−	++
Acute hepatitis	++	−	+/−	−	Liver only	++	+
Recovery (immunity)	−	++	−	+	−	+	−
Asymptomatic carrier state	++	−	−	+/−	−	++	+/−
Chronic active hepatitis	++	−	+	−	−	+	+/−

+ = Serum level raised.
*Presence implies high infectivity.

Persons at high risk for HCV include those who have:

* received blood from a donor who later tested positive for hepatitis C;
* ever injected illegal drugs;
* received a blood transfusion or solid organ transplant before about 1992;
* received a blood product for clotting disorders produced before about 1987;
* ever been on long-term renal dialysis;
* been MSM;
* evidence of persistently abnormal ALT (alanine transaminase) levels.

HCV is an RNA virus (Flaviviridae family) with a similar incubation period to hepatitis B (usually less than 60 but up to 150 days). Most acute infections (80–90%) are asymptomatic and anicteric but findings may include jaundice, malaise, fatigue, fever – usually a less severe and shorter acute illness than hepatitis B.

Many go on to chronic liver disease (75–85% of infected persons), and some develop liver cancer, or die (<3%). HCV infections in human populations show extreme genetic diversity; seven genotypes are known. The percentage of those with severe chronic infection is higher for patients who are co-infected with HIV.

Serological tests (ELISA) detect anti-HCV IgG after infection but usually not until 1–3 months (and may take up to a year). PCR can detect viral sequences.

There is no vaccine, but drugs used for HCV treatment include:

* Ribavirin plus.
* Interferon plus variously.
* First generation protease inhibitors:
  * telaprevir
  * boceprevir.
* Second generation protease inhibitors – simeprevir, faldaprevir or sofosbuvir.

Other inhibitors of viral replication include asunaprevir, beclabuvir, daclatasvir, dasabuvir, elbasvir, grazoprevir, ledipasvir, ombitasvir, paritaprevir.

Hepatitis D (HDV or delta agent [δ agent])

HDV is an incomplete virus carried within the HBV particle and only replicating in the presence of HBsAg, thus infecting patients with HBV. It is spread parenterally, mainly by shared hypodermic needles.

The incubation period is unknown, 90% of infections are asymptomatic but HDV infection does not necessarily differ clinically from hepatitis B though HDV can cause fulminant disease with a high mortality. HBV carriers with HDV superinfection are particularly likely to develop chronic liver diseases. HDV antigen and antibody can now be assayed. Drug treatment with alpha interferon is available.

Vaccination against HBV protects indirectly against HDV.

Liver non-infective diseases

Liver diseases fall into three broad groups:

- congenital;
- parenchymal; and
- extrahepatic;

but the main non-infective causes are autoimmunity and abuse of alcohol or other drugs (e.g. halothane, tetracyclines or paracetamol/acetaminophen).

Liver diseases can have many effects including jaundice, a bleeding tendency, and impaired drug and metabolite degradative and excretory activities (Table 5.27).

Diagnosis depends upon the history, physical examination, and evaluation of LFTs (Table 5.32).

Autoimmune hepatitis

Definition and classification

Liver damage produced by antibodies against self-antigens. Autoimmune disorders are either:

- *Type I*: antinuclear and/or anti-smooth muscle antibodies (SMA).
- *Type II*: anti-liver/kidney microsomes type 1 (LKMI) antibodies.

Table 5.27 Manifestations of liver diseases

Main causes	Consequences	Clinical features	Laboratory findings
Congenital hyperbilirubinaemia Extrahepatic obstruction	Impaired bilirubin metabolism	Jaundice	Hyperbilirubinaemia
Hepatocellular disease	Impaired bilirubin excretion	Jaundice Dark urine Pale stools	Hyperbilirubinaemia Bilirubinuria
Extrahepatic obstruction Hepatocellular disease	Impaired excretion of bile salts-causing malabsorption of fat and fat-soluble vitamins (especially vitamin K)	Pruritus Fatty stools Bleeding tendencies	Increased serum alkaline phosphatase and 5′ nucleotidase Prolonged prothrombin time
Hepatocellular disease	Impaired liver cell metabolism and impaired clotting factor synthesis Impaired albumin synthesis	Bleeding tendencies Oedema Coma or neurological disorders Impaired drug metabolism Portal venous hypertension Disorganized liver structure Cirrhosis Bleeding from oesophageal varices Splenomegaly	Prolonged prothrombin time Increased serum transaminases

Clinical presentation
- Acute hepatitis.
- Amenorrhoea.
- Fever, malaise, rash.
- Glomerulonephritis.
- Polyarthritis.

Diagnosis
- LFTs – abnormal.
- Serum autoantibodies – positive.
- Liver biopsy.

Treatment
Corticosteroids or azathioprine.

Liver cirrhosis

Definition and classification
Irreversible liver necrosis and fibrosis which can be:

- biliary (biliary obstruction)
- nutritional (alcohol abuse)
- post-necrotic (viral infection or toxins).

Aetiopathogenesis
Alcohol, autoimmune, biliary obstruction, chemicals, haemochromatosis, heart failure, HBV or HCV, or non-alcoholic steatohepatitis or NASH (seen increasingly in middle-aged, over-weight or obese patients with elevated blood lipids, and often diabetes). 30% of cases are cryptogenic (cause unknown).

Clinical presentation
May be asymptomatic or present with abnormal LFTs or:

- Skin signs – jaundice, leuconychia, clubbing, palmar erythema, Dupuytren's contracture, spider naevi.
- Gynaecomastia or testicular atrophy.
- Later signs – bleeding, oesophageal varices, ascites, peritonitis, encephalopathy, or hepatorenal syndrome. The risk of liver cancer (hepatocellular carcinoma) is increased. Most patients die in 5 to 10 years; cirrhosis is the third most common cause of death among adults.

Diagnosis
- Autoantibodies
- Hepatitis virus serology
- LFTs – abnormal
- Liver ultrasound
- Prothrombin time – increased
- Serum albumin – reduced.

Treatment
- Avoid alcohol and drugs
- Interferon alpha
- Low protein and low salt diet.

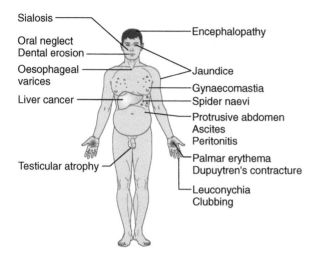

Sialosis

Encephalopathy

Oral neglect
Dental erosion

Oesophageal
varices

Jaundice

Gynaecomastia

Liver cancer

Spider naevi

Protrusive abdomen
Ascites
Peritonitis

Testicular atrophy

Palmar erythema
Dupuytren's contracture

Leuconychia
Clubbing

Figure 5.77 Liver failure features. Adapted from Scully et al. (2007) Special Care in Dentistry: Handbook of Oral Care. Churchill Livingstone, Elsevier.

Liver failure

Definition

Failure of normal liver functions – metabolism of drugs and toxins, and production of blood coagulation factors.

Aetiopathogenesis

- Drugs (alcohol, halothane, acetaminophen/paracetamol, many others)
- Infections (e.g. viral hepatitis)
- Other conditions.

Clinical presentation

- Encephalopathy
- Halitosis (hepatic foetor)
- Jaundice
- Tremor.

Diagnosis

- Abdominal ultrasound
- Blood glucose – reduced
- EEG – abnormal
- LFTs – abnormal
- Prothrombin time (and INR) – increased.

Treatment

- Dextrose IV
- Restrict protein intake
- Transplant if possible.

Drugs that can be hepatotoxic should be avoided (see Table 5.33). Aspirin and most NSAIDs such as indometacin – should also be avoided as they aggravate a bleeding tendency.

Table 5.28 Drugs contraindicated and alternatives in patients with liver disease

	Drugs contraindicated	Alternatives to use
Analgesics	Aspirin Codeine Indometacin Mefenamic acid Meperidine* NSAIDs Opioids Paracetamol/acetaminophen*	Codeine COX-2 inhibitors (celecoxib) Hydrocodone Oxycodone
Antimicrobials	Aminoglycosides Azithromycin Azole antifungals (miconazole, fluconazole, ketoconazole, itraconazole) Clarithromycin* Clindamycin* Co-amoxiclav* Co-tromoxazole Doxycycline Erythromycin estolate Metronidazole* Roxithromycin Talampicillin Tetracycline	Amoxicillin Ampicillin Cephalosporins Erythromycin stearate Imipenem Minocycline Nystatin Penicillins
Antidepressants	Monoamine oxidase inhibitors	SSRIs Tricyclics*
Muscle relaxants	Suxamethonium	Atracurium Cisatracurium Pancuronium Vecuronium
Local anaesthetics	Lidocaine*	Articaine Prilocaine
Anaesthetics	Halothane Thiopentone	Desflurane Isoflurane Sevoflurane
Central nervous system depressants	Barbiturates Diazepam* Midazolam* Phenothiazines Propofol*	Lorazepam* Oxazepam* Pethidine*
Corticosteroids	Prednisone	Prednisolone
Others	Anticoagulants Anticonvulsants Biguanides Carbamazepine Diuretics Liquid paraffin Lomotil Methyldopa Oral contraceptives	

*Or use in lower doses than normal.

IMMUNOLOGICAL

Allergies

Definition
An abnormal immune response to a protein (an allergen).

Aetiopathogenesis
Almost any substance or drug may produce reactions. Relevant allergens are shown in Table 5.29. Before an allergic reaction occurs, a person first has to be exposed to the allergen (though the patient may be unware of any exposure). The next time the allergen is contacted, it usually interacts with specific IgE antibody (on mast cells which then release histamine) and, within minutes to an hour, hypotension (anaphylaxis), urticaria or eczema, and bronchospasm may follow. Angioedema can be life-threatening if the swelling blocks the airway.

Classification
Allergic reactions are classified as:

- *Type I* (anaphylactic) – allergen reacts with mast cell IgE.
- *Type II* (cytotoxic) – allergen reacts with IgG or IgM on erythrocytes or platelets.
- *Type III* (immune complex) – allergen-IgE microprecipitates on blood vessel walls induce lysosome liberation from neutrophils.
- *Type IV* (cell-mediated or delayed hypersensitivity) – allergen reacts with sensitized T lymphocytes.

Clinical presentations
Clinical reactions may include:

- *Type I* – anaphylactic, with urticaria, bronchospasm and collapse.

Table 5.29	Common allergens
Allergens	**Main examples – in some**
Latex	Rubber gloves, bandages and tapes, local anaesthetic cartridges, suction tips, protective eyewear, latex ties on face masks, adhesive dressings, face masks, protective clothing, intubation tubes, catheters, tourniquets, sphygmomanometer cuffs, rubber surgical drains, stethoscopes
Foods	In children – eggs, milk and peanuts. In adults – shellfish, peanuts, other nuts, fish and eggs
Drugs	Penicillin, aspirin, ibuprofen, angiotensin-converting enzyme inhibitors (ACEI) and opioids
Animal allergens	Hair, dander
Materials	Mercury, gold alloys, methylmethacrylate, epoxy and composite resins, rubber base materials, essential oils, toothpastes, mouthwashes, iodides, chlorhexidine

- *Type II* – e.g. haematological disorders – including haemolytic anaemia, leukopenia and thrombocytopenia.
- *Type III* – e.g. erythema nodosum – often related to penicillin and sulfonamides; drug induced fever – sometimes with arthralgia, eosinophilia or rash; allergic exanthema or urticarial rash; or disseminated vasculitis.
- *Type IV* – usually contact reactions, e.g. to latex or cosmetics.

Diagnosis

History, diet diary, or an elimination diet are needed. Skin tests (prick and patch testing) may help but confirmation is by double-blind challenge. IgE levels (paper radio-immuno-sorbent test [PRIST] and radio-allergo-sorbent test [RAST]) may help. Testing is problematic since intradermal injection carries the potential risk of inducing anaphylactic shock.

For patients with Type I reactions, RAST can be carried out, but false positives are not uncommon. Patch testing for Type IV reactions is difficult to standardize.

Treatment

All allergies are best managed by allergen avoidance.

Latex can cause Type I (pruritus, urticaria and, rarely, anaphylaxis) or Type IV (contact dermatitis) reactions. The most common sensitizer is rubber in shoe soles, but latex products are common in the home (e.g. foam rubber, balloons, condoms, carpets, and textiles) and workplace. Latex allergy has increased since implementation of standard infection control procedures and now is an important occupational problem for healthcare workers; repeated rubber glove use, especially with abrasive handwashing, increases the risk. Latex is found in many healthcare items, including many:

- Adhesives and dressings and their packaging
- BP monitors
- Gloves
- Local anaesthetic cartridges
- Oral and nasal airways
- Oxygen masks and nasal cannulae
- Self-inflating bags.

Latex exposure can be via the skin, mucous membranes, or respiratory system via inhaled latex glove powder. Latex allergies are also common in patients frequently exposed to medical gloves during care, or chronically exposed from urethral catheterization (e.g. spina bifida). People with latex allergy can have cross-reactivity with some foods (e.g. apple, avocado, banana, carrot, celery, chestnut, kiwi, melons, papaya, raw potato and tomato).

Drugs can produce allergic reactions; some are 'high potential risk drugs' e.g. beta-lactams (e.g. penicillins or cephalosporins); others are 'low potential risk drugs' (e.g. erythromycin or lidocaine). Radio-contrast media, biologics and aspirin/NSAIDs are frequent

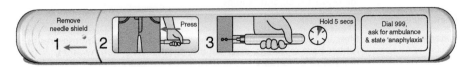

Figure 5.78 Adrenaline emergency injector.

causes of reactions, especially in people with asthma. Iodine, such as in some antiseptics may be allergenic. Parabens (a formerly used preservative) and sulphites (incorporated to prevent oxidation) have caused reactions to LAs. Metallic materials, notably nickel, can result in hypersensitivity reactions, as occasionally can chlorhexidine.

Food allergens are proteins not broken down by digestive acid or enzymes; peanuts, eggs and shellfish are common culprits.

Prevention of allergic reactions is essential – achieved by the healthcare team and the patient assiduously avoiding known allergens, and:

- Warning healthcare providers
- Wearing medical alert identification
- Carrying an adrenaline auto-injector for emergency
- Avoiding foods or drugs that may cross-react.

For penicillin – in allergic patients, alternative antibiotics such as clindamycin are recommended (cephalosporins cross-react in about 10%).

Treat urgently anaphylactic reactions (section 3) and angioneurotic oedema.

Main dental considerations

(*See also generic guidance under main dental considerations on page 63 top, and also Section 2).

Many drugs can cause an allergic reaction, and these must be discussed at the initial consultation and updated at subsequent visits. Never expose a patient to a known allergen. An emergency kit should always be readily available and staff trained in handling emergencies (Section 3). Common allergies are to penicillin (and other antibiotics), and NSAIDs. True allergy to amide local anaesthetics (e.g. lidocaine, articaine, mepivacaine, prilocaine or bupivacaine) is rare. Other allergies include reactions to latex, nickel, amalgam, resins, cobalt, mercury, acrylic and eugenol (see UK Medicines Information http://www.ukmi.nhs.uk/ukmi/about/default.asp?pageRef=1).

Immunodeficiencies (primary)

Definition
Congenital immune system defects.

Aetiopathogenesis and classification
Genetically determined or the result of development anomalies, and classified based on the predominant immune defect: B cell, T and B cell, complement or phagocytes (Table 5.30).

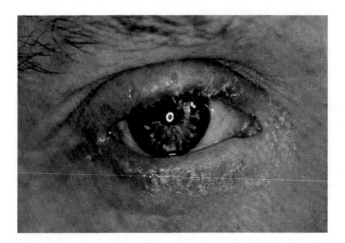

Figure 5.79 Blepharitis in immune defect.

Clinical presentation
Mainly an increased susceptibility to recurrent infections (Section 7) and to malignant disease.

- *B lymphocyte deficiency* – mainly:
  - Pyogenic infections (ear, respiratory, skin). Often pneumococci, meningococci or *Haemophilus influenza*;
  - Eczema and allergies;
  - Malignancies, mainly lymphomas.
- *T lymphocyte deficiency* – mainly serious or life-threatening infections:
  - Fungal – especially candidosis;
  - Viral – (e.g. HSV, VZV, CMV, EBV, KSHV);
  - Mycobacteria – tuberculosis or atypical mycobacteria.
- *Complement deficiencies* – mainly:
  - Autoimmune disease (especially lupus erythematosus);
  - Meningococcal and gonococcal infections;
  - Swelling of face and neck in hereditary angio-oedema only.
- *Granulocyte defects* – mainly:
  - Bacterial respiratory and skin infections, especially by *Staphylococcus aureus*, *Pseudomonas* spp. and *Serratia* spp.;

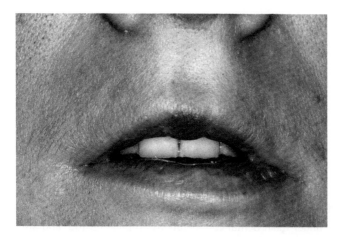

Figure 5.80 Herpes labialis (herpes simplex virus recurrence) in an immune defect.

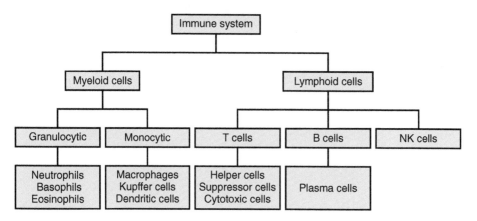

Figure 5.81 Main immunocytes (NK = natural killer).

- Lymph node and hepatic bacterial abscesses;
- Fungal infections by candida spp. and aspergillus.

Severe primary immune deficiencies cause early death – usually from pneumonia.

Diagnosis

Clinical, and:

- Complement levels and activity
- Delayed hypersensitivity skin tests
- Full blood picture
- Lymphocyte count
- Specific serum immunoglobulins
- T and B lymphocyte count and subtypes.

Treatment

- B cell defects – gammaglobulin (contraindicated in IgA deficiency)
- T cell defect – foetal thymus transplantation
- T and B cell defects – bone marrow transplant
- Granulocyte defects – granulocyte colony stimulating factor (G-CSF).

No operative treatment should be performed in patients with serum gamma-globulin levels below 20 mg/100 mL.

Antibiotic prophylaxis is indicated before any operative procedure likely to be associated with bleeding in patients with 500–1000 neutrophils/mL.

Patients with neutrophil counts <500 cells/mL should be treated in a hospital.

Main dental considerations

(*See also generic guidance under main dental considerations on page 63 top, and also Section 2.

The more severe congenital immune defects often cause early death, so they are not often relevant to dental care, except in so far as some are treated by bone marrow transplantation (Section 9). Infections and ulcers are the main oral manifestations; periodontal disease may be accelerated and minor oral infections may result in gangrenous stomatitis in severe cases. Surgical procedures should be covered with an antibiotic and attention should be paid to the possibility of haemorrhagic tendencies and to risks associated with corticosteroid treatment.

Table 5.30 Main primary immunodeficiencies

Predominant B cell defects

IgA deficiency (the most common primary immune defect)

Transient hypogammaglobulinaemia of infancy

X-linked infantile hypogammaglobulinaemia (XLA: Bruton syndrome)

Non-X-linked hyper IgM syndrome

X-linked hyper IgM syndrome

Common variable immunodeficiency

Hypogammaglobulinaemia after intrauterine viral infections, e.g. rubella

Wiskott–Aldrich syndrome (Thrombocytopenia, Immunodeficiency, Eczema; TIE)

IgG2 subclass deficiency

T and B cell defects

Congenital thymic aplasia (Di George syndrome)

Severe combined immunodeficiency

Deficiencies of MHC class II CD3, ZAP-70 or TAP-2

Immunodeficiency with ataxia telangiectasia

Late onset immunodeficiency

Complement deficiencies

Complement deficiencies C1, C2 or C4

C1, C3 or C5 deficiencies

C1 esterase inhibitor deficiency

Granulocyte defects

Interferon-gamma receptor (IFNGR) deficiency

Cyclical neutropenia

Chronic granulomatous disease

Myeloperoxidase deficiency

Chediak–Higashi syndrome (immune defect and albinism)

Leukocyte adhesion defect (LAD) 1

LAD defect 2

Papillon–Lefevre syndrome (cathepsin defect and keratoderma)

Job's syndrome (hyperimmunoglobulinaemia E: HIE)

Glycogen storage disease b

Schwachman syndrome (lazy leukocyte syndrome)

Lupus erythematosus (LE)

Definition
A multi-system connective tissue disease characterized by anti-nuclear antibodies (ANA) directed against double strand DNA (ds-DNA).

Aetiopathogenesis and classification
A defect in immune regulation, possibly virally-induced, in which antigen–antibody immune complexes deposited in blood vessels trigger vasculitis by activating complement.

- *Systemic lupus erythematosus (SLE)* – involves multiple organs and tissues. Drug-induced systemic lupus erythematosus – e.g. procainamide, hydralazine, gold, D-penicillamine, isoniazid and phenytoin.
- *Discoid lupus erythematosus (DLE)* – cutaneous or mucocutaneous variant.

Clinical presentation
Mainly:

- Musculoskeletal (pain, myopathy, arthritis).
- Renal (proteinuria, nephritis).
- Skin (rashes, alopecia, Raynaud phenomenon).

The most severe complications are lupus nephritis, pericarditis, CNS involvement, and Sjögren syndrome. Other features may include:

- mouth – ulcers, dryness
- pulmonary – pleurisy
- blood – pancytopenia
- lymphadenopathy
- fever
- cardiac – myocarditis which leads to cardiac failure, a higher risk of MI and a characteristic (Libman–Sacks) endocarditis.

Antibodies pass the placenta to cause foetal heart block.

Diagnosis
American College of Rheumatology (ACR) diagnostic criteria are based on presence of at least four of:

- Malar rash
- Discoid rash
- Photosensitivity
- Oral ulcers
- Arthritis
- Serositis (pleuritis or pericarditis)
- Renal disorder (proteinuria or cellular casts)
- Neurological disorder (seizures or psychosis)
- Haematologic disorder (anaemia, leukopenia or lymphopenia, thrombocytopenia)
- Immunologic disorder (positive LE cell, anti-DNA or anti-Sm, false-positive VDRL).

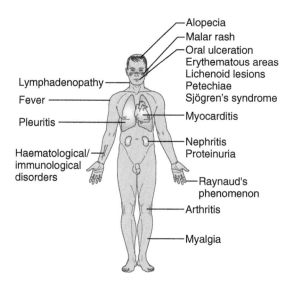

Alopecia
Malar rash
Oral ulceration
Erythematous areas
Lichenoid lesions
Petechiae
Sjögren's syndrome
Lymphadenopathy
Fever
Pleuritis
Myocarditis
Nephritis
Proteinuria
Haematological/
immunological
disorders
Raynaud's
phenomenon
Arthritis
Myalgia

Figure 5.82 Systemic lupus erythematosus – features. Adapted from Scully et al. (2007) Special Care in Dentistry: Handbook of Oral Care. Churchill Livingstone, Elsevier.

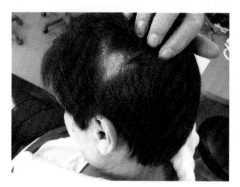

Figure 5.83 Alopecia in SLE.

Treatment

- Avoid sun exposure
- Hydroxychloroquine
- Immunosuppression (corticosteroids, methotrexate, azathioprine)
- NSAIDs.

Main dental considerations

(*See also generic guidance under main dental considerations on page 63 top, and also Section 2).

Oral manifestations in SLE may include xerostomia and ulceration. Defer elective care during acute SLE flare-ups or pulse therapy. Prescribe NSAIDs, aspirin with caution as bleeding may be increased. Use caution with drugs in patients with renal impairment; avoid tetracycline and cephalosporins): clindamycin is an alternative. Oral mucosal lesions can be a feature of DLE and may simulate lichen planus and may have some malignant potential.

Scleroderma

Definition
Degenerative changes and hypertrophy of collagen, with sclerosis of skin and other tissues.

Aetiopathogenesis
Autoimmune reactions, endocrine disorders and vascular and neural disturbances may play a role but genetics and some drugs have also been implicated.

Clinical presentation and classification
The main clinical findings may include:

- Arrhythmias and possibly cardiac failure
- Arthralgia
- Dysphagia
- Hypertension and possibly renal failure
- Neuropathy
- Pulmonary fibrosis
- Pigmentation (ivory colour) and telangiectasia
- Raynaud phenomenon
- Sclerodactyly (fibrosis and contracture of fingers)
- Sjögren's syndrome.

Limited cutaneous systemic sclerosis – CREST syndrome (calcinosis, Raynaud, esophageal hypofunction, sclerodactyly, telangiectasia of the face and extremities).

Diffuse cutaneous systemic sclerosis – causes renal, gastrointestinal, myocardial disease and malignant hypertension.

Localized scleroderma (morphoea) – rare and restricted.

Diagnosis
Clinical, confirmed by autoantibodies to:

- Centromeres.
- RNA polymerase.
- Topoisomerase (Scl-70).

Treatment
Para-aminobenzoic acid, chelating agents, dimethylsulphoxide, azathioprine and penicillamine have been used. Steroids may be useful in the early stages.

Main dental considerations
(*See also generic guidance under main dental considerations on page 63 top, and also Section 2).

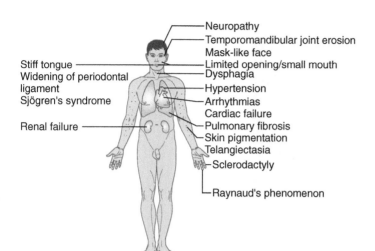

Neuropathy
Temporomandibular joint erosion
Mask-like face
Stiff tongue — Limited opening/small mouth
Widening of periodontal — Dysphagia
ligament
Sjögren's syndrome — Hypertension
Arrhythmias
Cardiac failure
Renal failure — Pulmonary fibrosis
Skin pigmentation
Telangiectasia
Sclerodactyly

Raynaud's phenomenon

Figure 5.84 Scleroderma – features. Adapted from Scully et al. (2007) Special Care in Dentistry: Handbook of Oral Care. Churchill Livingstone, Elsevier.

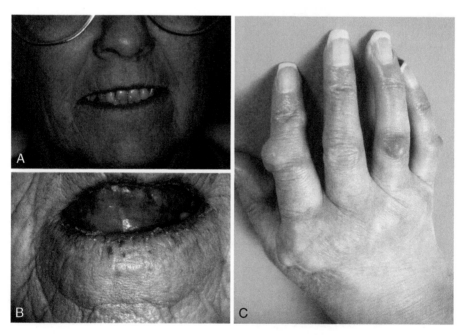

Figure 5.85 (A) Scleroderma face; **(B)** Scleroderma telangiectasia; **(C)** CREST syndrome;

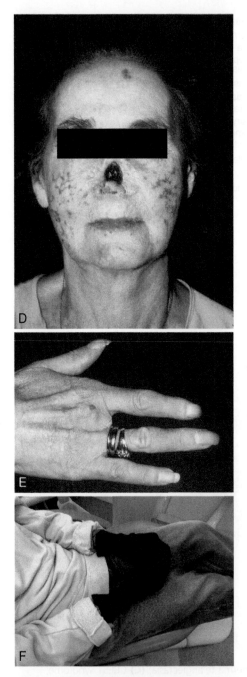

Figure 5.85, cont'd **(D)** Scleroderma telangiectasia and nasal destruction; **(E)** Scleroderma finger loss; **(F)** Cold hands due to Raynaud phenomenon in scleroderma.
Narrowing of the eyes and mask-like restriction of facial movement give a Mona Lisa-like face. The mandibular angle, condyle or coronoid process may be resorbed. Sjögren syndrome develops in a significant minority. A recognized but uncommon feature is widening of the periodontal membrane space without tooth mobility. Constriction of the oral orifice can cause progressively limited mouth opening – impeding access.

Sjögren syndrome (SS)

Definition
Autoimmune exocrinopathy, with progressive exocrine gland acinar destruction and often multi-system disease.

Aetiopathogenesis
Excessive B lymphocyte activity with autoantibodies against SS-A (Ro: Robair) and SS-B (La: Lattimer) antigens. Genetic predisposition (HLA -DR3, -B8 and -DQB genotypes), with IL-6 and TNFα gene polymorphisms, and hormones, drugs, and viruses have been implicated.

Clinical presentation and classification
The most common findings include:
- Dry mouth (hyposalivation) and dry eyes (keratoconjunctivitis sicca), and sometimes lacrimal or salivary gland swelling.
  - Hyposalivation effects can include:
    - Accelerated dental caries.
    - Ascending (bacterial) sialadenitis.
    - Difficulty in speaking or swallowing, or managing dentures.
    - Disturbed taste sensation.
    - Oral candidosis.
    - Xerostomia (sensation of dryness).
  - Dry eyes effects can include:
    - Blurred vision at end of day.
    - Difficulty wearing contact lenses.
    - Eye fatigue.
    - Light sensitivity.
    - Periods of excessive tearing.
    - Red eyes.
    - Stinging, or burning eyes.
    - Stringy mucus in or around eyes.
- Raynaud or other autoimmune phenomena.
- Multisystem features can include:
  - Cardiac – (pericarditis: in babies born to women with SS – congenital heart block).
  - Dryness – of skin, oesophagus, nose, larynx, trachea, bronchi, and lungs.
  - Gastrointestinal – (gastric reflux and chronic atrophic gastritis).
  - Hepatic – (primary biliary cirrhosis or autoimmune hepatitis).
  - Lymphoma – about 5% of people with SS develop MALT (mucosa-associated lymphoid tissue) lymphoma.
  - Nervous system – (central or peripheral) neuropathies in legs, feet, hands, arms, and even carpal tunnel syndrome is common.
  - Renal – (interstitial nephritis which can result in renal tubular acidosis, glomerulonephritis, nephrogenic diabetes insipidus and, if the bladder is involved, interstitial cystitis).

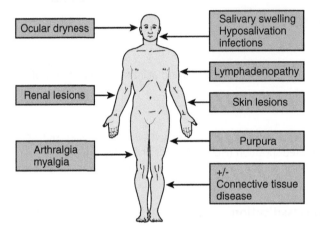

Figure 5.86 Sjögren's syndrome – features.

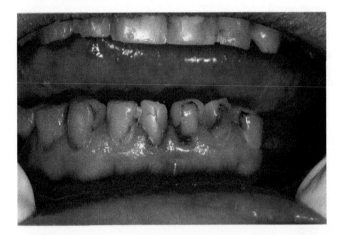

Figure 5.87 Sjögren syndrome: hyposalivation and resultant dental caries and repairs.

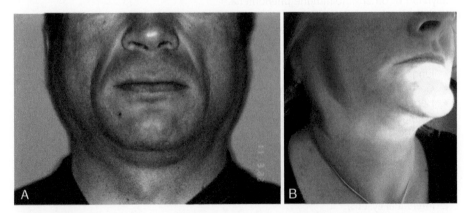

Figure 5.88 Sjögren syndrome. **(A)** Salivary enlargements (reprinted from Scully et al. (2007) Special Care in Dentistry: Handbook of Oral Care. Churchill, Livingstone Elsevier). **(B)** Sialadenitis.

- Reproductive – particularly vaginal dryness, with discomfort, painful sexual intercourse (dyspareunia), and infection.
- Thyroid – autoimmune thyroiditis.

Primary Sjögren syndrome (SS-1: 'Sicca syndrome') is the association of dry mouth with eyes in the absence of any connective tissue disease.

Secondary Sjögren syndrome (SS-2) refers to the association of dry mouth and dry eyes with a connective tissue disease, usually rheumatoid arthritis. The term 'Sjögren syndrome' often means SS-2.

Diagnosis

Other causes of hyposalivation – drugs, irradiation, and infections (e.g. hepatitis C, HIV, HTLV-1), should be ruled out.

No single investigation reliably establishes the diagnosis of SS, but tests which may be helpful include:

- Antinuclear antibodies SS-A and SS-B.
- Ophthalmological examination; Schirmer test shows impaired lacrimation.
- Salivary flow rates – confirm the presence and degree of hyposalivation.
- Salivary gland biopsy (often of labial glands).
- Salivary ultrasound and occasionally.
- Scintigraphy.
- Sialography.

Treatment

Management is largely symptomatic, though there have been attempts at immunosuppression (e.g. rituximab) to control the disease process.

Main dental considerations

(*See also generic guidance under main dental considerations on page 63 top, and also Section 2).

Oral involvement in SS results in poor salivary flow, with difficulty in speaking, swallowing, or managing dentures, disturbed taste sensation and accelerated caries, and susceptibility to oral candidosis and to ascending (bacterial) sialadenitis. Salivary gland swelling is seen in a minority. Late onset of salivary gland swelling, may indicate development of a lymphoma. Patients with SS who need dental treatment may not be good candidates for GA because of the tendency to respiratory infections.

Table 5.31 Diagnostic features of dementia

Multiple cognitive disturbances	Defects in: Language (aphasia) Motor activities (apraxia) organizing Planning Recognition (agnosia)
Memory impairment	

High level pathway
Awareness raising, understanding prevention and timely recognition:

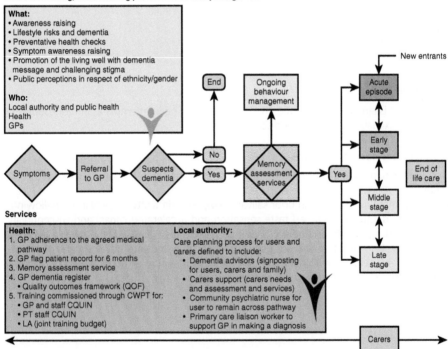

Figure 5.89 Alzheimer's disease: high level pathway. (Adapted from Living Well With Dementia. Coventry and Warwickshire. www.warwickshire.gov.uk).

MENTAL

Alzheimer disease (Alzheimer dementia; AD)

Definition

Acquired chronic organic brain disease characterized by amnesia, inability to concentrate, disorientation and intellectual impairment.

Main cause of dementia in older patients – affects >10% of those >65 years of age, 20% of those >80 and nearly half of those >85.

Aetiopathogenesis

A neurodegenerative disease, the hallmarks of which are neurofibrillary tangles and neuritic plaques consist of dying neurones clustered round deposits of amyloid. Tell-tale signs of AD are plaques of beta-amyloid and neurofibrillary tangles made of *tau*, loss of neuronal connections responsible for memory and learning; and atrophy of brain affected regions. Risk factors may include:

- Family history – if positive, predisposes.
- Head injury – or whiplash, or trauma over an extended period (e.g. boxing).
- Lifestyle – smoking, hypertension, low folate and high blood cholesterol.
- Genetic – mutations in amyloid precursor protein (APP) gene, or pre-senilins PS-1 or PS-2, or inheritance of apoplipoprotein E allele, are responsible for some cases. ApoE4 gene on chromosome 19 has been implicated in later onset AD. This and other genes involved in AD (e.g. TREM2, or Fad genes) seem responsible for abnormal processing of β-amyloid precursor protein (APP, betaAPP), and the subsequent generation, aggregation, and intracellular deposition of beta-amyloid (A beta: A beta 1-42) peptides which, as well as protein *tau*; may be the toxic factor or trigger neuronal death.
- *Suggested* risk factors also include insulin resistance, and herpes virus infection.

Clinical presentation

Gradual, progressive loss of cognitive activity, leading to inability to recognize family or friends, or carry out simple tasks; a general deterioration of motor skills; difficulties with decision-making and finding the right word; disorientation and grossly inappropriate or bizarre behaviour. AD eventually leads to irreversible mental impairment that destroys abilities to remember, reason, learn and imagine – ultimately severe mental dysfunction.

Diagnosis

Clinical. No definitive test is available, so it is crucial to exclude focal neurological deficits and other organic diseases (e.g. hypothyroidism, vitamin B_{12} deficiency). Investigations may include FBP, RFT (rod and frame test), LFT, vitamin B_{12} and folate levels, and syphilis serology. Additional studies may include neuropsychiatric tests, serial neuro-cognitive testing, neuroimaging (MRI – to show cortical atrophy and ventricular enlargement, single photon emission CT (neuroSPECT) to show brain blood flow and cell function), CSF assay of tau and beta-amyloid, and ApoE genotyping. Definitive diagnosis can be made only at autopsy.

Treatment

AD stage and treatment complexity will decide if the patient needs care in clinic, hospital or at home (chair or bed-ridden). Patients are best managed in the community if possible, although psycho-geriatric assessment is needed. Informed consent is a fraught issue.

In advanced AD, patients' inability to care for themselves leads to: difficulty eating, incontinence and health problems, such as aspiration pneumonia and other infections; urinary incontinence which may require catheterization, and the risks of falls and their complications. Prolonged immobilization, which may be needed to recover from injuries related to a fall, raises risks of VTE (venous thromboembolism).

Care may involve management of concurrent problems which may aggravate dementia (e.g. respiratory or urinary tract infections); social services (supportive interventions for both patients and carers); and drugs. Medications aim to help individuals by maintaining thinking, memory, or speaking skills, and can also help some of the behavioural and personality disturbances. They include acetylcholinesterase inhibitors (donepezil, rivastigmine, or galantamine), or memantine – a glutamate antagonist – or tacrine. Aspirin and gingka biloba may slow onset. Oestrogens, NSAIDs, and antioxidants (e.g. vitamin E) may improve cognition. Statins affect enzymes that generate A-beta-peptides. Sedatives and antidepressants help manage associated anxiety and depression.

Main dental considerations

(*See also generic guidance under main dental considerations on page 63 top, and also Section 2).

Oral manifestations may include poor oral hygiene, dry mouth and their consequences. Patients need an aggressive preventive dentistry programme. Treatment should, as far as possible, be carried out in the morning, when cooperation tends to be best, and with the usual carers present in a familiar environment with care to explain every procedure before it is carried out and to avoid discomfort. Complex dental procedures should be performed as soon as possible before the disease has reached the moderate to advanced stage. Patients with advanced dementia may be anxious, hostile, and uncooperative and difficult to treat. Access can be a serious handicap. Preoperative sedation with a short-acting benzodiazepine or haloperidol may be required. Use vasoconstrictors with caution in patients taking tricyclic antidepressants (e.g. desipramine) or serotonin–norepinephrine reuptake inhibitors (e.g. venlafaxine): increased risk of cardiovascular stimulation. Prescribe NSAIDs and antimicrobials (clarithromycin, erythromycin, ketoconazole) which may interact with donepezil with caution: risk of gastrointestinal side-effects. Antiplatelet effects of carbamazepine, venlafaxine, and divalproex when used concurrently with NSAIDs may increase the bleeding potential.

Attention deficit hyperactivity disorder (ADHD)

Also known as hyperkinesis or minimal brain dysfunction.

Definition

Gross behavioural abnormalities – inattention and hyperactivity and/or impulsivity which are excessive, long-term, and pervasive. Although people sometimes describe a badly behaved child as 'hyperactive', this is abuse of the term.

Aetiopathogenesis

Minor head injuries or undetectable brain damage, or refined sugar and food additives make some children hyperactive and inattentive. Overactivity can also be caused by external factors affecting parents, the child or the child–parent relationship.

Clinical presentation

One of the most common of childhood mental disorders, twice as common in boys, ADHD often continues into adolescence and adulthood. Features may include:

- being easily distracted
- blurting out answers prematurely
- difficulty waiting in a queue or for a turn
- failing to pay attention to details
- losing or forgetting things
- making careless mistakes
- rarely following instructions carefully
- restlessness, often fidgeting
- running, climbing, or leaving a seat.

Diagnosis

Clinical prerequisites for a diagnosis of ADHD, are that behaviours must appear before age 7 years, and continue for at least 6 months.

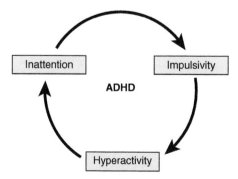

Figure 5.90 Attention deficit hyperactivity disorder.

Treatment

Specialized educational help, behavioural therapy, and emotional counselling. Stimulants (dextroamphetamine, methylphenidate, or pemoline) may help, as may antidepressants (e.g. atomoxetine – a selective noradrenaline re-uptake inhibitor, or imipramine or desipramine), or antihypertensive agents.

Main dental considerations

(*See also generic guidance under main dental considerations on page 63 top, and also Section 2).

Overactive children can often be almost impossible to manage in the dental surgery and frequently succeed in frustrating all concerned. Anxiolyitcs such as diazepam should be avoided as they usually exacerbate rather than depress overactivity. Visits should be scheduled for early morning, preferably 30–60 minutes after the patient has taken their medication. Dental treatment may not be possible without conscious sedation or GA. Since these patients commonly take medications that affect the CNS, sedation appointments can be challenging, and a medical consultation is advised. Inhalational sedation with nitrous oxide–oxygen may be the safest modality. LA containing adrenaline may interact with atomoxetine to increase blood pressure.

Autism

Definition

A spectrum of pervasive developmental disorders, which usually begin in the first 30 months of life, causing long-term disability. Asperger syndrome differs from classic autism in that typically language is usually intact, features appear later in childhood, and patients have a high intelligence quotient (IQ).

Aetiopathogenesis

Autism is three to four times more common in boys than girls. Cause – unknown.

Clinical presentation

Autists appear indifferent and remote and unable to form emotional bonds, avoid eye contact, may seem deaf and incapable of understanding other people's thoughts, feelings, and needs and act as if unaware of the coming and going of others. Obsessional desire for maintaining an unchanging environment and rigidity in following familiar patterns in their everyday routines makes them seem to prefer being alone. They may resist attention and affection or only passively accept hugs and cuddling, and they rarely seem upset when parent leaves, or show pleasure when the parent returns. They may physically attack and injure others without evident provocation. Characteristics can be:

- Inability to get along with people.
- Lack of interpersonal relationships.
- Ritualistic or compulsive behaviour with repetitive stereotyped activities, e.g. rocking or hand-flapping – or finger flicking near the eyes.
- Abnormal speech and language. May start developing language, then abruptly stop talking altogether. Often have echolalia, omit words, misuse pronouns and indicate consent by repeating a question.
- To cover their ears and scream at sounds.
- To simply scream or grab what they want.

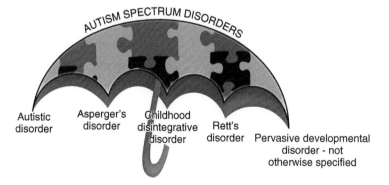

Figure 5.91 Autism umbrella. (Adapted from SciTech Daily. Available at: http://scitechdaily.com/scientists-reverse-autism-symptoms-in-mice/).

- To remain fixated on a single item or activity.
- To engage in self-harm.

Diagnosis

Clinical findings: it is essential to rule out other disorders such as hearing loss, speech problems, learning disability, neurological problems, and Rett syndrome (a progressive brain disease that affects only girls and causes repetitive hand movements, bruxism and loss of language and social skills).

Treatment

Patience and an empathetic approach are crucial. Some family member or a carer known to the patient, should be present. Develop a routine in which the child is not kept waiting, with a routine including always seeing the same staff. Patients may be disturbed by noise. Clomipramine, or SSRIs such as fluoxetine and beta-blockers may be helpful.

Main dental considerations

(*See also generic guidance under main dental considerations on page 63 top, and also Section 2).

It is essential to ensure the child is not kept waiting and has a short quiet visit with a routine that includes always seeing the same dental staff. Patients with autism may be disturbed by noise, such as a high-speed aspirator or air rotor, and it may be necessary to avoid their use. Autists may be unable to accept dental treatment under LA.

Body dysmorphic disorder (BDD)

Definition

A somatization disorder where a person becomes obsessively preoccupied with their appearance. BDD is estimated to affect 1–2% of people worldwide.

Aetiopathogenesis

BBD is an anxiety disorder that typically begins in the late teens or early 20s and is closely linked with a history of verbal and/or physical abuse or neglect. It may be comorbid with obsessive–compulsive disorder, depression and eating disorders.

Clinical presentation

The most common features that preoccupy people with BDD are the hair, skin and nose. They may:

- Repeatedly compare their looks with other people's.
- Spend a long time before a mirror, or at other times avoid mirrors altogether.
- Spend a long time concealing what they believe is a defect.
- Attempt to camouflage the perceived defect (e.g. covering mouth with hand).
- Excessively groom.
- Feel anxious when around other people and avoid social situations.
- Be secretive and reluctant to seek help.
- Excessively diet and exercise.
- Seek medical or surgical treatments for the perceived defect.

These patients have a significantly greater risk of depression and tendency to attempt and complete suicide, so recognition and appropriate referral is critical.

Diagnosis

Clinical. Individuals with BDD also often pursue and receive multiple dermatological, dental or surgical treatments but these may cause the disorder to worsen, leading to intensified or new preoccupations.

Treatment

Cognitive behavioural therapy and SSRIs are the treatments of choice.

Main dental considerations

(*See also generic guidance under main dental considerations on page 63 top, and also Section 2).

Oral manifestations may include an exaggerated dissatisfaction with the appearance of teeth and/or other facial aspects (e.g. nose, lips). Consider longer appointments to provide adequate time to address concerns the patient may have; it may be prudent to schedule appointments at the end of the day. Medications may need to be considered; NSAIDs may diminish SSRIs effect, and SSRIs may enhance NSAID antiplatelet effects. SSRIs can decrease benzodiazepine metabolism. SNRIs (e.g. venlafaxine) enhance epinephrine vasopressor effects. Carbamazepine should not be used in combination with SSRIs. Tramadol should be avoided in patients taking SSRIs, as they may induce serotonin syndrome (life-threatening disorder with high CNS serotonergic activity). Gabapentin and pregabalin should be used with caution, as psychomotor impairment may be increased.

Depression

Definition
A disorder that affects mood (the affect), and thoughts, which in turn influences the way a person eats and sleeps, feels about oneself, and thinks about things.

Classification
- *Bipolar disorder* – a psychosis of depression alternating with mania. May be regarded as a spectrum, with at one end severe depression, moderate depression and then low mood ('the blues') when brief but 'dysthymia' when chronic.
- *Dysthymic disorder* – a chronic, less intense depression.
- *Involutional melancholia* – appears in later life mainly in women.
- *Major depression* – severe depressive disorder.
- *Seasonal affective disorder* (SAD) – a chronic cyclic depression related to melatonin production, which appears as daylight hours shorten, and characterized by winter somnolence and carbohydrate craving.

Aetiopathogenesis
Cerebral amine (serotonin and norepinephrine/noradrenaline) levels are depleted and hyper-cortisolism common.

Some depression runs in families. Episodes can be triggered by life events such as a serious loss, difficult relationship, financial issues, or stressful life changes or diseases (mental health issues such as schizophrenia; viral infections [e.g. influenza, hepatitis, HIV/AIDS or infectious mononucleosis]; drug use [e.g. anti-depressants, benzodiazepines, corticosteroids, fenfluramine, ibuprofen, indometacin, levodopa, methyldopa, OCP, reserpine, or steroids]); or as a reaction to medical conditions (e.g. cancer; cardiac disease, endocrinopathies, HIV/AIDS, parkinsonism, stroke).

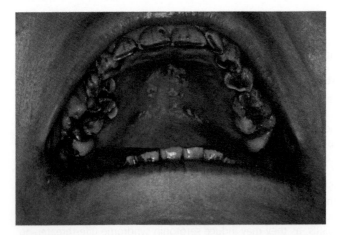

Figure 5.92 Depression: oral dryness from medications, and subsequent candidosis and tooth surface loss.

Clinical presentation

Effects appear related to changes in hypothalamic centres that govern food intake, libido, and circadian rhythms. They may include persistent:

- Anxiety, 'empty' mood, hopelessness, guilt, irritability, pessimism, sadness, worthlessness.
- Appetite changes (weight loss or gain or overeating).
- Chronic pain or other persistent bodily symptoms that are not caused by physical illness or injury.
- Decreased concentration, decision-making and energy.
- Loss of interest or pleasure in hobbies and activities that were once enjoyed, including sex.
- Sleep disturbance (early-morning awakening, insomnia, or oversleeping).
- Thoughts of suicide or death; suicide attempts.

Women appear to experience depression about twice as often as men; hormonal factors may contribute – particularly such factors as menopause, menstrual changes, miscarriage, pregnancy, and postpartum period.

Men are less likely to admit to depression, and doctors less likely to suspect it as it is often masked by anger or irritability, and may be suppressed by alcohol or drugs, or by the socially acceptable habit of excessive working.

Diagnosis

Diagnosed if five or more of the features above last most of the day, nearly every day, for 2 weeks or longer.

Treatment

The danger in depression is of suicide; the rate in men is four times that in women, though more women attempt it. Anyone thinking about committing suicide needs immediate attention from a psychiatrist. Important measures are to:

- ensure no access to drugs, weapons, or other items that could be used for self-harm;
- ensure the suicidal person is not left alone;
- call a doctor, or the emergency services.

Suicide/parasuicide may suggest self-harm is the same as wanting to kill oneself – but this is often *not* the case. Management of depression includes psychotherapy and antidepressants (drugs that raise brain levels of serotonin and norepinephrine) (Table 5.32).

Main dental considerations

(*See also generic guidance under main dental considerations on page 63 top, and also Section 2).

The most common oral complaint of depressed patients under treatment is of a dry mouth, especially as a result of the use of TCAs, MAOIs or lithium. Bodily complaints, often related to the mouth, are common in depression and the dental surgeon should appreciate the possibility of a psychological basis for the following painful disorders of the orofacial region:

- chronic facial pain
- burning mouth or sore tongue (oral dysaesthesia)
- occasionally temporomandibular pain dysfunction syndrome.

Other oral complaints may be delusional and include discharges (of fluid, slime or powder coming into the mouth), dry mouth or sialorrhoea despite normal salivary flow, spots or lumps, imagined halitosis, disturbed taste sensation.

Class	Type	Actions	Examples
Table 5.32 Antidepressants: types, actions, examples			
Tricyclic antidepressants	TCAs	Block norepinephrine & 5HT reuptake	Amitriptyline Dolesupin Doxepin
Serotonin norepinephrine reuptake inhibitors	SNRI	Block norepinephrine & 5HT reuptake	Duloxetine Venlafaxine
Selective serotonin reuptake inhibitors	SSRI	Block 5HT reuptake	Citalopram Fluoxetine Fluvoxamine
Noradrenaline reuptake inhibitors	NARI	Block norepinephrine reuptake	Reboxetine
Noradrenergic and specific serotonergic antidepressants	NASSA	Block norepinephrine, 5HT2 & 5HT3 reuptake	Mirtazapine
Serotonin reuptake inhibitors	SRI	5HT antagonists	Nefazodone
Monoamine oxidase inhibitors	MAOI	Inhibit MAO-A	Moclobemide

Tact, patience and a sympathetic, friendly manner are needed for dental treatment, which is preferably deferred until depression is under control. In patients taking TCAs, epinephrine in LA has not been shown clinically to cause hypertension. Acetaminophen/paracetamol can inhibit the metabolism of TCAs, and atropinics are potentiated by TCAs.

Patients on MAOIs are at risk from GA, since prolonged respiratory depression may result. Any CNS depressant, especially opioids and phenothiazines, given to patients on MAOIs (or within 21 days of their withdrawal) may precipitate coma. Pethidine is particularly dangerous. There is no evidence of any danger to patients on MAOI from epinephrine in LA.

Tricyclics and MAOIs can cause postural hypotension; patients using these should not be stood immediately upright if recumbent during treatment and the chair should be brought upright slowly.

SSRIs can potentiate benzodiazepines, carbamazepine, codeine and erythromycin. Sertraline (SSRI) metabolism may be impaired by antimicrobials (e.g. tetracycline; metronidazole), increasing serum levels. SSRI or SNRI taken in combination with another substance that raises serotonin levels, such as another antidepressant or St John's wort may lead to *Serotonin syndrome* – an uncommon, but potentially serious, reaction that can include: fever, confusion, agitation, muscle twitching or fits, sweating, shivering, arrhythmias and diarrhoea. Urgent hospitalization is indicated.

Eating disorders

Definition
Serious disturbances in eating behaviour, such as extreme and unhealthy reduction of food intake or severe overeating.

Aetiopathogenesis
Genetic, cultural, and psychiatric factors implicated.

Clinical presentation and classification
Usually develop during adolescence or early adulthood; seen most often in females; may co-exist along with other mental health issues (e.g. anxiety disorders, depression, substance abuse). Complications include anaemia, endocrine disturbances, peripheral oedema and electrolyte depletion (e.g. hypokalaemia), infrequent or absent menstrual periods, erosion of teeth (perimylolysis) from repeated vomiting. Eating disorders include:

- *Anorexia nervosa* (self-imposed starvation) – failure to eat, in the absence of any physical cause to extent that >15% of body weight is lost. Inadequate food intake and severe weight loss; intense fear of gaining weight or becoming fat, even though underweight; body image disturbance; attempts at weight control (e.g. intense and compulsive exercise, or purging by means of vomiting, or abuse of laxatives, or enemas). May be life-threatening from cardiac arrest, electrolyte imbalance, or suicide.
- *Bulimia nervosa* (binge eating and dieting) – often with self-induced vomiting and purgative abuse. Eating excessive food within a discrete period of time, plus recurrent inappropriate compensatory behaviour to prevent weight gain, such as self-induced vomiting or misuse of laxatives, diuretics, enemas, or other medications (purging); fasting; or excessive exercise. Prognosis poor because of suicide, severe psychiatric

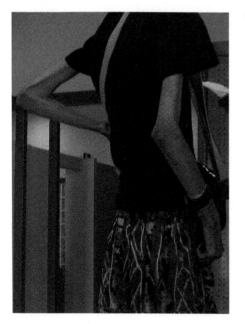

Figure 5.93 Anorexia nervosa.

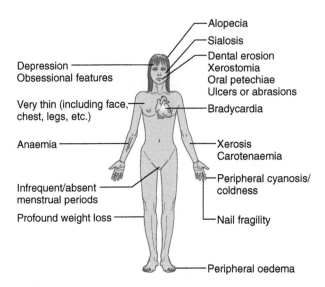

Alopecia
Sialosis
Dental erosion
Xerostomia
Oral petechiae
Ulcers or abrasions

Depression
Obsessional features

Very thin (including face, chest, legs, etc.)

Anaemia

Infrequent/absent menstrual periods

Profound weight loss

Bradycardia

Xerosis
Carotenaemia

Peripheral cyanosis/ coldness

Nail fragility

Peripheral oedema

Figure 5.94 Anorexia – features. Adapted from Scully et al. (2007) Special Care in Dentistry: Handbook of Oral Care. Edinburgh: Churchill Livingstone, Elsevier.

disturbances, aspiration, oesophageal or gastric rupture, hypokalaemia, cardiac arrhythmias, pancreatitis and cardiomyopathy.

Diagnosis

From clinical features.

Treatment

Correct malnutrition via psychosocial, medical, nutritional, counselling and interventions. Psychotherapy (cognitive-behavioural or interpersonal) can help. Selective serotonin reuptake inhibitors (SSRIs) helpful for weight maintenance and mood and anxiety symptoms. In some cases, intravenous feeding is needed.

Main dental considerations

(*See also generic guidance under main dental considerations on page 63 top, and also Section 2).
Oral manifestations can include tooth erosion (perimylolysis) after repeated vomiting. Parotid enlargement (sialosis) and angular stomatitis may develop as in other forms of starvation. Oral ulcers or abrasions in the soft palate, may be caused by fingers or other objects used to induce vomiting.

Defer elective dental care until the patient is stable from a cardiac standpoint – patients are at significant risk of cardiac arrhythmias secondary to electrolyte disturbances. Use vasoconstrictors with caution: increased risk for adverse outcomes in patients who have developed cardiac arrhythmia. Repeated doses of acetaminophen/paracetamol may be hepatotoxic in anorexia nervosa: doses should be kept to the minimum. NSAIDs may interact with fluoxetine (SSRI) increasing risk of postoperative bleeding. Sedatives (e.g. benzodiazepines) may interact with and enhance sedation from: lorazepam (benzodiazepine), phenelzine (MAOI), or fluoxetine (SSRI).

Mania

Definition and classification
A syndrome of elation, 'butterfly' thinking ('flight of ideas'), poor judgment, and extrovert social behaviour.

- Bipolar I disorder (mania with/without major depression) – classic mania, which usually also involves recurrent depressive episodes.
- Bipolar II disorder (hypomania with major depression) – lower mania level (hypomania), often with good functioning.

Aetiopathogenesis
Increased brain norepinephrine and decreased serotonin and dopamine.

Clinical presentations
- Abnormal or excessive elation, 'high,' overly good, euphoric mood
- Abuse of drugs, particularly cocaine, alcohol, and sleeping medications
- Denial that anything is wrong
- Distractibility
- Excessive sexual desire
- Excessive talking
- Grandiose notions and unrealistic beliefs in one's abilities and powers
- Inappropriate social behaviour
- Increased energy and provocative, intrusive, or aggressive behaviour
- Poor judgment
- Racing thoughts, jumping from one idea to another (butterfly mind)
- Spending sprees
- Less apparent need for sleep.

Untreated patients with bipolar disorder have a higher risk of hospitalizations and suicides than do patients with unipolar psychosis (major depression).

Diagnosis
Mania is diagnosed if the elevated mood comes with three or more of the other symptoms above, for most of the day, nearly every day, for 1 week or longer.

Treatment
Cognitive behavioural therapy (CBT) may be effective.

Lithium and valproate are the most useful drugs. Carbamazepine has also been successfully used. Drug interactions must be avoided.

Table 5.33 Potential interactions with lithium

Drug interacting	Consequences
Carbamazepine	Lithium toxicity
Diazepam	Hypothermia
Droperidol and other neuroleptics	Facial dyskinesias
NSAIDs	Lithium toxicity
Metronidazole	Lithium toxicity
Phenytoin	Lithium toxicity
SSRIs	Serotonin syndrome – life-threatening disorder with high CNS serotonergic activity
Suxamethonium and other muscle relaxants	Prolonged muscle relaxation
Tetracyclines	Lithium toxicity

Main dental considerations

(*See also generic guidance under main dental considerations on page 63 top, and also Section 2).

Manic-depressive patients may be treated with lithium and also antidepressants – with oral side-effects such as xerostomia.

An excited manic patient can be difficult to manage and dental treatment may have to be deferred until after stabilization. Most NSAIDs and metronidazole should be avoided as they can induce toxicity, but aspirin, acetaminophen/paracetamol and codeine are safe to use.

Lithium can interact with many drugs, and it may be advisable to stop lithium treatment 2–3 days before GA. Arrhythmias may be precipitated, particularly during GA.

Obsessive-compulsive disorder (OCD)

Definition
The urge to do or think certain things repeatedly.

Aetiopathogenesis
OCD is the fourth most common mental disorder, affecting 1–2% of the population and it appears to be increasing. The basal ganglia and striatum appear to be involved in OCD.

Clinical presentation
OCD strikes males slightly more commonly and usually starts in childhood, adolescence or early adulthood. OCD is comprised of thoughts (obsessions) that create anxiety, and things the patient does to reduce the anxiety (compulsions). Obsessional thoughts are those that come repeatedly into consciousness against the patient's will, are usually unpleasant, but always recognized as the patient's own thoughts. Typical obsessions are the repeated checking, questioning of decisions, hoarding, counting, religious compulsions, the fear of harm or harming, or the fear of dirtiness or contamination. These can dominate life, with obsessive activities consuming much of the day, causing significant disruption of life. The course of OCD is variable. Symptoms may come and go, may ease over time or they can grow progressively worse.

Diagnosis
Clinical.

Treatment
Treatment is often difficult, though OCD may respond to psychotherapy, or medication with antidepressants, especially SSRIs, clomipramine, and the tricyclic antidepressants, which are useful when there is also depression. The benzodiazepines may be useful when anxiety is predominant.

Main dental considerations
(*See also generic guidance under main dental considerations on page 63 top, and also Section 2).
It is questionable whether true obsessions often become centred on the mouth but they may, for example, result in compulsive toothbrushing. Occasional patients become obsessed with the imagined possibility of halitosis, or infections or cancer in the mouth.

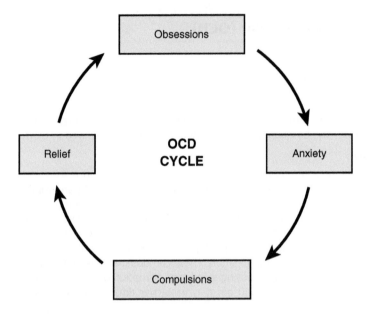

Figure 5.95 Obsessive-compulsive disorder (OCD).

Panic disorder

Definition

Term given to recurrent unpredictable attacks of severe anxiety with physical symptoms such as palpitations, chest pain, dyspnoea, paraesthesiae and sweating ('panic attacks').

Aetiopathogenesis

Usually develops in the twenties and it is approximately twice as common in women than in men. There are associations with mitral valve prolapse in 50%.

Clinical presentation

Panic attacks can come at any time, even during sleep. In an attack, there are features of catecholamine release – the heart pounds and the patient may feel sweaty, weak, faint or dizzy. Many or most of the symptoms then result from hyperventilation: the hands may tingle or feel numb, and there may be nausea, chest pain, a sense of unreality or fear of impending doom. An attack generally peaks in 10 minutes, but some symptoms may last longer. Panic disorder is often accompanied by other conditions such as depression, drug abuse or alcoholism and may lead to a pattern of avoidance of places or situations where panic attacks have struck. Many suffer intense anxiety between episodes, worrying when and where the next attack will strike.

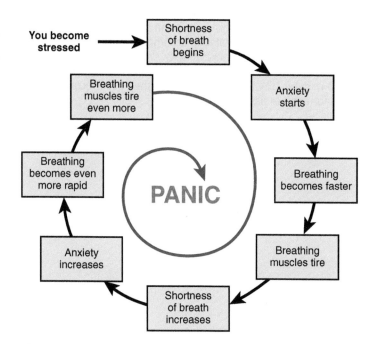

Figure 5.96 Panic disorder. (Adapted with kind permission from Heal Past Lives www.healpastlives.com/future/cure/crpanic.htm).

Diagnosis

Clinical.

Treatment

One of the most readily treatable mental disorders, it usually responds to psychotherapy, or medication with alprazolam or lorazepam, or tricyclic antidepressants. Patients should inform the Driver and Vehicle Licensing Agency (DVLA).

Main dental considerations

(*See also generic guidance under main dental considerations on page 63 top, and also Section 2).

Oral manifestations, such as facial arthromyalgia, dry mouth, lip-chewing or bruxism may be complaints in anxious people. Persons with clinically significant fear tend to have poorer perceived dental health, a longer interval since their last dental appointment, a higher frequency of past fear behaviours, more physical symptoms during dental injections, and higher percentage of symptoms of anxiety and depression. They may chatter incessantly, have a history of failed appointments, and appear tense and agitated ('white knuckle syndrome').

Anxiety is readily generated by dental or medical appointments. It is essential, therefore, not to dismiss patients who will not accept a proposed treatment as being 'phobic' or 'uncooperative'. Among fearful patients, increases in pulse rate and blood pressure are common. Early morning appointments, with pre-medication and no waiting, can help. The main aids are careful, painlessly performed dental procedures, psychological approaches, confident reassurance, patience and, sometimes, the use of pharmacological agents, for example anxiolytics such as oral diazepam, supplemented if necessary with sedation. Benzodiazepine metabolism is impaired by azole antifungals, and by macrolide antibiotics such as erythromycin and clarithromycin. Alcohol, antihistamines and barbiturates have additive sedative effects with benzodiazepines. The analgesic dextropropoxyphene should be avoided in patients taking alprazolam as it may cause toxicity.

If a panic attack occurs in the clinic it will probably peak in approximately 10 minutes and resolve after another 20–30 minutes. Discharge patient once they have recovered and reschedule the appointment for another day.

Phobias

Definitions
Extreme or irrational fear of, or aversion to, something.

Aetiopathogenesis and classification
The main types of phobia are:
- Agoraphobia – fear of being in public places.
- Claustrophobia – fear of closed spaces.
- Simple, or specific phobias (phobic neurosis).
- Social phobia – anxiety in normal social situations.

Clinical presentations
Extreme fear with blushing, profuse sweating, trembling, nausea, difficulty in talking, muscle tension, increased pulse, accelerated breathing, sweating, and stomach cramps.

Phobias may also be a minor part of an anxiety state, personality disorder or a more severe disorder such as depression, obsessive neurosis, or schizophrenia.

Diagnosis
Clinical.

Treatment
- Supportive or intensive psychotherapy: when phobias are centred on threats such as flying, anaesthetics or dental treatment, normal life is possible if threats are avoided.
- Drugs:
  - Anxiolytic drugs such as.
  - Benzodiazepines (e.g. diazepam, lorazepam, oxazepam or alprazolam) can be useful but are habituating. Buspirone is useful since it lacks psychomotor impairment, and dependency of benzodiazepines.
  - Antidepressants, especially tricyclics, are used if there is a significant depressive component.

Main dental considerations
(*See also generic guidance under main dental considerations on page 63 top, and also Section 2); see Panic disorders.

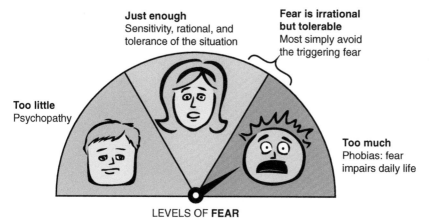

Just enough
Sensitivity, rational, and tolerance of the situation

Fear is irrational but tolerable
Most simply avoid the triggering fear

Too little
Psychopathy

Too much
Phobias: fear impairs daily life

LEVELS OF **FEAR**

Figure 5.97 Levels of fear.

Schizophrenia

Definition
A chronic, severe, disabling mental disorder with disorders of perception (hallucinations) and thought (delusions), causing inappropriate and incomprehensible thoughts and behaviour.

Aetiopathogenesis
Appears to be due to imbalance of brain dopamine and glutamate but aetiology is unclear. Genetic predisposition (involving chromosomes 5 and 10) and large, rare Copy Number Variants (CNVs) at genomic loci such as 22q11.2 are implicated in the risk. May develop in previously normal people – precipitated by organic disorders, stress or marijuana.

Clinical presentation and classification
Acute schizophrenia
May develop in previously normal individuals precipitated by organic disorders, drugs or external stress.

Chronic schizophrenia
This is more common. The first signs often appear as confusing, or even shocking, changes in behaviour, and the person's speech and behaviour can be so disorganized that they may be incomprehensible or even frightening to others because of (4 Ds):

- Diminished emotional expression and affect.
- Disordered thought processes.
- Disorders of perception (hallucinations) and thought (delusions) and illusions.
- Distorted perceptions of reality.

Some patients are strikingly paranoid, others have mainly motor symptoms (catatonia), a bizarre mixture of emotional, behavioural and thought disturbances (hebephrenia), or neuroses.

Some people have only one psychotic episode, others have many episodes during a lifetime, but lead relatively normal lives in the interim.

Diagnosis
Diagnosis is not easy since even healthy individuals may, at times, feel, think, or act in ways that resemble schizophrenia. There is considerable variation in the diagnostic criteria, but auditory hallucinations and ideas of a passive or irresistible response to external influences which may control or block the patient's thoughts, dictate, or control their behaviour to conspire to do them harm, are the most suggestive.

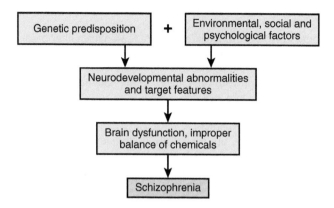

Figure 5.98 Schizophrenia. Adapted with kind permission from CC BY-SA 4.0. Source: Boundless. Explaining Schizophrenia. Boundless Psychology. Boundless. 03 Jul. 2014.

Table 5.34 Important antipsychotic drugs used to manage schizophrenia

Drug	Examples
Atypical antipsychotics	Clozapine, amisulpride, olanzapine, quetiapine, risperidone, sertindole, zotepine
Piperazine phenothiazines, with low sedative and antimuscarinic activity	Fluphenazine, perphenazine, prochlorperazine, or trifluoroperazine
Phenothiazines with low extrapyramidal effects, moderate sedative and antimuscarinic effects	Pericyazine or pipotiazine
Phenothiazines with pronounced sedative effects, but moderate antimuscarinic and extrapyramidal effects	Chlorpromazine, methotrimeprazine or promazine
Butyrophenones	Benperidol, droperidol or haloperidol
Thioxanthines	Flupenthixol/flupentixol and zuclopenthixol
Diphenylbutylpiperidines	Fluspirilene and pimozide

Treatment

- Drugs (antipsychotic neuroleptics or major tranquillizers) (Table 5.34) which alter basal ganglia dopamine/cholinergic balance so that extrapyramidal and anticholinergic effects are common. First line agents are the atypical antipsychotics (Table 5.34). Extrapyramidal features are more common with the piperazine phenothiazines, butyrophenones and depot preparations, and include:
  - Akathisia (restlessness)
  - Dystonia and dyskinesia (abnormal movements)
  - Neuroleptic malignant syndrome – a rare, but potentially life-threatening disorder
  - Parkinsonism
  - Tardive dyskinesia – involuntary movements most often affecting mouth, lips, and tongue, and sometimes the trunk or arms and legs.
- Family education.
- Psychotherapy.
- Rehabilitation.
- Self-help groups.

Main dental considerations

(*See also generic guidance under main dental considerations on page 63 top, and also Section 2).

Though schizophrenia has no specific oral features, some patients may have delusional oral symptoms, the treatment of which is beyond the expertise of dental staff, and then psychiatric help must be sought. The long-term use of neuroleptics can lead to hposalivation and xerostomia (with susceptibility to candidosis and caries, and, occasionally, ascending parotitis), oral pigmentation and severe extrapyramidal symptoms. Muscular rigidity or tonic spasms (facial dyskinesias) frequently involve the bulbar or neck muscles, with subsequent difficulties in speech or swallowing. Alternatively, there may be uncontrollable facial grimacing (orofacial dystonia). Haloperidol and clozapine can cause hypersalivation.

Communication can be challenging and often met by a response that indicates a failure to get through or interrupted by totally irrelevant remarks. Phenothiazines can cause epinephrine reversal in patients given a LA: there is vasodilatation instead of the anticipated vasoconstriction, but the practical importance of this in relation to LA is unclear. Haloperidol and phenothiazines may cause orthostatic hypotension. Patients should be raised slowly and carefully assisted from the dental chair. GA, especially with intravenous barbiturates, can lead to severe hypotension and should therefore be avoided if possible.

Self-harm

Self-harm (SH) includes self-injury (SI) and self-poisoning and is defined as the intentional, direct injuring of body tissue. Discrete from body art such as piercings/tattoos, self-harm is most common in adolescence and young adulthood, usually first appearing between the ages of 12 and 24.

Aetiopathogenesis

SH is seen more often in:

- Abused people who have experienced physical, emotional or sexual abuse during childhood.
- Asylum seekers, armed forces veterans and prisoners.
- Having a friend who self-harms.
- LGBT (lesbian, gay, bisexual and transgender) people: at least in part, due to stress of prejudice and discrimination.
- Women, usually young.

Self-harm may be classed as a coping mechanism which provides temporary relief of intense feelings such as anxiety, depression, stress, emotional numbness or a sense of failure or a borderline personality disturbance. A person will often struggle with difficulties for some time before they self-harm.

Clinical presentation

Common complaints expressed or not, may include feeling depressed, hopeless, isolated, alone, out of control or powerless, or abuse. The most common form of self-harm is skin-cutting but there is a wide range of behaviours including, harming themselves by:

- banging or punching
- burning
- hair pulling (trichotillomania)
- cutting
- overdosing
- sticking things in their body
- swallowing things (pica).

It is not often intended to be suicidal but that might result.
Self-harm may feature in:

- Mental issues (e.g. bipolar disorder, depression, schizophrenia). *Munchausen syndrome* (feign disease, illness, or psychological trauma to draw attention) – war avoidance behaviour; and attention-seeking may be involved.
- Rare genetic disorders (e.g. Lesch–Nyhan syndrome – congenital hyperuricaemia).
- Substance abuse or withdrawal.

Diagnosis

Clinical.

Treatment

Psychotherapy is indicated.

Main dental considerations

(*See also generic guidance under main dental considerations on page 63 top, and also Section 2).
Orofacial lesions may be seen.

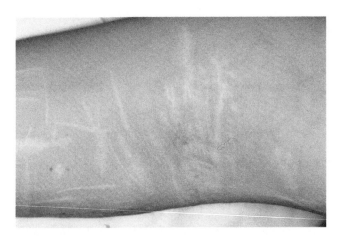

Figure 5.99 Scars from skin cutting in self-harm.

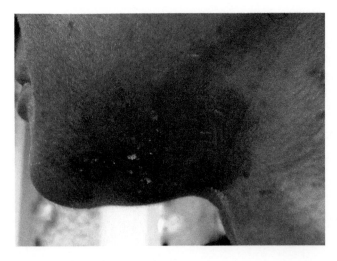

Figure 5.100 Self-induced abrasions.

MUCOCUTANEOUS

Main dental consideration

(*See also generic guidance under main dental considerations on page 63 top, and also Section 2).

The disorders apart from malignancy, may manifest with oral lesions and lesions of other mucosae (e.g. genital, and/or skin). Sometimes the oral lesions are the first manifestation.

Erythema multiforme (EM)

Definition

Mucosal and/or cutaneous lesions including virtually any rash. Sometimes recurrent.

Aetiopathogenesis

Uncertain – may be an immune complex disorder in which antigens can be various microorganisms or drugs (Table 5.35). Herpes simplex viruses may be involved in most cases affecting the mouth.

Clinical presentation and classification

Skin, ocular, genital or oral mucosae may be involved together or in isolation. The typical skin lesion is the target or iris in which there are concentric erythematous rings. Vesicles or bullae may also be seen. Typical oral features are swollen, crusted and blood-stained lips, and widespread oral ulceration. Severe EM with multiple mucosal involvement and fever are toxic epidermal necrolysis (TEN), or Stevens–Johnson syndrome (SJS).

Diagnosis

Clinical grounds. Biopsy useful to exclude serious diseases, such as pemphigus.

Table 5.35 Erythema multiforme: possible causes

Microorganisms	Drugs	Others
Herpes simplex virus	Barbiturates	Internal malignancy
Mycoplasma	Biologics	Irradiation
	Carbamazepine	Pregnancy
	Chlorpropamide	
	Codeine	
	Hydantoins	
	Penicillins	
	Phenylbutazone	
	Salicylates	
	Sulfonamides	
	Tetracyclines	
	Thiazides	

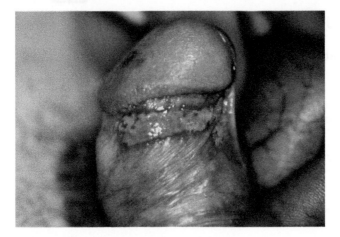

Figure 5.101 Erythema multiforme: penile erosions (Courtesy of Dr D Malamos).

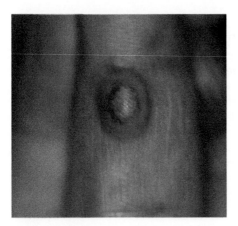

Figure 5.102 Erythema multiforme: skin target lesions.

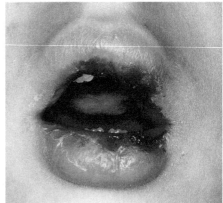

Figure 5.103 Erythema multiforme: lip swelling and blood-stained erosions.

Treatment

An ophthalmological opinion should be obtained if conjunctivae are involved. Mucosal lesions can be managed with topical corticosteroids, chlorhexidine or lidocaine. SJS and TEN may necessitate hospital admission for feeding; systemic corticosteroids are frequently given with little evidence base. Aciclovir is indicated for prophylaxis of recurrent EM, since HSV is often involved.

Lichen planus (LP)

Definition
A common idiopathic skin and/or mucosal disease.

Aetiopathogenesis
The immunopathogenesis includes a dense T-lymphocyte reaction to an unidentified provoking antigen.

Lesions clinically and histologically similar or identical to lichen planus (lichenoid lesions) can be related to dental restorations, and drugs, particularly to non-steroidal anti-inflammatory drugs (NSAIDs), gold, antimalarials, and beta-blockers. Similar lesions may be due to chemicals, such as photographic developing solutions, graft-versus-host disease, chronic liver disease and virus infections, such as hepatitis C or HIV.

Clinical presentation
Skin lesions are usually small polygonal, purplish, pruritic papules particularly affecting flexor surfaces of the wrists, but also elsewhere such as the shins or periumbilically – rarely, if ever, on the face. There is a fine lacy white network of striae (Wickham striae) on the papules. Mouth and genital lesions in LP include white striae, papules, plaques, or red atrophic areas or erosions. The nails or hair may be affected.

Diagnosis
Biopsy may help exclude leukoplakia, lupus erythematosus, chronic ulcerative stomatitis or keratoses.

Treatment
Topical corticosteroids or tacrolimus. Aloe vera may give symptomatic relief. Exceptionally severe LP sometimes responds only to systemic corticosteroids, vitamin A analogues (etretinate), dapsone, ciclosporin or biologics. Approximately 1% of cases of oral or genital LP may develop malignant change after 10 years.

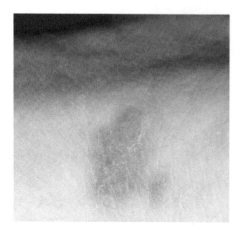

Figure 5.104 Lichen planus: papules.

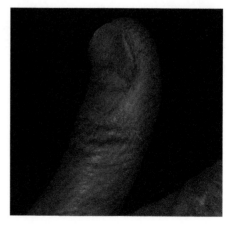

Figure 5.105 Lichen planus: nail lesions.

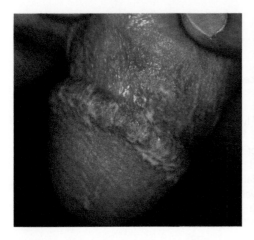

Figure 5.106 Lichen planus: penile Wickham's striae.

Figure 5.107 Lichen planus: rash.

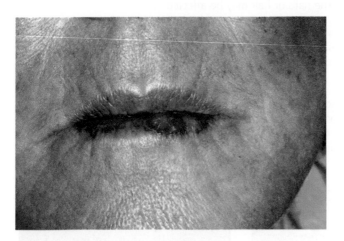

Figure 5.108 Lichen planus: lip lesions.

Pemphigoid

Definition
A group of subepithelial immune blistering diseases with autoantibodies directed to different epithelial basement membrane zone (EBMZ) proteins.

Aetiopathogenesis
Autoantibodies cause epithelium to lose attachment to connective tissue – and blisters. The common variant (mucous membrane pemphigoid; MMP) has antibodies against bullous pemphigoid antigen 2 (BP2) but types that mainly affect the mouth or eyes have integrin or epiligrin antibodies. Oral pemphigoid lesions have occasionally been reported with internal cancers or the use of certain drugs, such as penicillamine.

Clinical presentation
Predominantly affects women aged 50–70 years. Vesicles or bullae may appear on the skin, especially the abdomen, groin, and flexor surfaces of the extremities. Sometimes mucosae such as the mouth are affected and pemphigoid is an important cause of so-called 'desquamative gingivitis'. Scarring can be a serious complication in the eyes, larynx, genitalia or oesophagus.

Diagnosis
Confirmed by biopsy; IgG along the line of the EBMZ in 50% but complement components in 80%. Serum autoantibodies are rarely demonstrable by conventional techniques.

Treatment
Many lesions can be adequately controlled by potent topical corticosteroids. Dapsone or corticosteroids may be needed for severe cases. Recalcitrant lesions may respond to tacrolimus, mycophenolate mofetil, intravenous immunoglobulins, infliximab or other biologics. Ocular involvement needs systemic steroids.

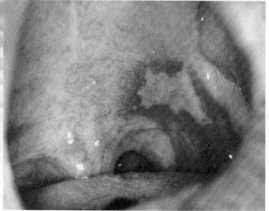

Figure 5.109 Pemphigoid erosions.

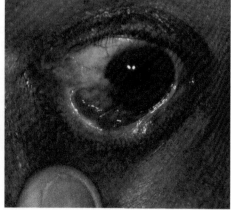

Figure 5.110 Pemphigoid conjunctival erosions have led to scarring (symblepharon).

Pemphigus

Definition
Autoimmune reaction against stratified squamous epithelium intercellular cement proteins (desmogleins).

Aetiopathogenesis
Common in Ashkenazi Jewish populations and Asians. HLA associations map to DRB1*0402 and DQB1*0503, or in Jews to HLA-G. Circulating IgG antibodies to desmogleins of epithelial cell intercellular attachments (desmosomes) cause cells to lose adherence to one another (acantholysis). There are pemphigus variants and rarely, pemphigus is drug-induced (e.g. captopril, penicillamine or rifampicin) or related to neoplasia (paraneoplastic pemphigus).

Clinical presentation
Pemphigus vulgaris (PV), the common variant, mainly affects middle-aged women, with widespread formation of mucocutaneous vesicles and bullae, followed by ulceration. Pemphigus is usually fatal in the absence of treatment.

Pemphigus may occasionally be associated with other autoimmune diseases, such as lupus erythematosus, inflammatory bowel disease, thymoma or myasthenia gravis.

Diagnosis
Stroking the skin or mucosa with a finger may induce vesicle formation in an apparently unaffected area or cause a bulla to extend (Nikolsky sign).

Confirmed by biopsy. The specimen should be halved to enable both light and immunofluorescent (IF) microscopy. Light microscopy on a paraffin section is usually distinctive showing suprabasal clefts containing free-floating acantholytic cells. IF examination shows IgG and C3 deposits intercellularly. It can be carried out by the direct method using fluorescein-conjugated anti-human IgG and anti-complement (C3) sera on the frozen specimen or on exfoliated cells. In the indirect method, the patient's serum is incubated with normal animal mucosa, which is then labelled with fluorescein-conjugated antihuman globulin. Antibodies to desmoglein 1 may be found with cutaneous lesions in PV, or pemphigus foliaceus; antibodies to desmoglein 3 may herald oral involvement.

Treatment
Immediate immunosuppressive treatment with high doses of systemic corticosteroids plus a steroid-sparer (e.g. azathioprine, cyclophosphamide, gold, methotrexate or mycophenolate mofetil). The anti-CD20 monoclonal antibody, rituximab, may be effective.

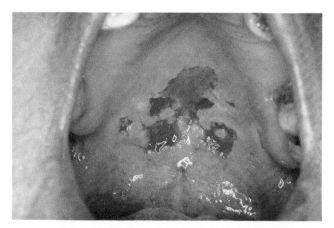

Figure 5.111 Pemphigus: mouth erosions.

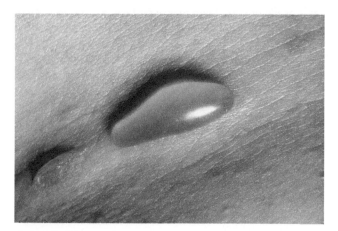

Figure 5.112 Pemphigus: early skin blisters.

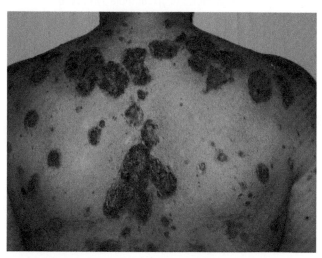

Figure 5.113 Pemphigus: late skin blisters with scabbing.

SKIN CANCERS

The three major types, all on the increase, are:

- basal cell carcinoma (BCC; rodent ulcer)
- melanoma (malignant melanoma)
- squamous cell carcinoma (SCC).

Cancers all develop mainly on sun-exposed skin: scalp, face, lips, ears, neck, chest, arms, hands, and legs. Nearly half of all men >65 years will develop a skin cancer. Risk factors are shown below under Melanoma.

Basal cell carcinoma

BCC is superficial, appearing as a pearly or waxy lump mainly on face, ears or neck, typically after middle age. In Gorlin syndrome (multiple keratocystic odontogenic tumours), BCC can appear in childhood.
  BCC respond well to excision, especially if found early.

Melanoma

Aetiopathogenesis
The incidence steadily rises with age and melanoma is now one of the most common cancers between the ages of 15–34 and is responsible for most skin cancer deaths. The highest incidence however, is in people >80 years. Melanocytes make melanin, colouring the skin and helping protect against the sun's ultraviolet light. Factors that increase the chances of developing melanoma include having:

- Multiple freckles or unusually shaped or large moles (atypical mole syndrome). A large mole is one >5 mm diameter. Even people with just one unusually shaped or large mole (atypical naevus) have a 60% increased risk of melanoma.
- Pale skin that burns easily.
- Family history of melanoma; 10% of melanomas may be genetic. Familial atypical multiple mole melanoma syndrome (FAMMM) due to the gene cdkn2a, also increases risk of pancreatic cancer.
- Inflammatory bowel disease.
- Parkinson's disease.
- Pesticide exposure (e.g. carbaryl, maneb, mancozeb or parathion).
- Red or blonde hair.
- Solar keratosis.
- Sunburns.
- UVA from sunbeds.

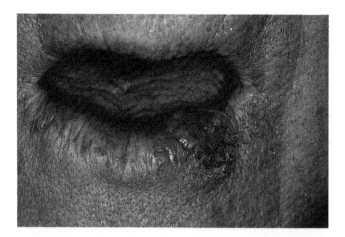

Figure 5.114 Lip cancer: mainly seen on lower lip in chronically sun-exposed older males who smoke tobacco.

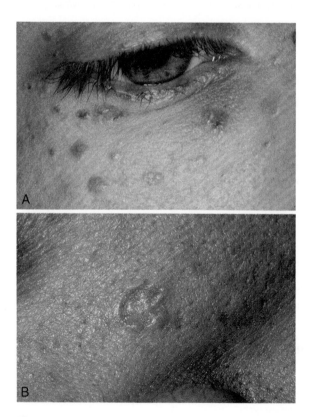

Figure 5.115 Basal cell carcinomas (Gorlin syndrome); **(A)** multiple cancers; **(B)** close-up.

Clinical presentation and classification

Melanoma affects the skin but also, rarely, the eye or mouth.

It typically appears on skin as a large brownish spot with darker speckles; a simple mole that changes in colour or size or consistency, or that bleeds or exhibits new growth; a lesion with an irregular border and red, white, blue or blue–black spots. The ABCDE method of melanoma diagnostic features stands for:

Asymmetry – irregular shape

Border – ragged, notched, or blurred

Colour – more than one colour in an individual mole

Diameter – bigger than 6 mm

Evolution – changing size, colour, or shape.

Types include:

Acral lentiginous melanoma – rare, most on palms and soles but the most common type in dark-skinned people.

Amelanotic melanoma – no, or little colour.

Superficial spreading melanoma – the most common type, mainly in middle-aged people and usually initially not at risk of spreading.

Nodular melanoma – usually a dark brown-black, or black raised area, seen in places only occasionally exposed to sun (e.g. chest or back). It develops rapidly, invading deeply.

Lentigo maligna melanoma – develops from very slow growing pigmented areas (Hutchinson's melanotic freckle or lentigo maligna), usually on the face.

Diagnosis

Dermatoscopy, biopsy.

Treatment

Malignant melanoma prognosis is usually poor as a consequence of late diagnosis and rapid spread: survival averages only 2 years but if the tumour is superficial the survival is 90% at 5-years. Treatment is usually excision, radiotherapy, chemotherapy (carmustine, dacarbazine, tamoxifen, temozolomide, vinblastine) or biologics (aldesleukin, bevacizumab, interferon, ipilimumab, vemurafenib).

Main dental considerations

(*See also generic guidance under main dental considerations on page 63 top, and also Section 2).

Immune checkpoint inhibitors (particularly ipilimumab) induce toxicities that share common features with graft-versus-host disease (GVHD; Section 9), particularly dry mouth.

Squamous cell carcinoma

SCC is superficial, slow-growing presenting as a firm, red nodule on the face, lip, ears, neck, hands or arms or a flat lesion with a scaly, crusted surface on the face, ears, neck, hands or arms. It usually responds to excision.

MUSCULOSKELETAL

Ankylosing spondylitis

Definition
A seronegative spondyloarthropathy.

Aetiopathogenesis
Genetic: family history may be positive and 90% of patients are HLA-B27.

Clinical presentation
Predominantly affects spine and sacroiliac joints, mainly in young males, with insidious low back pain (spondylitis) and stiffness followed by worsening sacro-iliac pain and tenderness (sacro-iliitis). Inflammation of ligament and tendon insertions is followed by ossification, which fuses adjacent vertebral bodies or other joints. The neck and back become fixed in extreme flexion, chest expansion becomes limited and respiration impaired. About 25% develop eye lesions (uveitis or iridocyclitis); about 10% develop cardiac disease (aortic incompetence or conduction defects).

Diagnosis
- ESR and PV are raised.
- HLA-B27 is often positive.
- Radiography shows progressive squaring-off of vertebrae with intervertebral ossification producing a bamboo spine appearance, calcification of tendon/ligament insertions (enthesitis) and obliteration of sacro-iliac joints.

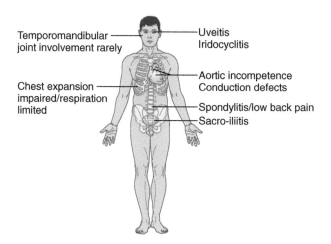

Figure 5.116 Ankylosing spondylitis – features.

Treatment
- Physiotherapy, and exercises
- Anti-inflammatory analgesics
- Rarely, spine radiotherapy (risk of leukaemia)
- Surgery is a final option, rarely indicated.

Main dental considerations

(*See also generic guidance under main dental considerations on page 63 top, and also Section 2).

Ankylosing spondylitis can affect the TMJ. Vision may be impaired. GA can be hazardous because of restricted mouth opening, and respiratory exchange.

Gout

Definition

A painful joint disease caused by sodium monourate crystal deposition.

Aetiopathogenesis and classification

Urate acid crystals in joints lead to lysozomal enzyme release from neutrophil leukocytes as they attempt phagocytosis of crystals. Hyperuricaemia predisposes and results from:
- accelerated purine metabolism;
- disturbed renal clearance of uric acid; or
- increased purine intake (Box 5.2).

Primary gout has a genetic basis, often associated with hypertriglyceridaemia, hypertension, atherosclerosis and diabetes.

Secondary gout is related to severe systemic diseases such as lymphoma, leukaemia and sickle cell anaemia.

Attacks of gout can be precipitated by:
- Diuretics (thiazides)
- Infection
- Starvation
- Trauma.

Clinical presentation

Acute gout presents with severe pain, redness and swelling, often in a single joint
– usually in males >50 years in the first metatarsophalangeal (big toe) joint (podagra).
The ankle, knee, wrist, and elbow may also be involved.

Chronic (tophaceous) gout presents with urate crystal deposits causing nodules on elbow
joint and/or ear. Kidney crystal deposits may cause calculi and renal disease.

Diagnosis

- Serum uric acid – typically raised.
- Synovial fluid – urate crystals.
- Radiology – juxta-articular radiolucencies.

Treatment

- Avoid purine-rich foods (Box 5.2), diuretics and obesity.
- Uricosuric agents such as allopurinol increase urate excretion.
- NSAID (indometacin not aspirin) or colchicine help acute gout.
- Probenecid has use in chronic gout.

Main dental considerations

(*See also generic guidance under main dental considerations on page 63 top, and also
Section 2).

Gout rarely affects the TMJ. Aspirin is contraindicated as it interferes with uricosuric drugs.

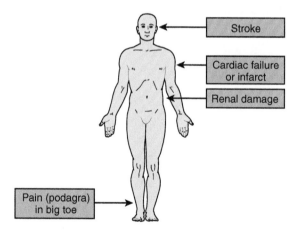

Figure 5.117 Gout – features.

Box 5.2   Foods to avoid in gout

- Alcohol
- Anchovies
- Asparagus
- Beans
- Herrings
- Kidney
- Mushrooms
- Mussels
- Peas
- Sardines

Osteoarthritis (osteoarthrosis; OA)

Definition
A very common degenerative joint disease especially seen in females >50 years.

Aetiopathogenesis
Primary osteoarthritis – no obvious predisposing factor.
Secondary osteoarthritis – usually follows joint trauma or instability, but also seen in metabolic diseases.
Pathogenesis includes:

- leukocyte degradative enzyme release
- proteoglycan dysfunction
- articular cartilage surface degradation
- bone metabolism alteration, sclerosis and compensatory thickening (osteophytes).

Clinical presentation
May affect any joint, especially those frequently used, weight-bearing or traumatized such as those in the fingers, hips, knees, lower back and feet.

Features may include pain, progressively diminished function and deformity, loss of joint flexibility, and bony lumps (osteophytes) on fingers, on middle (Bouchard's nodes) or terminal (distal intercarpophalangeal) joints (Heberden's nodes), or the 1st metacarpophalangeal joint at the thumb base. May also affect other joints:

- cervical spine
- lumbar spine
- knees.

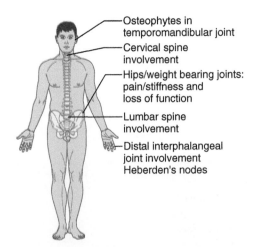

Osteophytes in temporomandibular joint

Cervical spine involvement

Hips/weight bearing joints: pain/stiffness and loss of function

Lumbar spine involvement

Distal interphalangeal joint involvement Heberden's nodes

Figure 5.118 Osteoarthritis – features. Adapted from Scully et al. (2007) Special Care in Dentistry: Handbook of Oral Care. Churchill Livingstone, Elsevier.

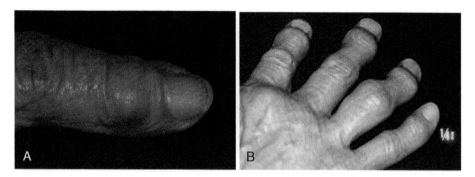

Figure 5.119 Osteoarthritis: **(A)** Heberden's nodes; **(B)** Heberden's and Bouchard's nodes.

Diagnosis

Clinical, with absence of systemic features (in contrast to RA), and normal FBP, ESR, and negative Rheumatoid factor, supported by imaging showing:

- Narrowing of the joint space.
- Marginal osteophyte formation (lipping).
- Subchondral bone sclerosis.
- Bone 'cysts' (rounded radiolucencies just beneath the joint surface).
- Deformity.

Treatment

Physical methods

- A walking aid
- Appropriate footwear
- Cold application
- Heat application
- Regular exercise
- Weight control.

Medical treatments

- Antidepressants, independent of antidepressant properties, can help lessen pain.
- Counter-irritant medications (e.g. methyl salicylate, menthol and camphor, or capsaicin).
- Glucosamine.
- Intra-articular corticosteroid or hyaluronate.
- Non-steroidal anti-inflammatory drugs.
- Topical analgesics (trolamine salicylate).

Surgical methods

- Arthroscopy – removes loose fragments that may cause pain or 'locking'.
- Joint replacement; hip, knee, shoulder, elbow, finger or ankle joints.
- Surgical bone repositioning to correct deformities, improve stability and reduce pain.

Main dental considerations

(*See also generic guidance under main dental considerations on page 63 top, and also Section 2).

Osteoarthritis may affect the TMJ, typically painlessly and symptoms do not correlate with the radiographic severity. Age and immobility may influence ability to maintain adequate oral hygiene and access to dental care. Since joint stiffness tends to improve during the day, short appointments in the late morning or in the early afternoon are recommended. Depending on which joints are involved, a sitting or semisupine chair position is recommended. There is no reliable evidence of a need for antibiotic prophylaxis before dental treatment in most patients with prosthetic joints, and risks from adverse reactions to antibiotics probably exceed any benefit. Patients who have compromised immune systems (diabetes mellitus, rheumatoid arthritis, cancer, chemotherapy, chronic steroid use) might be at greater risk for implant infections and might wish to consider antibiotics before dental procedures. Management may be complicated by a bleeding tendency if the patient is anticoagulated or takes high doses of aspirin.

Osteogenesis imperfecta (OI)

Definition
A rare, inherited condition characterized by brittle bones that are susceptible to fracture.

Aetiopathogenesis
Underlying autosomal dominant defect appears to be in type I collagen formation and, although osteoblasts are active, the amount of bone formed is small and mostly woven in type. This rare disorder has several variants. The gene for dentinogenesis imperfecta, one of the more common heritable defects of the teeth, is closely related – and some patients (OI types I and IV) have both conditions.

Clinical presentation
Bones are fragile and minimal trauma can cause multiple fractures; healing is rapid but often with distortion, so the ultimate effect in severe cases can be gross deformity and dwarfism. The long bones are normal in length, with epiphyses of normal width, but slender shafts, giving a trumpet-shaped appearance. The parietal regions of the skull may bulge outwards causing eversion of the upper part of the ear. Other features are blue sclerae, deafness, easy bruising and weakness of tendons and ligaments causing loose-jointedness and often hernias.

Cardiac complications such as mitral valve prolapse or aortic incompetence may be present.

Diagnosis
Clinical and imaging.

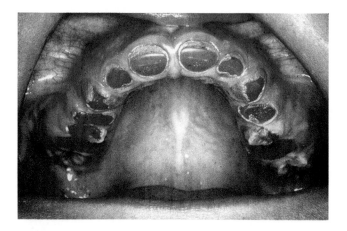

Figure 5.120 Osteogenesis imperfecta: dentinogenesis imperfecta is seen in some types. Reprinted from Scully C et al. (2012) Pocketbook of oral disease. Elsevier Churchill Livingstone with permission from Elsevier.

Treatment

Care to avoid fractures.

Main dental considerations

(*See also generic guidance under main dental considerations on page 63 top, and also Section 2).

When dentinogenesis imperfecta is associated, the teeth may have abnormal translucency, brown or purplish colour and readily wear. Dentinogenesis imperfecta can appear as an isolated abnormality without OI. It is important not to confuse children with OI with those subjected to physical abuse. Management problems relate to bone fragility and careful handling of the patient.

Osteoporosis

Definition

A loss of bone mineral density characterized by reduced mineralized bone mass.

Aetiopathogenesis

This metabolic bone disease results from an imbalance in osteoblastic and osteoclastic activities.

Primary osteoporosis is caused by androgen–oestrogen deficiency, lack of vitamin D and lack of exercise.

Secondary osteoporosis is caused by chronic liver disease, diabetes, drugs, hyperparathyroidism, hyperthyroidism or malabsorption.

Medications responsible may include androgen deprivation therapy used to treat prostate cancer, anticonvulsants, corticosteroids, thyroid hormone, and some drugs given to organ transplant patients, or used in cancer chemotherapy.

Clinical presentation

Especially common in older women, osteoporosis is usually asymptomatic. Increased bone fragility may lead to vertebral crush fractures or femoral neck fractures, often causing persistent lower back pain, kyphosis and loss of height. The rate of death in osteoporotic patients who fracture their hip is 20% within one year – often because of resultant pneumonia.

Diagnosis

- Bone densitometry – reduced
- Radiography
- Serum alkaline phosphatase – normal or low
- Serum calcium – normal
- Serum phosphorus – normal or low.

Prevention

Exercise, calcium supplementation, hormone replacement therapy (HRT), avoiding risk factors.

Treatment

Bisphosphonates (BPs), HRT or vitamin D. Bisphosphonates are used for treatment as they are adsorbed on to hydroxyapatite and can prevent or significantly slow osteoclastic activity leading to a 50% reduction in fractures (including hip and spine) compared with women taking calcium only.

Main dental considerations

(*See also generic guidance under main dental considerations on page 63 top, and also Section 2).

There seems to be a correlation between osteoporosis and alveolar bone loss in older patients. Patients with osteoporosis may have any of the problems of older people (Section 4). They may be at risk during GA if there has been vertebral collapse and chest deformities.

Agents such as BPs may induce anti-resorptive osteonecrosis of the jaws (ONJ). Monoclonal antibodies against RANKL (denosumab and bevacizumab), and the multikinase inhibitor sunitinib are also potent inhibitors of osteoclastic bone resorption. *Osteonecrosis of the jaw (ONJ: osteoclast modifier-related osteonecrosis of the jaws [OMRONJ]; bisphosphonate related or induced ONJ [BRONJ; BIONJ]),* defined as the presence of exposed bone in the mouth that fails to heal after appropriate intervention over a period of 6–8 weeks, has been reported in about 5% of patients with cancer receiving high-dose *intravenous*

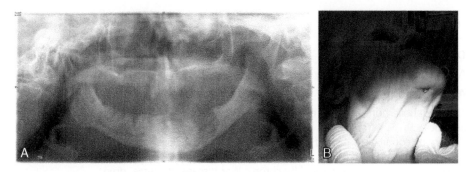

Figure 5.121 Osteonecrosis of mandible discharge to skin. From New England Journal of Medicine, Scully C, Brooke AE. Halitosis and sensory loss. 367: 551 ©2012 Massachusetts Medical Society. Reprinted with permission from Massachusetts Medical Society.

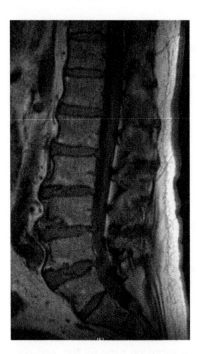

Figure 5.122 Vertebral crush fracture.

bisphosphonates in an attempt to reduce the hypercalcaemia seen in some malignant or other diseases. Oral bisphosphonates such as alendronate and risedronate, used in osteoporosis prophylaxis, result in an incidence of ONJ of only about one case per 1500 patients to two cases per 100,000 patient years. Bisphosphonates remain in bone for years and have an extremely long-lasting effect.

Most ONJ cases are preceded and probably precipitated by tooth extraction. Preventive dentistry prior to initiation of high-dose anti-resorptive therapy is thus crucial in patients with cancer. Prevention of most ONJ is by avoiding elective oral surgery. If dental extractions become unavoidable in a patient taking bisphosphonates, prophylactic antibiotics may be considered, but there is no evidence to support their use. If surgery is essential, the dentist must counsel the patient about the risks of use of intravenous, or oral bisphosphonates taken for more than 3 years. NSAIDs may increase the adverse effects of bisphosphonates.

Paget disease of bone

Definition
Disorder of excessive bone turnover, causing remodelling and enlargement of skull, pelvis and long bones.

Aetiopathogenesis
Unclear but a slow virus and endocrinopathies have been implicated.

Clinical presentation
In osteolytic phases bone resorption predominates, and in osteosclerotic phases there is appositional bone growth. May be asymptomatic, or bone pain and swelling. Leg deformities, kyphosis and loss of height, enlarged skull with headache, deafness or visual impairment may be seen. Bone arterio-venous shunting can cause cardiac failure.

About 1% of patients may develop an osteosarcoma.

Diagnosis
- Bone scintigraphy
- Radiography
- Plasma calcium and phosphorus levels – normal
- Serum alkaline phosphatase level – raised
- Urinary hydroxyproline level – raised.

Treatment
- Analgesia
- Bisphosphonates
- Calcitonin.

Main dental considerations
(*See also generic guidance under main dental considerations on page 63 top, and also Section 2).

The maxilla is involved occasionally and the mandible rarely. Typically, maxillary enlargement causes symmetrical malar bulging (leontiasis ossea). The intraoral features are gross symmetrical widening of the alveolar ridges, loss of lamina dura and hypercementosis often forming enormous craggy masses which may become fused to the surrounding bone. Pulpal calcification may be seen. Serious complications follow efforts to extract severely hypercementosed teeth. Prophylactic antibiotics may help prevent postoperative infection. Use of bisphosphonates may predispose to BRONJ (see above).

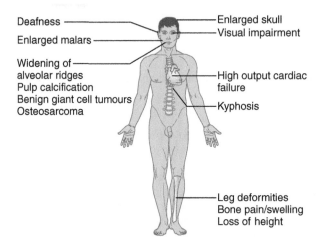

Figure 5.123 Paget disease – features. Adapted from Scully et al. (2007) Special Care in Dentistry: Handbook of Oral Care. Churchill Livingstone, Elsevier.

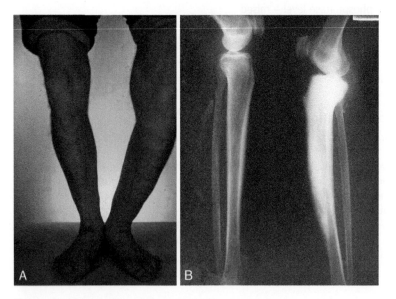

Figure 5.124 Paget disease bowed tibias.

Rheumatoid arthritis (RA)

Definition

A common chronic disease, of persistent, symmetrical, deforming peripheral arthropathy.

Aetiopathogenesis

A multi-system autoimmune disease associated with HLA-DR4, in which an autoantibody (rheumatoid factor [RF] – an IgM antibody directed against abnormal IgG) – forms immune (antigen–antibody) complexes that activate complement, causing synovial inflammation and articular cartilage destruction.

Clinical presentation

RA affects mainly females aged 30–50 years as an insidious chronic symmetrical polyarthritis of small joints of the wrists, hands and feet, with increasing stiffness of hands or feet, worse in the morning. The meta-carpo-phalangeal and interphalangeal joints typically ache, swell, become red, tender, limited in movement and become spindle-shaped as a result of joint swelling with muscle wasting on either side. Ulnar deviation of the fingers may develop. Later also, elbows, ankles and knees are often involved.

Other manifestations may include tenosynovitis, subcutaneous rheumatoid nodules, lymphadenopathy, and Sjögren syndrome.

Juvenile rheumatoid arthritis (Still disease) is a variant affecting children and characterized by chronic synovitis with or without extra-articular involvement.

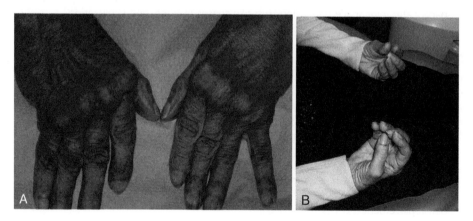

Figure 5.125 Rheumatoid arthritis deformities.

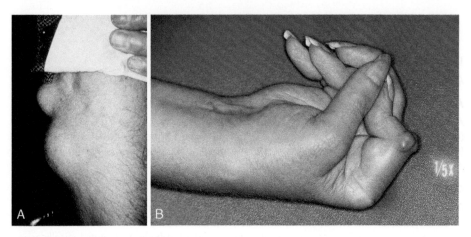

Figure 5.126 Rheumatoid nodules.

Diagnosis

Diagnosed if at least four of the following are present:

- Arthritis affecting more than three joint areas.
- Arthritis of hand joints.
- Morning joint stiffness.
- Positive rheumatoid factor (RF).
- Radiographic; soft tissue swelling, juxta-articular osteoporosis and widening of joint space. Later joint space narrowing, cyst-like spaces in bone, and subluxation. Ultimately severe bone destruction, deformity, but no ankylosis.

Treatment

- Rest, in acute phases.
- Medications:
  - *Symptom-modifying drugs* – usually NSAIDs or COX-2 inhibitors.
  - *Disease-modifying anti-rheumatic drugs* (DMARDs) – relieve painful, swollen joints and slow joint damage (mainly sulphasalazine, or gold, hydroxychloroquine, minocycline or penicillamine). For severe arthritis – azathioprine, ciclosporin, corticosteroids, cyclophosphamide, leflunomide, methotrexate, or biological response modifiers (e.g. tofacitinib, tocilizumab, certolizumab, adalimumab, abatacept, rituximab, golimumab, anakinra, etanercept or infliximab).
- Joint replacement – occasionally needed.

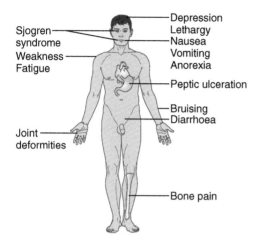

Figure 5.127 Rheumatoid arthritis – features. Adapted from Scully et al. (2007) Special Care in Dentistry: Handbook of Oral Care. Churchill Livingstone, Elsevier.

Main dental considerations

(*See also generic guidance under main dental considerations on page 63 top, and also Section 2).

Patients with RA may have restricted manual dexterity, which may compromise their ability to maintain adequate oral hygiene. Sjögren syndrome is the most common oral complication of RA. The TMJ may be affected, but though there may be limitation of opening or stiffness, these are often painless. Since joint stiffness tends to improve during the day, short appointments in the late morning or in the early afternoon are recommended for patients with arthritis. Supine positioning may be uncomfortable for them, and they may need neck and leg supports. Intubation for GA can be difficult. In some patients, dislocation of the atlantoaxial joint or fracture of the odontoid peg can readily follow sudden jerking extension of the neck, as a result of weakness of the ligaments. Biologic treatment may need to be stopped in consultation with the rheumatologist a month prior to surgery. Patients with joint prostheses because of RA may possibly require antibiotic cover before surgical procedures since they are regarded as mildly immunocompromised.

Rickets and osteomalacia

Definition
Normal amount of bone but low mineral (calcium and phosphorus) content, caused by vitamin D deficiency.

Aetiopathogenesis
Vitamin D deficiency may be due to:
- Dietary deficiency; chappatis contain phytates that bind vitamin D
- Lack of sunlight exposure
- Liver disease reducing 25-hydroxy vitamin D
- Malabsorption
- Renal disease causing deficiency of 1,25 di-hydroxycholecalciferol
- Vitamin D resistance.

Clinical presentation
Rickets – starts in the period of bone growth; patients usually show knock-knees and bow legs, and rarely seizures due to hypocalcaemia.
Osteomalacia – starts after bone growth ceases, and is characterized by bone pain, fractures and myopathy.

Diagnosis
- Blood tests:
  - Low calcium
  - Low phosphate
  - High alkaline phosphatase.
- Radiographic changes.
  - Low bone density with thin cortical bone and hypomineralization lines:
    Children:
      - epiphyseal cupping/widening
      - long bones bowing
      - transverse radiolucent (Looser's) lines
      - skull flattening
      - costal cartilages enlarge (rachitic 'rosary')
      - dorsal kyphosis.
    Adults:
      - Osseous changes in osteomalacia are similar but less evident than those in children.
      - Milkman pseudofractures or Looser lines; focal collections of osteoid may produce ribbon-like transverse zones of incomplete radiolucency, particularly notable on concave side of long bones, medial side of the femoral neck, the ischial and pubic rami, ribs, clavicles, and axillary borders of scapulae.

Treatment
Vitamin D, sunlight exposure and calcium.

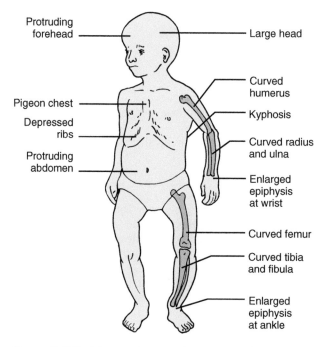

Protruding forehead

Large head

Curved humerus

Kyphosis

Pigeon chest

Depressed ribs

Curved radius and ulna

Protruding abdomen

Enlarged epiphysis at wrist

Curved femur

Curved tibia and fibula

Enlarged epiphysis at ankle

Figure 5.128 Rickets and osteomalacia. Clinical findings are related to the involved skeletal site. Adapted from van Rijn RR, McHugh K (2013) Rickets imaging. Medscape. Online. Available at: http://emedicine.medscape.com/article/412862-overview.

Main dental considerations

(*See also generic guidance under main dental considerations on page 63 top, and also Section 2).

Dental defects are seen only in unusually severe cases, but eruption may be retarded. The jaws may show abnormal radiolucency. In vitamin D-resistant rickets (familial hypophospha-taemia), the skull sutures are wide and there may be frontal bossing. Dental complaints frequently bring attention to the disease, since the teeth have large pulp chambers, abnormal dentine calcification, and are liable to pulpitis and multiple dental abscesses.

NEUROLOGICAL

Brain tumours

Definition
Primary brain tumours – rare, start in brain and remain there, not spreading to the body elsewhere.
Secondary brain tumours – cancers that have spread from another part of the body (metastases) – are far more common.

Aetiopathogenesis
Primary tumour causes are uncertain but may include: previous radiotherapy to the head; or genetic syndromes (e.g. tuberous sclerosis, Von Hippel–Lindau [a hereditary cancer predisposition], Li–Fraumeni [a hereditary cancer syndrome related to defect in *p53* tumour supressor gene], Turcot [mismatch repair cancer syndrome], neurofibromatosis, or Gorlin [nevoid basal cell carcinoma syndrome]).
Secondary tumours almost always arise from bladder, breast, lung, kidney, or skin cancer – but rarely prostate or colon or may be a cancer of unknown primary (CUP) origin.

Clinical presentations

Symptoms from raised intracranial pressure (ICP)
ICP: increased pressure in the skull. Can cause headaches – often dull, constant, occasionally throbbing, maybe worse at night, on coughing, sneezing, bending or with physical work. Nausea and vomiting – may be worse in morning or on sudden position changes. Some people have seizures, drowsiness or coma. Other features may be visual changes (blurred vision, 'floating objects' tunnel vision) or problems with balance.

Symptoms connected with the tumour's location
- Brainstem – unsteadiness; uncoordinated walking; facial weakness; diplopia; difficulty speaking and swallowing.
- Cerebellum – uncoordination; dysarthria; unsteadiness; nystagmus; vomiting, neck stiffness.
- Frontal lobe – personality and intellect changes; uncoordinated walking or unilateral weakness; anosmia; speech difficulties.
- Meninges – headaches, nausea and sight problems.
- Occipital lobe – loss of vision to one eye.
- Parietal lobe – difficulty speaking, understanding words, writing, reading, simple calculations, coordinating movements, unilateral numbness or weakness.
- Pituitary – various symptoms (e.g. tunnel vision; irregular periods; infertility; weight gain; lethargy; hypertension; diabetes; mood swings; and enlarged hands and feet).
- Temporal lobe – seizures; feelings of fear or intense familiarity (déjà vu), strange smells or blackouts; speech difficulties; or memory problems.

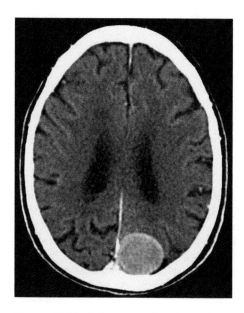

Figure 5.129 Brain tumour imaging. Left parasagittal occipitoparietal meningioma. Courtesy Mr A Kalantzis (Manchester).

Diagnosis

Electroencephalogram (EEG); brain MRI, PET (positron emission tomography), SPECT (single photon emission CT); CT chest, abdomen and pelvis; mammogram; lumbar puncture (LP); angiography; biopsy; blood tests.

Treatment

Steroids, surgery, radio- or chemotherapy.

Main dental considerations

(*See also generic guidance under main dental considerations on page 63 top, and also Section 2).

Ionizing radiation is a risk factor for meningioma, the most common primary brain tumour. Dental bitewing examinations and panorex films may be associated with an increased risk of meningioma. The American Dental Association's statement on the use of dental radiographs (American Dental Association Council on Scientific Affairs. The use of dental radiographs: update and recommendations. J Am Dent Assoc. 2006;137:1304–1312) highlights the need for dentists to examine the risk/benefit ratio associated with the use of dental X-rays.

Epilepsy

Definition

A tendency to recurrent seizures; only when a person has had two or more seizures are they considered likely to have epilepsy.

Classification

International League Against Epilepsy classifies three main seizure groups – generalized, partial, and other (Table 5.36).

Aetiopathogenesis

Temporary brain dysfunction with disturbances of nerve cell activity produces symptoms that vary depending on which part (and extent) of the brain is affected. Febrile convulsions may be seen in children with a high fever. Most cases of epilepsy are idiopathic. Symptomatic or secondary epilepsy is most prevalent in the young and in the mentally or physically impaired and can arise from brain injury, tumours or infections: hypoxia; metabolic abnormalities such as hypoglycaemia; or drugs or their withdrawal (alcohol, amphetamines, anticonvulsants, barbiturates, benzodiazepines, cocaine, opioids and psychotropics).

Clinical presentation

Seizures may produce changes in awareness or sensation, involuntary movements, or other behavioural changes, lasting from a few seconds to a few minutes. The most recognizable seizure is generalized tonic-clonic seizure, often called grand mal, when sufferers may cry out, lose consciousness, fall to the ground, and have rigidity (tonus) and muscle jerks

Table 5.36	Epilepsy: different types	
Seizures	**Sub-type**	**Main features**
Generalized	Tonic–clonic (Grand mal)	Loss of consciousness Tonic phase Clonic phase Tongue biting Incontinence Seizure lasts <5 minutes
	Absences (Petit mal)	Brief period of unresponsiveness Episode lasts <30 seconds
Partial	Simple (Jacksonian)	Motor, sensory, autonomic or psychic features
	Complex (Temporal lobe)	Impaired consciousness Automatic repetitive acts

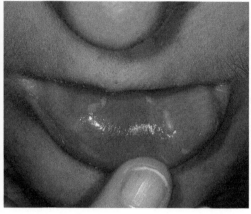

Figure 5.130 Epilepsy: lip trauma after a seizure.

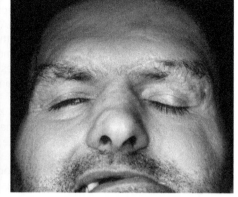

Figure 5.131 Facial scarring from trauma in seizures.

Table 5.37 Anticonvulsant treatment of epilepsy

Type of epilepsy	First choice drugs	Second choice drugs
Grand mal	Carbamazepine Valproic acid Gabapentin	Primidone
Petit mal	Valproic acid Ethosuximide	Clonazepam
Focal or partial complex seizures	Carbamazepine	Primidone

(clonus) for up to a few minutes, with an extended period of confusion and fatigue afterward. Usually, no trigger is apparent for epileptic attacks but seizures may sometimes be triggered by factors such as:

- drugs (illicit drugs, alcohol, antipsychotics, chlorpromazine, flumazenil, fluoxetine, enflurane, ketamine, methohexitone, tramadol, tricyclic anti-depressants)
- hormones (e.g. menstruation or pregnancy)
- hunger
- illness
- lack of sleep
- sensory stimuli (e.g. light flashes, sounds, touch).

Diagnosis

History; electroencephalography (EEG). CT or MRI and sometimes lumbar puncture (spinal tap) and CSF analysis may be indicated, as may be:

- Blood chemistry, especially glucose
- Full blood picture
- Liver function tests
- Renal function tests.

Treatment

Treat cause, if identifiable. Prophylaxis of epilepsy is with anticonvulsants; (see Table 5.37) which act on gamma amino butyric acid (GABA) or its receptor, or with neuronal inhibitors. Carbamazepine and sodium valproate are the most widely used but newer drugs are used more frequently either in monotherapy (lamotrigine) or as adjuncts (gabapentin, tiagabine, topiramate, vigabatrin). With certain types of partial epilepsy, especially when seizures consistently arise from a single area of brain (the 'seizure focus'), surgical removal of that focus may be effective.

Other supplemental treatments include ketogenic diet – a high fat, low carbohydrate diet with restricted calories, and vagus nerve stimulation therapy (VNST); this involves the use of an implantable electronic device to intermittently stimulate the vagal nerve in the neck.

People with epilepsy face legal restrictions, notably in driving and employment, being prohibited from specific occupations (e.g. pilots, ambulance drivers, military, etc.).

Main dental considerations

(*See also generic guidance under main dental considerations on page 63 top, and also Section 2).

Convulsions may have craniofacial sequelae such as lacerations, haematomas and fractures of the facial skeleton, or fractures, devitalization, subluxation or loss of teeth (a chest radiograph may be required), TMJ subluxation, or lacerations or scarring of the tongue, lips or buccal mucosa. Anticonvulsants in pregnancy, particularly phenytoin, are potentially teratogenic and can cause foetal anticonvulsant syndrome (FACS) of cleft palate and distinctive facial features (prominent forehead, broad flattened nasal bridge, thin upper lip, medial deficiency of the eyebrows and infraorbital grooves). Valproate depresses platelet numbers and function to produce a bleeding tendency. In the past, particularly, gingival swelling due to phenytoin was common. Dental treatment should be carried out in a good phase of epilepsy, when attacks are infrequent. Drugs that can be epileptogenic or interfere with anticonvulsants, or can themselves be changed by anticonvulsant therapy may be contraindicated. Aspirin, azoles and metronidazole can interfere with phenytoin. Antimicrobials (e.g. erythromycin, clarithromycin, tetracycline) can increase blood levels of carbamazepine, leading to toxicity. Benzodiazepines are anti-epileptogenic, but occasionally fits have been recorded in epileptics undergoing intravenous sedation with midazolam. Flumazenil, the antidote however, can be epileptogenic.

Migraine

Definition
A common recurrent headache combined with autonomic disturbances.

Aetiopathogenesis
Usually associated with increased cerebral and extracranial blood flow possibly caused by serotonin (5 hydroxytryptamine; 5HT) adsorbed to blood vessel walls. This may cause the trigeminal nerve to release neuropeptides; the combination of serotonin and bradykinin may cause blood vessels to become dilated and inflamed, either widening or narrowing of extracranial and intracranial arteries. The prodrome is usually accompanied by diminished cerebral blood flow, possibly the result of a neuronal trigger mechanism in the trigemino-vascular nucleus. Migraine triggers can include:

- alcohol (red wine mainly)
- aspartame
- botulinum toxin A injections
- bright lights, loud noises, or strong odours
- caffeine (excess or withdrawal)
- drugs (e.g. cimetidine, fenfluramine, nifedipine and theophylline)
- hypoglycaemia
- intense exertion, including sexual
- mealtime changes, skipped meals or fasting
- menstrual cycle hormone changes
- MSG (monosodium glutamate)
- nitrates or nitrites (cured meats)
- sleep deprivation
- stress, anxiety, or relaxation after stress
- tobacco
- tyramine (aged cheeses, soy products, fava beans, hard sausages, smoked fish, bananas, citrus fruits, nuts, beer, red wine or chocolate, or fermented, pickled or marinated foods)
- weather, season, altitude, or time zone changes.

Clinical presentation
Severe unilateral headache (hemicrania) for hours or days. Several types of migraine are recognized; migraine without aura is the most frequent – presenting with unilateral headache. Classical migraine is preceded by an aura (warning symptoms) of visual (fortification spectra), sensory (paraesthesia or anaesthesia – usually of the contralateral upper limb, or face and mouth), motor (weakness – again of the contralateral upper limb) or speech disturbances. Photophobia and sometimes phonophobia, nausea and sometimes vomiting may occur. Obvious vascular phenomena may be associated and range from facial flushing and oedema to temporary hemiplegia. The number, frequency, intensity and duration of migraine attacks vary widely, but they tend to diminish in frequency and intensity with increasing age. Spontaneous remissions are not uncommon and migraine tends to improve in pregnancy.

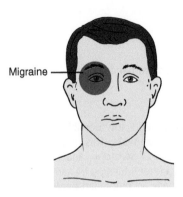

Figure 5.132 Migraine – location of pain.

Diagnosis

Clinical; no diagnostic tests are available.

Treatment

Avoid precipitating factors. Patients in an attack usually prefer to lie in a quiet, dark room. Aspirin or ibuprofen can be effective but triptans (5HT1 receptor agonists), e.g. sumatriptan, are effective in up to 80% if given within 1 hour. Antiemetics (e.g. metoclopramide, domperidone or buclizine) may help. A beta-blocker or serotonin antagonist (ergotamine, pizotifen, cyproheptadine) or calcium-channel blockers such as verapamil or nifedipine, may be useful prophylaxis.

Main dental considerations

(*See also generic guidance under main dental considerations on page 63 top, and also Section 2).

Dental procedures, such as tooth extraction, amalgam removal or the use of occlusal splints, are of no proven value in the management of true migraine. Temporomandibular disorders can cause tension headaches, which are in the differential diagnosis for migraine.

Motor neurone disease (MND)

Definition
A group of uncommon lethal neuro-degenerative diseases affecting especially males in old age, causing motor neurone damage (especially anterior horn cells) and weakness.

Aetiopathogenesis
May be viral, or due to exposure to heavy metals, immunologic abnormalities or biochemical deficiencies.

Clinical presentation and classification
Muscle atrophy, weakness, and spasticity, but no sensory or intellectual defects. Three MND subtypes:

- *Progressive muscular atrophy* – affects anterior horn below foramen magnum with lower motor neurone lesions causing wasting and weakness which start in the hands and spreads proximally. Best prognosis.
- *Amyotrophic lateral sclerosis* (ALS) – the most common sub-type, and with poor prognosis, affects anterior horn and pyramidal tract, damaging upper and lower motor neurones resulting in wasting and weakness of the hands and spasticity of the legs. Early signs and symptoms of ALS include:
  - Difficulty swallowing, speaking or breathing.
  - Fatigue.
  - Impaired chewing, swallowing, speaking and breathing.
  - Muscle cramps/twitching initially in arms, shoulders and tongue.
  - Slow loss of strength and coordination in one or more limbs.
  - Weakness in feet and ankles.
  - Brainstem involvement leads to pseudobulbar palsy – bulbar palsy with emotional lability (involuntary weeping or laughing).
- *Progressive bulbar palsy* – affects anterior horn cells of brainstem and thus cranial nerve motor neurones arising in the medulla (IX–XII inclusive). Characterized by wasting, weakness and fasciculation of muscles of pharynx, tongue, palate, sternocleidomastoid and trapezius, it has the worst prognosis.

Diagnosis
Clinical and:

- Electromyography (EMG).
- Nerve conduction studies.

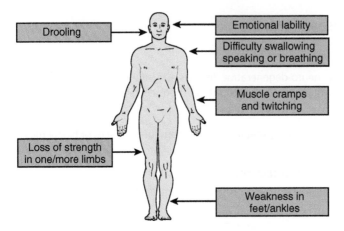

Figure 5.133 Motor neurone disease – features.

Treatment

Riluzole may slow the progress of ALS.
 Also sometimes needed are:

- Breathing assistance
- Nutritional support
- Physical and occupational therapy
- Speech therapy.

Airway protection may be impaired. Because of respiratory paralysis, few patients survive over 5 years. Morphine or pethidine may be needed for terminal care.

Main dental considerations

(*See also generic guidance under main dental considerations on page 63 top, and also Section 2).

Weakness or paralysis in the neck and head can lead to dysphagia and drooling. Protection of the airway may also be impaired and can lead to inhalation (aspiration) pneumonia.

Multiple sclerosis (MS); disseminated sclerosis (DS)

Definition
A chronic relapsing demyelinating CNS (brain and spinal cord) disease affecting mainly the corticospinal tract. The most common neurological disease.

Aetiopathogenesis
Perhaps viral, possibly human herpes virus 6 (HHV-6), this autoimmune disease is directed against myelin sheath proteins, resulting in inflammation and damage with multiple areas of scarring (sclerosis), which slow or block muscle coordination, visual sensation and other nerve signals.

Clinical presentation and classification
MS is a progressive disorder causing multifocal plaques of demyelination, leading to neurological disturbances ranging from:

- decreased conduction velocity
- differential rate of impulse transmission
- partial conduction blocking
- complete failure of impulse transmission.

MS has been classified based on the clinical course (Table 5.38). It varies in severity, ranging from a mild illness to one that results in permanent disability with widespread paralysis and loss of sphincter control and urinary incontinence, and eventually paralysis.
   Some common early presentations include:

- Cerebellar symptoms (diplopia/ataxia)
- Leg weakness
- Limb paraesthesia/anaesthesia
- Unilateral optic neuritis (rapid visual deterioration and pain on eye movement).

Symptoms, disseminated in site and time, may include:

- Brief pain, tingling or electric-shock sensations
- Dizziness
- Fatigue
- Impaired vision
- Numbness, weakness or paralysis in a limb
- Tremor, lack of coordination or unsteady gait.

Remissions, complete and partial, are common. More than 75% of patients survive 25 years. Occasionally there are fulminant cases.

Diagnosis
- Clinical findings during acute attack.
- CSF examination by lumbar puncture – increased IgG and oligoclonal bands.
- Delayed visual evoked response potentials (VEPs).
- MRI to show demyelinating plaques in the CNS.

Treatment
There is no specific treatment but acute episodes may be ameliorated by beta interferons, glatiramer, or mitoxantrone and relapses by natalizumab.

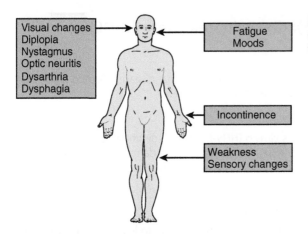

Figure 5.134 Multiple (disseminated) sclerosis – features.

Table 5.38 Multiple sclerosis subtypes

Subtypes	Frequency (% of patients)	Features
Relapsing-remitting	80	Short acute attacks about once a year
Primary progressive	10	Progressive deterioration from outset
Secondary progressive	40 of patients with relapsing-remitting MS	Progressive deterioration in patients with relapsing-remitting MS, after ~10 years
Progressive-relapsing	Rare	Relapses in patients with primary progressive MS

Symptomatic care may include:
- Physical and occupational therapy
- Counselling
- Corticosteroids
- Methotrexate
- Muscle relaxants (e.g. baclofen and tizanidine)
- Antidepressants such as fluoxetine.

Main dental considerations

(*See also generic guidance under main dental considerations on page 63 top, and also Section 2).

MS should always be considered in a young patient presenting with trigeminal neuralgia, particularly if bilateral, or if there have been other neurological disturbances, or if the pain lasts minutes or hours. Other presentations of MS may include abnormal speech; abnormal perioral sensation; facial palsy, myokymia or hemispasm. Atropinics used in treatment of bladder dysfunction may cause dry mouth, as may tizanidine. Glatiramer may cause facial oedema.

Limited mobility and psychological disorders may interfere with routine dental treatment. Schedule short, stress-free morning appointments when the patient is more relaxed and well rested. Patients with severe MS are best not treated supine, as respiration may be embarrassed. Treatment is best carried out under LA if possible.

Myasthenia gravis (MG)

Definition
An autoimmune disorder characterized by muscular weakness, affecting mainly adult females.

Aetiopathogenesis
Auto-antibodies to acetylcholine receptors result in their progressive loss, and poor neuromuscular transmission. MG may be aggravated by:
- Beta-blockers
- Emotion
- Pregnancy
- Some antimicrobials (gentamicin, tetracyclines).

Clinical presentation and classification
Based on main muscles involved, there are bulbar, ocular and generalized forms. Initially there is usually bulbar and extraocular weakness, with:
- Facial (jaw drop)
- Limbs weak
- Neck weak
- Quiet speech.

There is an increased risk of aspiration and ventilatory problems. MG sometimes is associated with a connective tissue disease, hyperthyroidism or thymic tumour.

Diagnosis
Clinical plus:
- Acetylcholine receptor antibodies
- Edrophonium test (a brief action anticholinesterase)
- CT mediastinum (for thymus enlargement)
- Neurophysiology.

Treatment
- Anticholinesterase (e.g. pyridostigmine – a long-acting agent)
- Corticosteroids
- Thymectomy.

Main dental considerations
(*See also generic guidance under main dental considerations on page 63 top, and also Section 2).
The most obvious orofacial features are facial weakness, diplopia, ptosis and voice changes. Weakness of masticatory muscles may cause the mouth to hang open (hanging or lantern jaw sign). Dental treatment is best carried out during a remission, best early in the day, within 1–2 h of routine medication with anticholinesterases, and with short appointments, since weakness increases during the day and fatigue or emotional stress may precipitate a myasthenic crisis. LA is preferred: lidocaine, prilocaine or mepivacaine can safely be used but minimal doses should be given. Pemphigus or Sjogren syndrome may be associated.

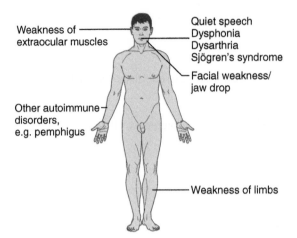

Weakness of extraocular muscles

Quiet speech
Dysphonia
Dysarthria
Sjögren's syndrome

Facial weakness/
jaw drop

Other autoimmune disorders,
e.g. pemphigus

Weakness of limbs

Figure 5.135 Myasthenia gravis – features. Adapted from Scully et al. (2007) Special Care in Dentistry: Handbook of Oral Care. Churchill Livingstone, Elsevier.

A small oral dose of a benzodiazepine may be given if the patient is anxious, but intravenous sedation must not be given in the dental surgery since bulbar or respiratory involvement impairs respiration. GA is an issue; opioids, barbiturates, suxamethonium, curare or anaesthetic agents are potentiated by or aggravate the myasthenic state. Postoperative respiratory infection can result and may also cause myasthenia to worsen. Drugs that can also worsen myasthenia and should be avoided include beta-blockers, lithium, phenytoin, and some antimicrobials (aminoglycosides, clindamycin, lincomycin, quinolones, sulfonamides, tetracyclines). Occasionally, aspirin has caused a cholinergic crisis in those on anticholinesterases; acetaminophen/paracetamol and codeine do not have this disadvantage.

Parkinsonism

Definition
A common progressive degenerative neurologic disorder characterized by tremor, rigidity, and shuffling gait.

Aetiopathogenesis
Primary Parkinson's disease – degeneration of dopamine neurones in brain basal ganglia, substantia nigra, or dopamine blocking.
Secondary Parkinson's disease may follow exposure to:
- Cerebrovascular disease.
- Drugs (e.g. phenothiazines) or toxins (e.g. pesticides) or the illicit drug MPTP [1-methyl-4-phenyl-1,2,3,6-tetrahydropyridine]).
- Encephalitis.
- Recurrent head trauma (e.g. boxing).

Clinical presentation
- Depression.
- Facies – mask-like with paucity of blinking.
- Rigidity – throughout movements ('lead pipe' rigidity).
- Slowness (bradykinesia).
- Speech slow, monotonous.
- Tremor – pill-rolling of thumb over fingers, worst at rest.
- Walking – difficulty starting/stopping (festinant gait).

Usually starts >age 50 years. There is a slow progression over many years and patients may also develop gradual dementia, manifesting with confusion, paranoia, and visual hallucinations. Emotional lability and constipation are common.

Diagnosis
Clinical findings.

Treatment
Parkinsonism due to drugs is virtually always reversible.
Other forms are usually managed with one or two of:
- Dopaminergic drugs:
  - Dopamine precursor (levodopa).
  - Dopa-decarboxylase inhibitors (benserazide or carbidopa).
  - Dopamine agonists (apomorphine, pramipexole, ropinirole), including those derived from ergot (bromocriptine, cabergoline, lisuride, pergolide).
- Catechol O methyl transferase (COMT) inhibitors (entacapone and tolcapone).
- Antimuscarinic drugs (benzatropine, orphenadrine, procyclidine, rivastigmine, trihexylphenidyl).
- Selegeline – a monoamine oxidase inhibitor.
- Apomorphine or dopa by pump.
- Stereotactic surgery (deep brain stimulation) – improves the tremor.

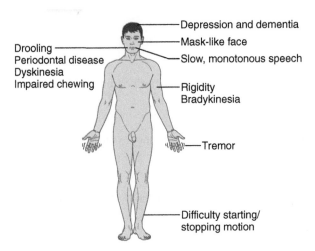

Depression and dementia
Mask-like face
Slow, monotonous speech
Drooling
Periodontal disease
Dyskinesia
Impaired chewing
Rigidity
Bradykinesia
Tremor
Difficulty starting/
stopping motion

Figure 5.136 Parkinson's disease – features. Adapted from Scully et al. (2007) Special Care in Dentistry: Handbook of Oral Care. Churchill Livingstone, Elsevier.

Main dental considerations

(*See also generic guidance under main dental considerations on page 63 top, and also Section 2).

Drooling of saliva may be troublesome. Orofacial involuntary movements (dyskinesia), such as 'flycatcher tongue' and lip pursing, are side-effects of levodopa and bromocriptine and may make the use of rotating dental instruments more hazardous. Sympathetic handling is particularly important, as anxiety increases tremor. Short, early morning appointments should begin approximately 90 minutes after administration of anti-Parkinson agents. Patients should be raised upright only cautiously and carefully assisted out of the dental chair, since parkinsonism, L-dopa and some other agents may cause hypotension. Levodopa in combination with a dopa-decarboxylase inhibitor may interact with epinephrine to cause tachycardia, arrhythmias and hypertension. Epinephrine may interact with COMT inhibitors (tolcapone, entacapone) to cause tachycardia, arrhythmias and hypertension; therefore, LA without epinephrine should be used in these patients. Antimicrobials (e.g. ampicillin, erythromycin) may interact with entacapone or pramipexole.

Trigeminal autonomic cephalgias (TACs)

Activation of the autonomic nervous moiety of the trigeminal nerve in the face, TACs include migrainous neuralgia and short-lasting unilateral neuralgia with conjunctival injection and tearing (SUNCT).

Migrainous neuralgia

(Periodic migrainous neuralgia, cluster headaches, Horton neuralgia, superficial petrosal neuralgia, histamine cephalgia, Sluder headaches.)

Definition

Unilateral excruciatingly severe pain attacks in the ocular, frontal and temporal areas, recurring in bouts with nightly or almost nightly attacks for weeks, usually with ipsilateral lacrimation, conjunctival injection, photophobia, nasal stuffiness and/or rhinorrhoea.

Aetiopathogenesis

First-degree relatives are more likely to have migrainous neuralgia and there is a significant association with the HCRTR2 gene. Attacks are sometimes precipitated by alcohol, histamine and nitroglycerine, heat, exercise, solvents and disrupted sleep.

Clinical presentation and classification

Less common than migraine. Males are mainly affected and attacks often begin in middle age. Attacks of migrainous neuralgia commence at night (classically at around 02.00), last less than 1 h (often 30–45 min), and often terminate suddenly, but may recur from 1–8 times a week. Autonomic features include flushing and/or sweating of the ipsilateral face with lacrimation, conjunctival injection and nasal congestion, and sometimes Horner syndrome (interruption of the sympathetic nerve supply to the eye – characterized by miosis [i.e., constricted pupil], ptosis [eyelid droops], and loss of hemifacial sweating [i.e., anhidrosis]). Occasionally, similar pain is due to ocular disease, lesions of the trigeminal nerve, brainstem or in the middle cranial fossa, such as lesions involving the craniospinal junction, cavernous sinus, circle of Willis or pituitary. Presentation may then be atypical.

Diagnosis

Clinical but CT/MRI are indicated to exclude other pathologies.

Treatment

Precipitants should be avoided and oxygen inhalations can help. Other therapies include butorphanol tartate nasal spray; capsaicin; ergotamine; lidocaine intranasally; melatonin; pizotifen; and triptans (e.g. eletriptan, naratriptan, rizatriptan, sumatriptan, zolmitriptan). Preventive medications include amitriptyline, diltiazem, cyproheptadine, ergotamine, lithium carbonate, prednisolone, propranolol, or verapamil. Neurosurgery or deep brain stimulation may help those with intractable neuralgia.

Main dental considerations

(*See also generic guidance under main dental considerations on page 63 top, and also Section 2).
Migrainous neuralgia must be distinguished from migraine, and from dental pain by the characteristic history and confirmation of the absence of a dental cause.

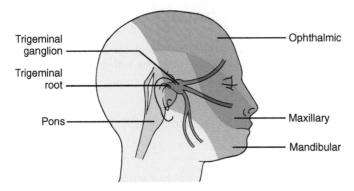

Trigeminal ganglion

Trigeminal root

Pons

Ophthalmic

Maxillary

Mandibular

Figure 5.137 Trigeminal nerve. Adapted from Scully (2010) Medical Problems in Dentistry, 6e.

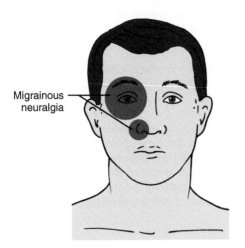

Migrainous neuralgia

Figure 5.138 Pain in migrainous neuralgia.

Trigeminal neuralgia (TN)

Definition
A painful, unilateral affliction of the face, characterized by brief electric-shock, lightning-like (lancinating) pains lasting only seconds and limited to one or more trigeminal nerve divisions.

Aetiopathogenesis and classification
Idiopathic TN cause may possibly be demyelination of trigeminal nerve roots caused by arteriosclerotic blood vessels in posterior cranial fossa pressing on them (TN typically affects people >50 years, and many have hypertension or arteriosclerosis).

Secondary TN causes include posterior cranial fossa lesions, particularly aneurysms or tumours (acoustic neurinomas, carcinomas or meningiomas), brainstem ischaemia or infarction in cerebrovascular disease, multiple sclerosis or neurosyphilis.

Clinical presentation
TN pain has the following characteristics; it is:

- Confined to the trigeminal area of one side, usually the maxillary or mandibular division or occasionally both.
- Severe and sharply stabbing (lancinating), of only a few seconds' duration, but paroxysms may follow in quick succession.

Triggers may be features; these are mild stimuli, which, applied to trigger zones within the trigeminal area, typically provoke an attack, and may include:

- brushing teeth
- drinking a hot or cold liquid
- eating
- encountering a cold breeze
- putting on cosmetics
- shaving
- stroking or touching the face
- talking.

Idiopathic TN is likely the diagnosis if the pain started when >40 years age, when there is an intact corneal reflex, no abnormal neurological signs, no objective sensory loss in the area and no other defined neurological deficit.

Secondary TN is more likely the diagnosis if the pain started when <40 years age, if there is predominant forehead and/or orbit pain (i.e. trigeminal nerve first division), if the pain is bilateral, if there are abnormal trigeminal reflexes, or if there are physical signs such as facial sensory or motor impairment or other disorders noted above.

Diagnosis
Clinical organic disease must be excluded by neurological examination, skull radiographs, MRI or CT brain scans, and occasionally CSF examination, or neurophysiological tests (e.g. trigeminal evoked potentials and corneal reflex latency). The main differential diagnoses are from glossopharyngeal neuralgia, idiopathic facial pain, Raeder paratrigeminal syndrome and Frey syndrome (sweating while eating [gustatory sweating] and facial flushing).

Treatment

Initially this is with anticonvulsants, particularly carbamazepine, which change GABA (gamma amino butyric acid) levels in the central pain-inhibiting systems. Some Asians and others metabolize carbamazepine poorly and can thus suffer from overdose or other adverse events, so they should be screened for HLA-B*1502 allele which is strongly correlated with carbamazepine-induced Stevens–Johnson syndrome (SJS) and toxic epidermal necrolysis (TEN) in Han Chinese and other Asian populations, or HLA-A*3101 allele in people of Northern European ancestry. Carbamazepine is contraindicated in pregnancy and porphyria, and should be used with caution in persons with hepatic, renal, cardiac (especially atrioventricular conduction defects) or bone marrow disease. Monitoring of blood carbamazepine levels, BP, blood urea and electrolytes, LFTs, platelet and white cell counts and FBC is helpful.

If a patient presumed to have TN does not respond to carbamazepine in 24–48 h, then the initial diagnosis should be reconsidered. Should carbamazepine in maximum dosage fail to control TN, baclofen, gabapentin, lamotrigine or oxcarbazine are second choices. Additional agents that may be added or replace carbamazepine include topical capsaicin, or phenytoin, tizanidine, or valproate. If medical therapy fails or adverse effects are intolerable, surgery (surgical division, cryosurgery, injections of alcohol or phenol) to the trigeminal nerve branches involved is usually needed. If these treatments fail, the intracranial neurosurgery available includes:

Gamma knife radiosurgery (GKR) – is non-invasive, can be successful in eliminating pain in up to 80% but pain recurs in more than half the cases.

Microvascular decompression (MVD), – an invasive procedure via a suboccipital craniotomy, may be effective but occasionally results in damage to the VIIth or VIIIth cranial nerves and also carries a small mortality.

Percutaneous radiofrequency trigeminal (retrogasserian) rhizotomy (PRTR) – is the most widely used technique and is minimally invasive involving inserting a needle, but has morbidity and some mortality.

Percutaneous trigeminal ganglion (Fogarty balloon) *compression* (rhizotomy) – is minimally invasive, and often effective; 60% of patients are pain-free 8 years after surgery. Over 50% of patients have mild to moderate postoperative numbness, but no corneal numbness.

All destructive surgical procedures can result in a sensory deficit, relapse is common beyond 2 years and the more peripheral the procedure, the greater the risk of recurrence.

Neurosurgical techniques can occasionally be followed by continuous facial pain (anaesthesia dolorosa) that responds poorly to treatment.

MVD provides the longest-lasting pain relief but involves risks of major neurological complications; gamma-knife is the least invasive and safest procedure – but pain relief may take one month or so to develop.

Main dental considerations

(*See also generic guidance under main dental considerations on page 63 top, and also Section 2).

Orofacial pain is the main feature. Patients may be reluctant to brush their teeth or attend for dental treatment.

RESPIRATORY

Asthma

Definition

Bronchial asthma is a common state of generalized reversible bronchial narrowing, caused by excessive bronchial smooth muscle tone (bronchospasm), mucosal oedema and congestion, and mucus hypersecretion, from bronchial hyper-reactivity.

Classification

Allergic or extrinsic, and idiosyncratic or intrinsic types (Table 5.39).

Aetiopathogenesis

Hypersensitivity to either known precipitants (extrinsic asthma) or unknown stimuli (intrinsic asthma). Airways obstruction is caused by bronchial smooth muscle contraction – due to histamine and leukotrienes-inflammation and oedema – due to IgE-mediated mast cell and basophil degranulation releasing inflammatory mediators with mucus production.

Table 5.39	Types of asthma	
Type	**Extrinsic**	**Intrinsic**
	Allergic	Idiosyncratic
Frequency	Most common	Least common
Associations	Atopy, eczema, hay fever, drug sensitivities	–
Pathogenesis	IgE-mediated mast cell degranulation releasing histamine, leukotrienes, prostaglandins, bradykinin and platelet activating factor	Mast cell instability
Age of onset	Child	Adult
Triggers	Allergens in house dust, animal dander, feathers, animal hairs, moulds, milk, eggs, fish, fruit, nuts, non-steroidal anti-inflammatory agents (NSAIDs) and antibiotics. Infections (especially viral, mycoplasmal or fungal)	Emotional stress. Gastro-oesophageal reflux. Infections (viral, mycoplasmal or fungal). Cigarette smoke. Air pollution. Exercise. Cold air. Weather changes. Foods such as nuts, shellfish, strawberries or milk; food additives such as tartrazine; some drugs, particularly NSAIDs, beta-blockers, and ACE inhibitors.

Table 5.40 Asthma severity

Severity of asthma	Symptom duration	Attacks per week	Other comments	Typical therapy
Mild	<1 h	<2	Attacks follow exercise or exposure to trigger	Beta agonist as required
Moderate	days	>2	Activity restricted	Beta agonist plus steroid
Severe	persists	persists	Audible wheezing. Tachypnoea. Activity and sleep severely restricted	Beta agonist plus steroid plus theophylline

Episodes of either type of asthma can sometimes be initiated by allergens; emotional stress; infections; irritating fumes including air pollution, cigarette smoke; exercise, climate changes; food additives; or drugs, particularly aspirin and other NSAIDs.

Clinical presentation

Most common in males, usually begins in childhood or early adult life with wheeze, cough, dyspnoea, and use of accessory muscles in respiration (Table 5.40).

Diagnosis

History, physical examination, chest radiographs, spirometry – lowered peak expiratory flow rate (PEFR), blood gas analysis, skin tests for allergens and blood examination (usually raised total IgE and specific IgE antibody concentrations).

Treatment

- Avoid identifiable irritants and allergens.
- Drug treatment, based on the PEFR reduction (Table 5.41):
  - Beta 2 agonist (e.g. salbutamol) inhaled
  - Corticosteroids
  - Leukotriene receptor antagonists.

Prognosis is usually good, especially when asthma appears first during childhood. In a few adults asthma may progress to respiratory failure.

Rarely, a prolonged and often life-threatening attack refractory to treatment starts which, if persisting >24 hours, is termed *status asthmaticus* and potentially lethal.

Reassurance and prophylactic bronchodilator use may be a useful and sensible precaution. Acute attacks are usually self-limiting or respond to medication such as a beta-agonist inhaler (salbutamol 5 mg). If an asthmatic attack is severe, hydrocortisone 200 mg intravenously plus prednisolone 20 mg orally should also be given.

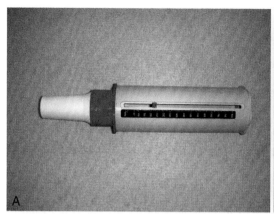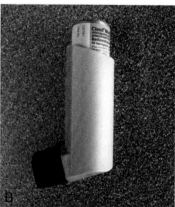

Figure 5.139 (A) Spirometer; **(B)** inhaler (steroid).

Table 5.41 Medical management of asthma

Drug group	Examples	Comments
Beta agonists	Salbutamol (albuterol), terbutaline, fenoterol, rimiterol, pirbuterol, reproterol, tulobuterol Bambuterol, salmeterol or eformoterol	Safest and most effective bronchodilators with little cardiac effect Effect lasts 3–6 hours. Effect lasts at least 12 hours
Antimuscarinic bronchodilators	Ipratropium or oxitropium bromide	Useful for those with asthma associated with bronchitis. Effect lasts up to 8 hours
Methylxanthines	Theophylline preparations	Prolonged action useful in nocturnal asthma
Corticosteroids	Beclomethasone, betamethasone valerate, budesonide or fluticasone aerosol	Can cause adrenal suppression
Mast cell stabilizers	Cromoglicate or nedocromil	Used as prophylaxis, particularly
Leukotriene receptor antagonists. 5-lipoxygenase inhibitor	Montelukast Zafirlukast Zileuton	May impair liver function and increase INR
Recombinant humanized monoclonal anti-IgE antibody	Omalizumab	Effective in allergic asthma

Main dental considerations

(*See also generic guidance under main dental considerations on page 63 top, and also Section 2).

Asthmatic attacks are occasionally precipitated by fear.

It is important to attempt to lessen fear by gentle handling and reassurance. To minimize the risk of an asthma attack, schedule late morning or late afternoon appointments. Minimize stress of appointment with oral or intravenous sedation.

Asthmatic patients should be asked to bring their usual medication with them when coming for dental treatment. Elective dental care should be deferred in severe asthmatics until they are in a better phase; this can be advised by their own general practitioner.

LA is best used: occasional patients may react to the sulphites present as preservatives in vasoconstrictor-containing LA, so it may be better, where possible, to avoid solutions containing vasoconstrictor. Epinephrine may theoretically enhance the risk of arrhythmias with beta-agonists and is contraindicated in patients using theophylline as it may precipitate arrhythmias. Sedatives in general are better avoided as, in an acute asthmatic attack, even benzodiazepines can precipitate respiratory failure. Relative analgesia with nitrous oxide and oxygen is preferable to intravenous sedation. GA is best avoided as it may be complicated by hypoxia and hypercapnia, which can cause pulmonary oedema even if cardiac function is normal, and cardiac failure if there is cardiac disease. Allergy to penicillin may be more frequent in asthmatics. Acute asthmatic attacks may be precipitated by aspirin (Samter triad syndrome; of aspirin-induced asthma, nasal polyposis or sinusitis) and other drugs, and anxiety. Acute asthmatic attacks are usually self-limiting or respond to the patient's usual medication such as a beta-agonist inhaler but status asthmaticus is a potentially fatal emergency (see Section 3).

Gastro-oesophageal reflux is not uncommon, with occasional tooth erosion. Periodontal inflammation is greater in asthmatics. Those using steroid inhalers may develop oropharyngeal candidosis or, occasionally, angina bullosa haemorrhagica (localised purpura) in mouth or pharynx.

Chronic obstructive pulmonary disease (COPD)

Also termed chronic obstructive airways disease [COAD]

Definition

Chronic progressive, essentially irreversible, airways obstruction, consisting of either, or both chronic bronchitis and emphysema.

Chronic bronchitis is the excessive production of mucus and persistent cough with sputum production for more than 3 months in a year over more than two consecutive years. It leads to excessive, viscous mucus, which obstructs and stagnates, and becomes infected especially with *Strep. pneumoniae, Moraxella catarrhalis,* and *Haemophilus influenzae.* Areas of lung alveolar collapse can result.

Emphysema is dilatation of air spaces distal to the terminal bronchioles with destruction of alveoli.

Aetiopathogenesis

Tobacco smoking, air pollution, environment contamination, respiratory infections, and familial predisposition (e.g. alpha-1-antitrypsin deficit).

Clinical presentation

Dyspnoea (breathlessness), wheeze (airways obstruction), cough, and sputum production lead to progressively low oxygen saturation, accumulation of carbon dioxide (hypercapnia), acidosis, and eventual respiratory failure or right sided-heart failure (cor pulmonale). Affected people are ultimately dyspnoeic at rest and especially when recumbent (orthopnoea).

Some, especially those with chronic bronchitis fail to maintain hyperventilation, lose the CO_2 drive, become hypercapnic and hypoxic, but the chronic hypoxaemia leads to central cyanosis which, in association with ankle oedema and raised jugular venous pressure of cor pulmonale, gives rise to a 'blue bloated' appearance. Others, patients with emphysema, manage to maintain normal blood gases by hyperventilation to produce a 'pink panter or pink puffer' who is severely breathless and pink from vasodilatation caused by CO_2 retention.

Respiratory failure may be:

- **Hypoxaemic (type I)**: caused by ventilation-perfusion mismatch with either/both:
  - Under-ventilated alveoli (e.g. pulmonary oedema, pneumonia or acute asthma).
  - Venous blood bypasses ventilated alveoli (e.g. right to left cardiac shunts).

Hyperventilation increases CO_2 removal without increasing oxygenation: PaO_2 is <60 mm Hg (8 kPa) with a normal or low $PaCO_2$.

- **Hypercapnic (type II)**: ventilation-perfusion mismatch affects PaO_2 and therefore inadequate alveolar ventilation with hypoxaemia is common: $PaCO_2$ is >50 mmHg (6.5 kPa).

Diagnosis

Blood gases analysis – PaO_2 (partial pressure of oxygen in arterial blood) lowered. Lung function tests (forced expiratory volume and forced vital capacity) – impaired.

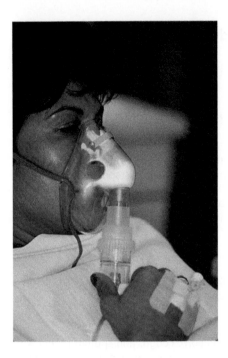

Figure 5.140 Oxygen therapy in COPD. Courtesy Dr N Kumar.

Treatment

Stop smoking. Exacerbations of bronchitis are managed with antibiotics and mucolytics such as carbocisteine. Breathing may benefit from bronchodilators – ipratropium bromide, others (tiotropium), or beta-agonists, or occasionally low dose inhaled or systemic corticosteroids or theophylline. Long-term oxygen therapy (LTOT) may be needed (but not in blue bloaters). Severe cases are occasionally treated with surgery – bullectomy, or lung transplantation.

Main dental considerations

(*See also generic guidance under main dental considerations on page 63 top, and also Section 2).

Proceed with caution in patients with severe lung function impairment and in those who use oxygen at home as they are sensitive to effects of any sedatives, are prone to desaturation, and require oxygen saturation monitoring during procedures. Defer elective care if the patient is short of breath at rest, or has a productive cough, fever, upper respiratory infection or an oxygen saturation level less than 91%. Avoid the use of a rubber dam in patients with severe COPD. Patients with COPD are best treated in an upright position at mid-morning or early afternoon, since they may become increasingly dyspnoeic if laid supine. LA is preferred for dental treatment, but bilateral mandibular or palatal injections should be avoided. Conscious sedation with diazepam and midazolam should not be used as benzodiazepines are respiratory depressants. Patients with COPD should be given relative analgesia only in hospital after full preoperative assessment. Patients should be given GA only if absolutely necessary; postoperative respiratory complications are more prevalent. Interactions of theophylline with drugs, such as epinephrine, erythromycin, clindamycin, clarithromycin or ciprofloxacin, may result in dangerously high levels of theophylline.

Lung cancer

Definition

The most common cancer in high-income countries in adult, urban, males. 95% is bronchogenic carcinoma. Other tumours are usually metastases.

Aetiopathogenesis

Risk factors include:

- Exposure to:
  - air pollution;
  - asbestos, certain metals (e.g. chromium or arsenic), toxic chemicals;
  - radon, a radioactive gas which seeps into buildings from natural breakdown of uranium in soil and rock;
  - tobacco smoke.
- Family history of lung cancer.
- History of oral or upper aerodigestive tract cancer or pre-cancer.
- Men who have had tuberculosis.

Metastases from other cancers are frequent to the lungs.

Clinical presentation

Recurrent cough, haemoptysis (blood in sputum), dyspnoea, chest pain and recurrent chest infections are the predominant features.

Local infiltration may cause pleural effusion, lesions of the cervical sympathetic chain (Horner syndrome), brachial neuritis, recurrent laryngeal nerve palsy or obstruction of the superior vena cava with facial cyanosis and oedema (superior vena cava syndrome).

Metastases from bronchogenic cancer are common and typically form in the brain (which may manifest with headache, epilepsy, hemiplegia or visual disturbances), liver (hepatomegaly, jaundice or ascites) or bone (pain, swelling or pathological fracture).

Non-metastatic extrapulmonary effects of bronchogenic (or other) carcinomas include, for example, weight loss, anorexia, finger-clubbing, neuromyopathies, thromboses (thrombophlebitis migrans), muscle weakness, various skin manifestations and ectopic hormone production (of antidiuretic hormone, adrenocorticotropic hormone, parathyroid hormone, or thyroid-stimulating hormone).

Diagnosis

Clinical plus CT and MRI, sputum cytology, bronchoscopy and biopsy. Spiral CT detects tumours at an early stage. Synchronous or metachronous second primary tumours (SPTs) elsewhere in the aerodigestive tract must always be ruled out.

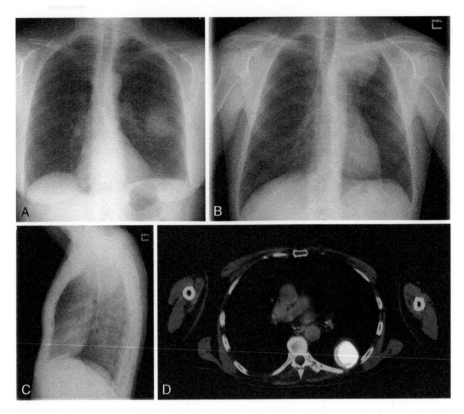

Figure 5.141 Lung (bronchogenic) cancer.

Treatment

Radiotherapy is the most common treatment. Only ≈25% of patients are suitable for surgery but, even then, the 5-year survival is only about 25%. Chemotherapy has been disappointing except in small cell carcinomas. Overall 5-year survival rate is only 8%.

Main dental considerations

(*See also generic guidance under main dental considerations on page 63 top, and also Section 2).

Lung cancer metastases may occasionally affect the jaws. Lung cancer may be associated with potentially malignant lesions or second primary tumours in the aerodigestive tract, including the mouth.

Pneumonia

Definition
Inflammation in the air sacs in one or both lungs, usually from infection. The air sacs may fill with fluid or pus.

Aetiopathogenesis and classification
Pneumonia may be viral, bacterial, or rarely, fungal.

Primary pneumonia – occurs in a previously healthy individual, is usually lobar pneumonia and causes are mainly pneumococcus (*Strep. pneumoniae*), *Haemophilus pneumoniae*, or *Moraxella catarrhalis*.

Secondary pneumonia – results from some other disorder and is usually bronchopneumonia. Pneumonia is the second most common nosocomial (hospital-acquired) infection in critically ill patients, affecting up to 25%.

Causes of bronchopneumonia include:

- Aspiration of foreign material or microorganisms. Nosocomial pneumonias are 80% associated with mechanical ventilation (ventilator-associated pneumonia [VAP]). hospital-acquired pneumonia (HAP) is often early on associated with *Strep. pneumoniae* or *Haemophilus influenzae*, but later, polymicrobial infections or meticillin-resistant *Staphylococcus aureus* (MRSA) are particular hazards.
- Community-acquired pneumonia (CAP) is often associated with *Str. pneumoniae* or *H. influenzae* or Enterobacteriaceae, such as *Klebsiella* species, *Escherichia coli* and *Pseudomonas aeruginosa,* especially in the very old and infirm.
- Impaired immunity (e.g. alcoholism, HIV/AIDS or immunosuppression).
- Lung disease (bronchiectasis or carcinoma).
- Previous lower respiratory viral infections.

Clinical presentation
Pneumonia causes cough, fever, rapid respiration, breathlessness, chest pain, dyspnoea and shivering. Complications can include lung abscess or empyema (pus in pleural cavity). It is potentially lethal.

Diagnosis
Clinical, pulse oximetry, imaging and microbiology.

Treatment
Fluids, analgesics, antipyretics and, if bacterial, broad-spectrum antimicrobials (usually include a macrolide [azithromycin, clarithromycin or erythromycin], quinolone [moxifloxacin, gatifloxacin or levofloxacin]), or doxycycline for outpatients. For inpatients, cefuroxime or ceftriaxone plus a macrolide. Most otherwise healthy people recover in one to three weeks, but pneumonia can be life-threatening. Pneumonia prophylaxis includes immunization against influenza and pneumococci – especially important in older people.

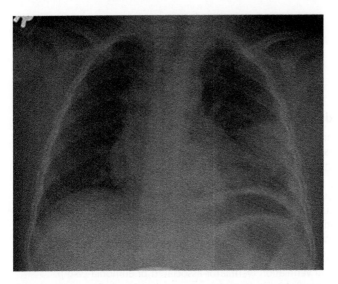

Figure 5.142 Lobular pneumonia. Reprinted from Townsend CM, Beauchamp RD, Evers BM, Mattox KL (2012) Sabiston Textbook of surgery: the biological basis of modern surgical practice, 19e. Elsevier Saunders with permission from Elsevier.

Main dental considerations

(*See also generic guidance under main dental considerations on page 63 top, and also Section 2).

The major route for acquiring endemic VAP is oropharyngeal colonization by endogenous flora or by exogenously acquired pathogens from ITU (intensive care units). The Health-care Infection Control Practices Advisory Committee of the Centers for Disease Control and Prevention guidelines for prevention of VAP include strategies aimed at preventing aspiration of contaminated oral or gastric material (e.g. raising the head of the bed and draining subglottic secretions), and interventions to alter bacterial colonization of stomach (e.g. stress ulcer prophylaxis and selective digestive decontamination), and mouth – oral hygiene, suctioning, and providing moisture to lips and oral mucosa plus tooth brushing.

Sarcoidosis

Definition
A multisystem granulomatous disorder.

Aetiopathogenesis
Seen most commonly in young adult females in northern Europe, especially in people of African heritage, the aetiology is unclear but bacteria such as *Propionobacterium acnes, P. granulosum* and *Mycobacterium paratuberculosis* have been implicated – as has exposure to inorganic particles, insecticides, moulds; and occupations, such as firefighting and metal working. T helper 1 (Th1) cells release IL-2 and IFN-gamma, and augment macrophage Tumour Necrosis Factor alpha (TNF-alpha) release. Granulomas form. CD25 regulatory T cells cause limited impairment of cell-mediated immune responses (partial anergy), but no obvious special susceptibility to infection. Sarcoidosis is associated with HLA-DRB1 and DQB1, and a butyrophilin-like 2 (BTNL2) gene on chromosome 6.

Clinical presentation
Protean manifestations; can involve virtually any tissue but the thorax in 90%. Most typically causes Löfgren syndrome (arthralgia – especially of the ankles, bilateral hilar lymphadenopathy, erythema nodosum, fever). Other common presentations may include pulmonary infiltration and impaired respiratory efficiency, or acute uveitis.

Diagnosis
Clinical; helpful investigations may include raised serum angiotensin-converting enzyme (SACE – released by epithelioid cells of granulomas), C reactive protein, and calcium (from extrarenal vitamin D production); chest imaging (enlarged hilar lymph nodes); positive gallium-67 citrate, gadolinium or FDG positron emission tomography (PET) scans; and biopsy for non-caseating epithelioid cell granulomas (lesional, salivary gland or bronchial).

Treatment
Half the patients with sarcoidosis remit within 3 years and two-thirds by 10 years. Patients with only minor symptoms usually need no treatment. Corticosteroids, or azathioprine, etanercept, hydroxychloroquine, infliximab, methotrexate, or tetracyclines may be given for active organ disease (ocular, lung, cerebral or hypercalcaemia).

Main dental considerations
(*See also generic guidance under main dental considerations on page 63 top, and also Section 2).
Sarcoidosis can involve any of the oral tissues but has a predilection for salivary glands, cervical nodes, and less frequently deposits in the lips or elsewhere. The association of salivary and lacrimal gland enlargement with fever and uveitis is termed uveoparotid fever (Heerfordt syndrome). Facial palsy and other cranial neuropathies may be seen.

Biopsy of the minor salivary glands may be helpful in obviating more invasive diagnostic procedures.

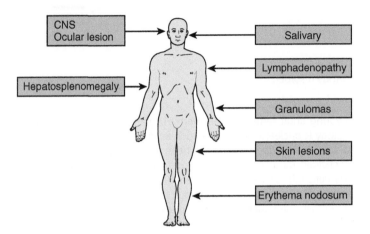

Figure 5.143 Sarcoidosis – features.

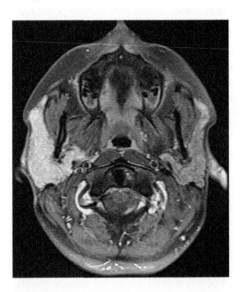

Figure 5.144 Sarcoidosis of right parotid – diffuse pattern with enlargement of gland and homogenous contrast enhancement. Reprinted from Zenk J, Iro H, Klintworth N, Lell M (2009) Salivary gland infections diagnostic imaging in sialadenitis. Oral and Maxillofacial Surgery Clinics 21(3): 275–292 with permission from Elsevier.

6 Trauma

Facial trauma

Aetiopathogenesis

Trauma is increasing; injuries are a leading cause of death in children and men up to age 35. Violence (assaults or fights) and road traffic accidents (RTAs) are major causes, with alcohol or drugs frequent cofactors. Domestic violence including child abuse, spousal and old people abuse, and abuse of the disabled is the single most common type of violence.

Males are more likely to be admitted with fractures but not soft tissue injury only, more likely to be assaulted with a weapon, and more likely to be involved in an altercation, gang violence, arrest, or robbery.

Females are more prone to domestic violence and sexual assaults and less prone to involvement in criminal violent activity or gang association.

Clinical presentation and classification

Trauma is potentially life-threatening especially if involving the face, head, spine, airway or heart/major vessels. Maxillofacial trauma is the single most common injury in RTAs. Industrial accidents, sport, falls, epilepsy and non-accidental injuries (child abuse) are other causes. Sports injuries arise in contact sports mainly, but also from bicycling, skating, and gymnastics, especially on trampolines. Falls are a major cause of trauma to face, jaws and teeth in children and older adults. Orofacial injuries are common from toddlers falling with a bottle or pacifier in their mouth. Falls may indicate underlying pathology or simple locomotor inadequacy and are especially common after age 80 years. Trauma can leave significant impairments.

Diagnosis

Clinical and imaging.

Treatment

All patients with facial injuries must be urgently assessed using the ABC system (Airway and cervical spine, Breathing and bleeding, and Chest injuries) since damage to the head, cervical spine, chest, liver or spleen can be immediately life-threatening. Maxillofacial trauma demands special attention since it may damage sight, breathing, hearing, smelling, eating and speech – especially in middle third facial fractures (particularly Le Fort III fractures).

Dental considerations

Trauma to face, jaws and teeth needs consideration after head and other serious injuries have been addressed. The bones most commonly fractured are the nasal, zygoma, mandible and maxilla. See www.rad.washington.edu/academics/academic-sections/msk/teaching-materials/online-musculoskeletal-radiology-book/facial-and-mandibular-fractures

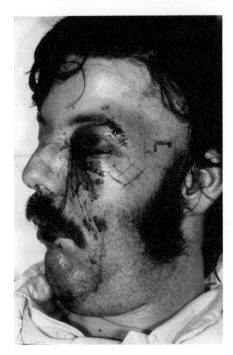

Figure 6.1 Fractured zygoma (marked '#' on skin), and facial lacerations.

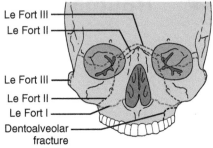

Figure 6.2 Le Fort fractures.

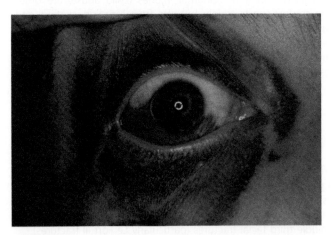

Figure 6.3 Haematoma and circumorbital and subconjunctival haemorrhage after trauma.

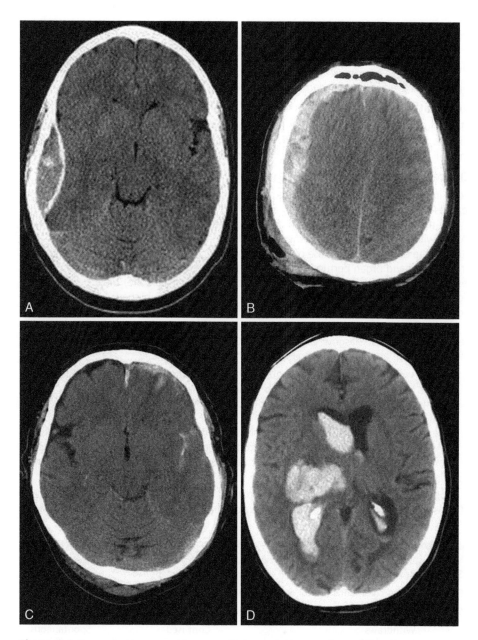

Figure 6.4 Computed tomographic scans of intracranial haemorrhage. **(A)** Epidural; **(B)** subarachnoid; **(C)** subarachnoid; **(D)** intracerebral. Reprinted from DeLee JC, Drez Jr D, Miller MD (1994) Delee & Drez's Orthopaedic sports medicine: principles and practice, 3e. Philadelphia, WB Saunders. With permission from Elsevier.

Head injury

Definition
Injury that may involve brain damage.

Aetiopathogenesis
Most injuries are in fit young males: RTAs, assaults and war injuries are the main causes. Patients are often multiply injured with hazards to other areas including airway, spine, eye, chest, liver, spleen, kidneys, long bones or bladder and are at risk of death.

Clinical presentation and management
Head injuries are a major cause of death – almost 50% of which occur before the patient reaches hospital.

Life-threatening injuries to immediately be addressed are – Airway, Breathing, Circulation (ABC), with care to avoid further neurological damage if cervical spine injury is possible. Stabilise the neck. Shock because of bleeding leading to hypovolaemia should be prevented or controlled and organ perfusion ensured by intravenous fluids. Vital signs (pulse rate, BP, respiratory rate, urine output and fluid balance and conscious state) must be monitored closely. The Advanced Trauma Life Support Manual (ATLS; published by The American College of Surgeons) has fuller details.

An essential step is to immediately assess, record, monitor and act upon the consciousness level using the Glasgow Coma Scale (GCS; Table 6.1), which records Eye opening, Motor response and Verbal response (EMV).

- Patients with a GCS score of <8 require immediate neurosurgical attention. 85% of patients with score of 3 or 4 succumb within 24 h.
- Patients who score <15 points should be admitted to hospital for observation – even if drugs or alcohol are suspected causes.
- Patients who are fully alert and otherwise well, with a full and unchanging score of EMV 15 and no neurological signs or symptoms, and no skull fracture or intracranial haemorrhage on CT or MRI scan, do not need hospital admission for observation – unless for other reasons.

A good history must be obtained from the patient, if conscious, and from witnesses. Loss of consciousness, amnesia, nausea, vomiting or headache must be noted, as well as the

Table 6.1 Glasgow Coma Scale (GCS)

Scale	Best motor response	Verbal response	Eye opening
6	Obeys commands (motor, verbal, eyes)		
5	Movement localized to stimulus	Orientated	
4	Withdraws	Confused	Spontaneous
3	Abnormal muscle bending and flexing	Inappropriate words	To speech
2	Involuntary muscle straightening and extending	Incomprehensible sounds	To pain
1	None	None	None

www.rayur.com/hemiplegia-defintion-causes-symptoms-diagnosis-and-treatment.html

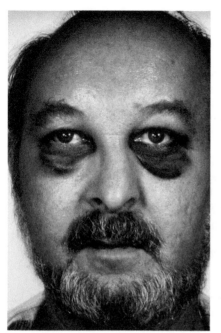

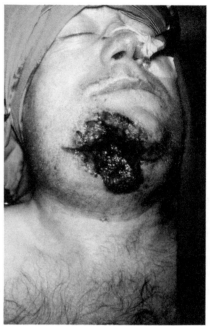

Figure 6.5 Le Fort type II, blood pooling behind skin under eyes.

Figure 6.6 Gunshot wound to chin before debridement.

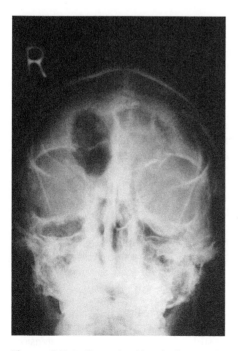

Figure 6.7 Radiograph of head after gunshot, front view; showing air in frontal lobe.

medical and drug history. The brain is invariably damaged in those who lost consciousness for however briefly, and sometimes in those who have not. Amnesia is common. Many patients are confused, concussed or comatose, though 30% of patients with ultimately fatal head injuries may talk after injury and some are completely lucid for a time. Maintenance of consciousness does not guarantee no brain injury, but the extent of retrograde amnesia is a rough measure of its severity. Concussion, an immediate but transient loss of consciousness, is always associated with some amnesia and brain damage, even if not detectable from neurological testing, cerebrospinal fluid (CSF) examination, CT or MRI. Consciousness is almost invariably impaired after diffuse brain damage, and there is usually amnesia for the traumatic event, and after (post-traumatic amnesia). Consciousness may not be lost if brain damage is local (e.g. skull penetration by a sharp object).

After trauma, patients must be carefully and regularly observed for intracranial bleeding and other complications. CT scans are essential to exclude skull fractures, bleeding and brain lesions. MRI can provide better images but cannot always be used.

- *Deterioration of consciousness* is the most important sign, sometimes with worsening restlessness, headache and vomiting.
- *Pupil size and reaction* must be checked for localizing signs of neurological damage. A dilated fixed (unreactive to light) pupil often indicates rising intracranial pressure (ICP) – usually a serious sign.
- *BP* that is low or falling with rising pulse rate is indicative of haemorrhage or shock, which can lead to fatal cerebral anoxia or renal failure. A high or rising BP with bradycardia, by contrast, is indicative of raised ICP secondary to cerebral oedema or haemorrhage.
- *A skull fracture* greatly increases the risk of brain damage and an intracranial haematoma; but the brain can be fatally damaged without any skull fracture.
- *CSF leaks* risk meningitis.
- *Epidural (extradural) bleeding* (between skull and dura mater) – usually due to middle meningeal artery tearing after a temporal bone fracture evolves rapidly and compresses the brain and raises ICP. The typical story is of a heavy blow followed by loss of consciousness. There is usually then a period of apparent recovery (lucid interval) followed by signs of rising ICP. This is an emergency requiring neurosurgical skull burr holes to drain the clot and ligate the bleeding vessel to avoid death from respiratory arrest.
- *Subdural bleeding* – between dura and leptomeninges, often caused by a tear in the arachnoid – is venous and associated with brain contusion. Acute subdural haematoma is and may be associated with laceration or contusion of the brain. Clinically, there is a latent interval after the injury, followed by progressive deterioration of consciousness and development of symptoms similar to those of an extradural haematoma. Evacuating the clot through burr holes improves survival. Chronic subdural haematoma can be caused by a very mild injury usually in an older person, who after several weeks, or even months, develops symptoms such as headache, dizziness, slowness of thinking, or confusion and disturbance of consciousness. Treatment is neurosurgery. Intracerebral (sub-arachnoid) bleeding may not be amenable to surgical intervention.

Head injury sequelae

Approximately 50% of patients have paralyses, speech loss, impaired vision, epilepsy, personality disturbances or mental defects. Management goals are to detect damage and prevent or reverse secondary insults to the brain, such as from hypoxaemia, hypotension and intracranial bleeding or haematoma – to allow recovery of as much damaged brain tissue as possible. Medical complications of head injuries can include: cardiovascular (neurogenic hypertension, myocardial dysfunction, arrhythmias or deep vein thrombosis); respiratory (neurogenic pulmonary oedema, infections, embolism); coagulopathy (disseminated intravascular coagulopathy); electrolyte imbalance (hyponatraemia, hypernatraemia or hypokalaemia); endocrine (inadequate or inappropriate secretion of ADH); gastrointestinal (stress gastritis and haemorrhage); fat embolism (mainly after long bone fractures); or infections (of wounds, foreign bodies, CSF, intravenous lines, intracranial pressure monitoring devices, sinuses and lungs). Tetanus can be an issue. Since 60% of coma patients are drug users or alcoholics, these need management.

Long-term sequelae

These may include: intracranial haematomas; epilepsy; infection; mental or physical disability; compensation neurosis; or post-traumatic syndrome or damage to the cochlear–vestibular apparatus). Complaints include temporary headache, irritability, inability to concentrate, short temper, loss of confidence, vertigo and hyperacusis. If symptoms persist, psychiatric advice should be sought.

Dental considerations

Trauma to face, jaws and teeth needs consideration after head and other serious injuries have been addressed.

Further reading

http://intranet.tdmu.edu.te.ua/data/kafedra/theacher/stomat_hir/stojanno/English/Recommendation%20
    for%20preparing%20practical%20classes/4%20course/13.%20Zygomatic%20and%20nasal%20
    bones%20damages.htm

Non-accidental injury (NAI; see also Section 4)

Definition
Any act of omission or commission that endangers or impairs the physical or emotional health or development of an individual.

Aetiopathogenesis
Families living in adverse social environments (e.g. poverty, social isolation or poor housing), are mainly involved. People with disabilities are much more at risk of experiencing abuse.

Injuries are usually inflicted by an adult, often a parent or parent's partner or an older sibling. Young or single parents, parents with learning difficulties, those who themselves have had adverse childhoods and those with mental health problems (including drug or alcohol abuse) are all more at risk of abusing their children. In the case of older people, most abuse is perpetrated against those over age 70, and a quarter of abusers are their children. Staff in care homes or visiting carers may also abuse.

Clinical presentation
A person is considered to be abused if treated in a way that is unacceptable in a given culture at a given time. Abuse and neglect are described as physical, emotional, sexual and neglect, but some level of emotional abuse is involved in all ill-treatment. Physical abuse may involve hitting, shaking, throwing, poisoning, burning or scalding, drowning, suffocating or otherwise causing physical harm. The head and face are the areas most commonly affected. Some suffer significant neurological, intellectual or emotional damage. Psychological trauma can cause sleep disturbances, eating disorders, developmental growth failure, and nervous habits such as lip and fingernail biting and thumb sucking. Effects may also include chronic under-achievement and poor peer relationships.

Diagnosis
Recognition of abuse is important since there is a high risk of further assaults, or death (Box 6.1). After genuine accidents, victims are usually immediately taken for medical attention but, when abused, there is often considerable delay. Abuse should also be suspected if any injuries are incompatible with the history. Take care to exclude disease which may cause similar injuries (e.g. osteogenesis imperfecta). See also, Section 10; vulnerable groups.

Management
Healthcare professionals are obliged to know and follow local procedures. Full records must be kept (www.cpdt.org.uk/). The victim must be fully and immediately examined to exclude

---

Box 6.1 Findings suggestive of non-accidental injury

- Cowed person
- Long interval before attendance for treatment
- Evidence of previous injury (or a previous history of injury)
- Injuries often committed at night
- Multiple injuries incompatible with history at unusual sites.

serious injury, especially subdural haematomas or intraocular bleeding, and must therefore be admitted to and kept in hospital until the diagnosis is confirmed. A skeletal radiographic survey should be undertaken to reveal both new and old injuries. All injuries must be carefully recorded, with photographs.

The main charitable and government-sponsored organizations that offer support include police, hospitals, general medical practitioners, carer organizations, social services/social work departments, and social care inspection bodies. Be clear about whether the person knows you are reporting your concerns; whether the person is confused or lacks the capacity to make informed decisions about his/her life; who you think is being abused (name, address, age); what you think is happening to that person; and give reasons/examples to illustrate why you think abuse is occurring.

Dental considerations

Trauma to face, jaws and teeth need consideration after head and other serious injuries have been addressed. Injuries in abuse can be varied and often multiple, including bites, bruises, black eyes, torn fraenum, hair loss, laceration, wheals, marks from a ligature or gag, burns and scalds. Child abuse is of particular concern because >65% of cases involve head and oral–facial trauma: dentists are required to report suspected cases and, in the young child, head injury is the most common cause of death. Ensure that there are not other issues such as bruising in thrombocytopenia that may mimic abuse.

Spinal trauma

Spinal cord injury (SCI) usually begins with a blow that fractures or dislocates the vertebrae, and causes damage when pieces of vertebrae tear into the cord. The level at which the spinal cord is injured, and type of injury to the cord (complete or partial) determine the extent of neurological deficits – sensory and motor (Table 6.2). With a complete spinal cord injury there is paralysis below the injury but with an incomplete injury, some movement and sensation are retained below the injury.

The most dangerous are higher spinal cord injuries which may cause:

- impaired ventilation
- reduced gag and cough reflex
- difficulty controlling oral fluids.

Most patients with lumbar injuries or below become wheelchair-independent and may be able to walk independently with long leg braces and crutches.

Diagnosis

- Clinical
- CT
- MRI.

Treatment

SCI is an emergency: immediate treatment can reduce long-term effects. Protect the airway and neck, give oxygen and call an ambulance. In patients involved in RTAs, movement of

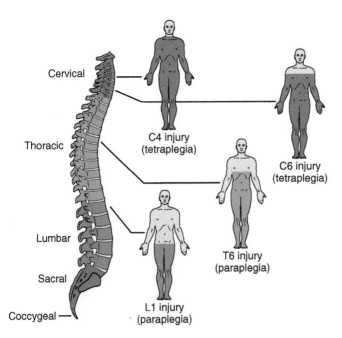

Figure 6.8 Cord injuries.

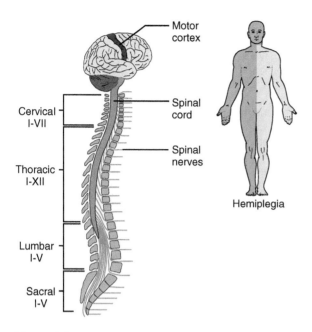

Figure 6.9 Hemiplegia; typically a result of damage to motor cortex.

Table 6.2	Effects of spinal cord injuries at different levels
Level	**Features**
C1–C5	Quadriplegia (tetraplegia) or death
C5–C6	Paraplegia, hands paralyzed Arms paralyzed except for abduction and flexion
C6–C7	Paraplegia. Hands, but not arms, paralyzed
T1	Paraplegia. Normal hand function. All functions of a non-injured person, except standing and walking
T2–T5	Paraplegia. Patients have partial trunk movement and may be able to stand, with long leg braces and a walker, and may be able to walk short distances with assistance
T6–T12	Paraplegia, but have partial abdominal muscle strength, and may be able to walk independently for short distances with long leg braces and a walker or crutches
T11–T12	Paraplegia, and sensory loss at T12 and below
T12–L1	Legs paralyzed below knees
L2	Patients have all movement in the trunk and hips
L3	Patients have knee extension
L4	Patients have ankle dorsiflexion
L5	Patients have extensor hallucis longus function, are able to walk independently with ankle braces and canes
S1–S2	Patients have gastrocnemius and soleus function and walk independently on all surfaces, usually without bracing

the neck if damaged may cause serious cord damage, spastic quadriplegia or death. The neck must never be extended or rotated; a support collar should be fitted prophylactically. Hospitalization is needed. Treatments may include, braces or traction to stabilize the spine, and surgery. Diaphragmatic pacemakers and mechanical ventilation may be needed.

Dental considerations

Cervical spine injury is potentially fatal and may be symptomless whilst the patient is conscious due to protective muscle spasm which 'stabilizes' the spine. After trauma, avoid any movement of the spinal column, and establish and maintain proper immobilization with the use of an appropriate neck splint until vertebral fractures or spinal cord injuries have been carefully ruled out. GA is very dangerous, as this protective muscle spasm is abolished on induction. Patients with spinal injuries may be unable to respond protectively. Many are chairbound and can sometimes be treated in their wheelchair or using a double-articulating headrest, but otherwise, transfer them to the dental chair by carrying them, using a hoist, or by sliding them across a 'banana' transfer board, or tilt their wheelchair. Bowel and bladder are best emptied before dental treatment. There is a high prevalence of latex allergy and some are on anticoagulants or other medication. Postural hypotension is likely, and thus the patient is best not treated supine.

7 Infections

A range of infections

Microorganisms important in healthcare worldwide are mainly bacterial, fungal or viral. Malaria is a huge issue, especially in the tropics. Space precludes discussion of other parasites and infections that currently are seen mainly in people in and from resource-poor regions. Infections are increased among immune- and medically compromised patients and this includes children in whom immunity has yet to develop naturally or by immunization, and older people whose immunity is declining with age or illness.

Aetiopathogenesis

Infection transmission is by direct contact with mucosae, body fluids, aerosols, air drops, or instruments which are contaminated. Some infections are particularly important because of the risk of cross-infection in healthcare. Universal (standard) infection control measures must always be used. Standard Infection Control Precautions (SICP) are designed to prevent cross-transmission from recognized and unrecognized sources of infection. These sources of (potential) infection include blood and other body fluid secretions or excretions and any equipment or items in the care environment which are likely to become contaminated. Measures necessary include (adapted from NHS Professionals: Standard Infection Control Precautions):

- Hand hygiene
- Respiratory hygiene
- Personal protective equipment
- Occupational exposure management including sharps
- Management of care equipment
- Safe care of linen including uniforms
- Control of environment
- Safe waste disposal.

Viral, bacterial, fungal and parasitic infections that are transmitted mainly through sexual contact are considered sexually transmitted or shared diseases or infections (STDs or SSIs). These infections can often be transmitted by direct contact with a lesion, blood, genital fluids or saliva, so appropriate precautions are always indicated. Worldwide rates of STDs are increasing, with young people (16–24 years) accounting for 50% of all cases. Common STDs include:

- **Viral**
  - Epstein–Barr virus (EBV)
  - Hepatitis B (HBV)
  - Herpes simplex virus (HSV)-1 and HSV-2

- HIV/AIDS
- HPV (human papillomaviruses)
- **Bacterial**
  - *Chlamydia trachomatis* (chlamydia)
  - *Haemophilus ducreyi* (chancroid)
  - *Mycoplasma genitalium* (non-gonoccocal urethritis; NGU)
  - *Neisseria gonorrhoeae* (gonorrhoea)
  - *Treponema pallidum* (syphilis)
  - *Ureaplasma urealyticum* (non-gonococcal urethritis; NGU)
- **Fungal**
  - *Candida* (thrush or candidiasis)
- **Parasites**
  - *Phthirus pubis* (pubic lice, 'crabs')
  - *Sarcoptes scabiei* (scabies)
  - *Trichomonas vaginalis* (trichomoniasis).

Table 7.1 Bacterial infections

Infecting organism	Main features	Treatment
Bacillus anthracis	Anthrax	Penicillin
Borrelia burgdorferi	Lyme disease	Doxycycline, amoxicillin, cefuroxime axetil
Brucella, melitensis, suis and *abortus*	Brucellosis	Tetracycline with streptomycin
Clostridium perfringens (Cl. welchii), Cl. sporogenes, Cl. oedematiens, Cl. septicum	Gas gangrene	Antitoxin Penicillin
Clostridium tetani	Tetanus	Antitoxin Penicillin
Legionella pneumophila	Legionellosis	Antibiotics
Mycobacterium avium-intracellulare	Skin/respiratory	Antibiotics
Mycobacterium leprae	Leprosy	Antibiotics
Mycobacterium tuberculosis	Tuberculosis	Antibiotics
Mycoplasma hominis and *pneumoniae*	Pneumonia	Tetracyclines
Neisseria gonorrhoea	Gonorrhoea	Ceftriaxone with either azithromycin or doxycycline
Neisseria meningitidis	Meningitis	Penicillin
Salmonellae typhi, paratyphi, choleraesuis and *enteritidis*	Typhoid and paratyphoid fever	Co-trimoxazole Ampicillin
Streptococcus pyogenes	Pharyngitis Cellulitis Scarlet fever Erysipelas	Penicillin
Treponema pallidum	Syphilis	Penicillin

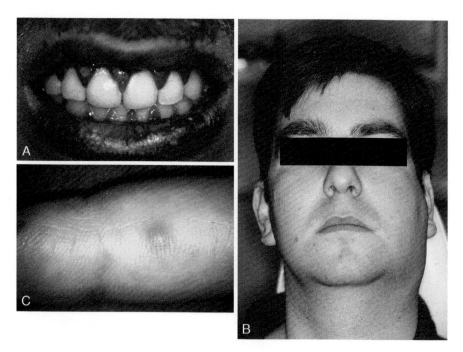

Figure 7.1 A range of viral infections: **(A)** herpes simplex stomatitis; **(B)** mumps, swelling on left side of face; **(C)** hand, foot and mouth disease.

Diagnosis

Clinical findings and sometimes specific cultures and microbiological identification, increasingly employing nucleic acid technology.

Treatment

Treatment of the main infections is shown in Tables 7.1–7.3.

Dental considerations

Elective dental care may be deferred in cases of active infection.

Table 7.2 Viral infections

Infecting organisms	Main features	Treatment
Coxsackie viruses	+/– rash	Symptomatic
Cytomegalovirus (CMV)	Glandular fever	Ganciclovir Foscarnet Valganciclovir
ECHO viruses	+/– rash	Symptomatic
Epstein–Barr virus (EBV)	Glandular fever	Aciclovir Ganciclovir
Haemorrhagic fever viruses (e.g. Ebola) – often lethal	Bleeding	Symptomatic
Hepatitis viruses	See Section 5	See Section 5
Herpes simplex viruses (HSV-1 and HSV-2)	Stomatitis or genital infection	Aciclovir Famciclovir
	Recurrent lesions at mucocutaneous junctions	Penciclovir Aciclovir Famciclovir Valaciclovir
Herpes varicella virus (VZV)	Chickenpox (varicella)	Aciclovir Valaciclovir
	Zoster (shingles)	Famciclovir Valaciclovir
HIV (human immunodeficiency virus)	HIV disease/AIDS (acquired immune deficiency syndrome)	Anti-retrovirals
Human herpesvirus-8 (Kaposi sarcoma herpesvirus, or KSHV)	Kaposi's sarcoma	Anti-retrovirals Symptomatic
Human papillomaviruses (HPV)	Warty lesions Carcinomas (ano-genital and oro-pharyngeal)	Removal or imiquimod
Influenza virus	Respiratory infection	Amantadine Oseltamivir Rimantadine Zanamivir
Measles virus	Exanthem (rash)	Symptomatic
Mumps virus	Sialadenitis	Symptomatic
Respiratory syncytial virus (RSV)	Respiratory infection	Symptomatic
Rhinoviruses	Common cold	Symptomatic
Rubella virus	Exanthem	Symptomatic
Zika virus	Birth and neurological defects	Symptomatic

Candidosis (candidiasis)

Definition

Candida albicans is a ubiquitous fungus found mainly on oral or genital mucosae.

Aetiopathogenesis

Carried commonly as a commensal, *Candida* species may become opportunistic pathogens causing infection (candidosis) typically where the local ecology is disturbed (from appliances, hyposalivation, or the local use of immunosuppressants or antimicrobials), or where there is a systemic immune defect (e.g. HIV/AIDS) or immunosuppression.

Candidosis is a 'disease of the diseased'.

Clinical presentation and classification

White and/or red painful or painless mucosal lesions may be seen. White patches that resemble milk curds on the surface of the mucosa characterize thrush and can be wiped off to reveal a raw erythematous and sometimes bleeding base. White adherent lesions may be found in chronic hyperplastic candidosis. Red (erythematous) areas are also characteristic of candidosis. Thrush (acute pseudomembranous candidosis) is the term used for the multiple white-fleck appearance of acute candidosis. *Chronic hyperplastic candidosis* typically presents as a leukoplakia often at the angles of the mouth or on the tongue, and it has a malignant potential.

Chronic mucocutaneous candidosis (CMC) is a group of rare syndromes, in which persistent mucocutaneous candidosis with persistent skin and mucosal lesions respond poorly to topical treatment.

Generally, the more severe the candidosis, the greater the likelihood that immunologic defects (particularly of cell-mediated immunity) can be identified.

Diagnosis

Usually based on physical examination alone. Candida stains poorly by haematoxylin and eosin, so Gram, periodic acid–Schiff (PAS), Gridley, or Gomori methenamine silver (GMS) stains are often used. PCR (polymerase chain reaction) or restriction fragment length polymorphism (RFLP) tests may be used.

Treatment

Antifungals are used, such as *Polyenes* – amphotericin, nystatin, and pimaricin – or *Azoles* including imidazoles (e.g., clotrimazole, miconazole, econazole, ketoconazole) and triazoles (e.g., fluconazole, itraconazole, voriconazole).

Dental considerations

Manifestations are typically red or white mucosal lesions.

Table 7.3   Fungal infections*

Disease	Organism	Source	Endemic	Main features
Aspergillosis	*Aspergillus fumigatus Aspergillus flavus Aspergillus niger* Others	Ubiquitous	Worldwide	Allergic bronchopulmonary, pulmonary, disseminated aspergilloma
Blastomycosis	*Blastomyces dermatiditis*	Soil	Mississippi and Ohio valleys in USA, Canada, North Africa and Venezuela	Cavitary pulmonary, disseminated, others
Candidosis	*Candida* spp., *albicans, tropicalis, glabrata, parapsilosis, krusei, lusitaniae, kefyr, guilliermondii, dubliniensis*	Ubiquitous	Worldwide	Mucocutaneous candidosis may respond to topical antifungals (nystatin, amphotericin or an azole) except in disseminated forms
Coccidioidomycosis	*Coccidioides immitis*	Soil	Southwestern USA, Mexico, Latin America	Acute pulmonary, disseminated, chronic pulmonary, meningitis
Cryptococcosis	*Cryptococcus neoformans*	Soil, pigeon droppings	Worldwide	Pneumonia, meningitis, disseminated, crypto-coccoma
Histoplasmosis	*Histoplasma capsulatum*	Soil, bird and bat droppings	Mississippi and Ohio valleys in USA, Latin America, Africa, India, Far East, Australia	Benign pulmonary, disseminated, chronic pulmonary, cutaneous
Mucormycosis	*Mucor, Rhizopus* and *Absidia*	Ubiquitous	Worldwide	Rhinocerebral, pulmonary, gastrointestinal
Paracoccidioidomycosis (South American blastomycosis)	*Paracoccidioides brasiliensis*	Soil	South America, esp. Brazil	Pulmonary, disseminated
Pneumocystosis	*Pneumocystis carinii (jiroveci)*	Ubiquitous	Worldwide	Pulmonary, disseminated
Sporotrichosis	*Sporothrix schenkii*	Thorny plants, wood, sphagnum moss	Worldwide	Lympho-cutaneous, localized cutaneous, pulmonary, disseminated

*Systemic treatment is usually with fluconazole or another azole (e.g. ketoconazole, miconazole, itraconazole, voriconazole).

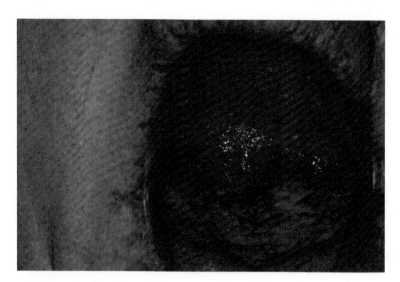

Figure 7.2 Candidosis (thrush).

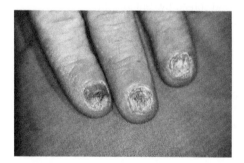

Figure 7.3 Chronic candidosis.

Creutzfeldt–Jakob disease (CJD)

Definition

A progressive lethal degenerative brain disease characterized by microscopic vacuoles in the CNS grey matter, giving a sponge-like (spongiform) appearance – a transmissible spongiform encephalopathy (TSE).

Aetiopathogenesis and classification

Animal TSEs are several, including bovine spongiform encephalopathy (BSE – 'mad cow disease'), and scrapie in sheep and goats. TSEs are associated with an abnormal form of a host-encoded protein termed a prion (proteinaceous infectious particle) – PrP, originally termed 'slow virus' though no virus has ever been associated. A protease resistant isoform (PrPsc) which fails to evoke a protective immune response, accumulates in the brain in prion diseases especially in the CNS and posterior orbit – tissues which are most likely to be infective. Some TSEs are transmissible from animal to man.

Human TSEs exist in acquired, inherited (familial) or sporadic forms (Table 7.4), and are often referred to collectively as Creutzfeldt–Jakob disease or CJD:

- *Acquired CJD* forms include:
  - *Variant* CJD (vCJD) – seems to be a variant of BSE, recognized in UK in 1986, spread by use of meat and bonemeal in cattle food. In 1996, vCJD first appeared in humans, linked to ingestion of BSE-infected bovine offal but is now rare.
  - *Kuru* – an acquired spongiform encephalopathy which was endemic among the Fore ethnic group in Papua New Guinea and spread by cannibalism.
  - *Iatrogenic* CJD (iCJD) can be transmitted mainly by exposure to:
    - cadaver-derived growth hormone;
    - pituitary gonadotropins;
    - dura mater homografting;
    - corneal grafts; or
    - inadequately sterilized neurosurgical equipment.

Recipients of human growth hormone were excluded from blood donation in 1989, and recipients of other human-derived pituitary hormones have been excluded since 1993, to avoid the possibility of prion transmission.

There is concern over use of human dura mater grafts since theoretically they might contain prions.

- *Familial CJD* (fCJD) – rare autosomal dominant disorders that do not manifest until adult life.
- *Sporadic CJD* (sCJD), where no source is identifiable (85% of all CJD cases).

Clinical presentation

All TSEs have prolonged incubation periods of months to years. Psychiatric symptoms (severe depression) and behavioural issues together with persistent paraesthesias and dys-aesthesias, are followed by dementia, cerebellar and other neurological signs, myoclonus or other involuntary movements, and finally akinetic mutism, gradually increasing in severity and leading to death over months or years.

Diagnosis

Clinical, and investigations that can include:

- Blood tests; genetic mutations related to vCJD and raised neurone-specific enolase (NSE)
- CSF analysis

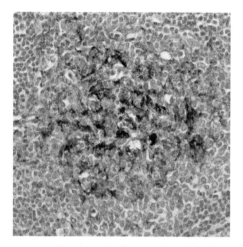

Figure 7.4 Tonsil biopsy in variant CJD. Prion Protein immunostaining. By Sbrandner (own work) [GFDL (www.gnu.org/copyleft/fdl.html) or CC-BY-SA-3.0-2.5-2.0-1.0 (http://creativecommons.org/licenses/by-sa/3.0)], via Wikimedia Commons.

Table 7.4 Creutzfeldt–Jakob disease types

Type	Abbreviation	Comments
Sporadic	sCJD	–
Familial	fCJD	Autosomal dominant
Kuru	–	Ritualistic cannibalism
Iatrogenic	iCJD	Contaminated surgical instruments. Dura mater grafts or pituitary hormones
Variant	vCJD or nvCJD	Consumption of BSE-infected material

- EEG
- MRI
- Psychometric tests
- Tonsillar biopsy.

Treatment

No effective therapy is available.

Dental considerations

PrPsc is uniquely resistant to inactivation by heat, disinfectants, ionizing, ultraviolet and microwave radiations – a significant infection control challenge.

Effective cleaning (to remove adherent tissue) coupled with autoclaving produces a significant reduction in infectivity levels on instruments if a non-porous load steam sterilizer is used at 134–137°C for a single cycle of 18 minutes, or six successive cycles of 3 minutes.

Concentrated bleach does appear to inactivate prions; 20,000 ppm available chlorine of sodium hypochlorite for 1 hour, or 2 M sodium hydroxide for 1 hour are considered effective. Copper-hydrogen peroxide may be effective. There are significant restrictions to blood donations in order to protect the blood supply.

Endocarditis (see Cardiovascular disease)

See Section 5, Cardiovascular.

Gonorrhoea

Definition
Infection by the bacterium *Neisseria gonorrhoeae* predominantly of the urethra or endocervix; sometimes of the rectum, oro-pharynx or conjunctivae.

Aetiopathogenesis
A sexually shared infection (SSI), less common than most, but about 15 times more common than syphilis. Transmission is by genital–genital, genital–anorectal, oro-genital or oro-anal contact or by mother-to-child transmission at birth. The highest incidence of gonorrhoea is in young adults with a disproportionate prevalence in ethnic minority groups and MSM (men who have sex with men).

Clinical presentation and classification
Rectal and pharyngeal infections in either gender are mostly asymptomatic. Genital tract infections are asymptomatic in 50% women and up to 10% in men. In females, endocervical and urethral infection may cause increased or altered vaginal discharge, intermenstrual bleeding, dysuria and menorrhagia. In males, acute urethritis with urethral discharge and dysuria is the main symptomatic presentation. Since gonorrhoea in all sites is often asymptomatic, it increases risk of transmission.

An important complication of genital gonorrhoea is urethral stenosis. Infection can also ascend the genital tract to cause pelvic inflammatory disease (PID) and epididymo-orchitis or disseminate in bacteraemia.

Diagnosis
Diagnosis is established by identification of *N. gonorrhoeae* in secretions. Culture allows confirmatory identification and antimicrobial susceptibility testing. Nucleic Acid Amplification Tests (NAATs) are generally more sensitive than culture. Serology is uninformative.

Treatment
A single dose of a cephalosporin (oral cefixime or injectable ceftriaxone) is recommended, but since cefixime is becoming less effective, the extended-spectrum cephalosporin (ESC) ceftriaxone intramuscular (IM), in combination with an oral antibiotic (azithromycin or doxycycline) is increasingly used.

The gonorrhoea H041 strain resistant to ceftriaxone is spreading.

Co-infection with *Chlamydia trachomatis* is common in young heterosexuals with gonorrhoea; this is also treated (ceftriaxone and doxycycline or azithromycin).

Dental considerations
Oral manifestations may include inflammation, pseudomembrane formation, pustules, tonsillar inflammation/infection.

Healthcare associated infections

Main dental considerations

(*See also generic guidance under main dental considerations on page 63 top, and also Section 2).

Infection control is as always, essential. Surgery and trauma may lead to wound infections – a type of healthcare associated infection (HCAI). Tetanus can follow contaminated wounds.

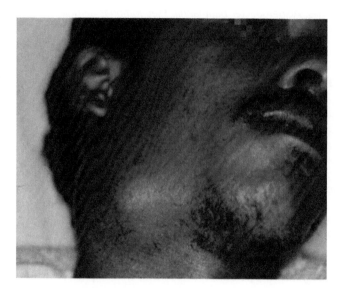

Figure 7.5 Infected intrao-oral wound.

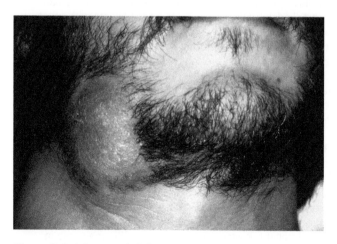

Figure 7.6 Odontogenic infection.

HCAI or nosocomial infections are increasing globally and may affect wounds (surgical site infections), skin, respiratory tract, gastrointestinal tract, urinary tract, catheters, ventilators or any implanted device. Catheter-associated urinary tract infections, and ventilator-associated pneumonia (VAP) account for about two-thirds of all *non-surgical site* HCAIs.

Several microorganisms can be involved in HCAI, usually bacteria, and many are antimicrobial-resistant ('super bugs'). The main examples of these antibiotic-resistant infections are methicillin-resistant *Staph. aureus* (MRSA), and clindamycin-resistant *Clostridium difficile* (*C. diff*) but there are several others, and the most important are discussed, alphabetically, below. Six of these bacteria have been dubbed ESKAPE (*Enterococcus faecium, Staph. aureus; Klebsiella* species, *Acinetobacter baumannii, Pseudomonas aeruginosa* and *Enterobacter* species). Some of these infections are with multi-drug resistant organisms (MDRO).

Drug resistant infectious agents

Acinetobacter are common in soil and water; infections in the community are rare, and most strains are sensitive to antibiotics. Infections are usually HCAIs – typically in intensive care units, in very ill patients and with resistant organisms. *Acinetobacter baumannii* accounts for about 80% of infections and these include pneumonia, bacteraemia, wound infections, and urinary tract infections – often resistant to antibiotics and increasingly difficult to treat. Carbapenems (imipenem, meropenem, or doripenem) are most important options for serious infections caused by multidrug-resistant *A. baumannii*.

Burkholderia cepacia is a group of bacteria found in soil and water, often resistant to common antibiotics, but posing little risk to healthy people. They can cause infections in people with immune defects or chronic lung disease (particularly cystic fibrosis/bronchiectasis). Treatment typically needs multiple antibiotics and may include ceftazidime, doxycycline, piperacillin, meropenem, chloramphenicol or co-trimoxazole.

Clostridium difficile (also called C. diff, and CDI) is the major reason for antibiotic-associated diarrhoea and colitis, usually caused by expanded-spectrum and broad-spectrum cephalosporins and clindamycin; mostly affects older patients with other underlying diseases in hospital environments. The disease usually develops after cross-infection from another patient, or via healthcare staff, or a contaminated environment. Metronidazole and vancomycin are the treatments of choice, but some strains are now resistant.

Clostridium sordellii is a rare bacterial cause of pneumonia, endocarditis, arthritis, peritonitis, and myonecrosis typically susceptible to β-lactams, clindamycin, tetracycline, and chloramphenicol but resistant to aminoglycosides and sulfonamides.

Extended-spectrum beta-lactamase (ESBL) producers are Gram-negative enteric bacilli (Enterobacteriaceae) most commonly *Escherichia coli* and *Klebsiella pneumonia*. ESBL infection may originate in infected chicken meat and outbreaks have originated in hospitals, nursing homes, and the community, typically as urinary tract infections and bacteraemia. The vast majority of Enterobacteriaceae, including ESBL producers, remain susceptible to carbapenems. However, carbapenem-resistant Enterobacteriaceae (CRE) or glycopeptide resistant enterococci (GRE) may arise in *Klebsiella* species and *E. coli* – most commonly in patients receiving treatment involving devices such as catheters or ventilators, and in those who are on long antibiotic courses.

Methicillin-resistant *Staphylococcus aureus* (MRSA) is resistant to beta-lactam antibiotics (methicillin [meticillin] and other more common antibiotics such as oxacillin, flucloxacillin, penicillin, and amoxicillin). MRSA is usually spread through person-to-person contact with someone who is colonized or who has an MRSA infection. It can also spread through contact with towels, sheets, clothes, dressings or other objects that have been used by someone with MRSA. *Staph. aureus* can also survive on objects or surfaces such as door handles, sinks, floors and cleaning equipment. MRSA infections are most commonly hospital-associated (HA-MRSA). Community-associated MRSA infections (CA-MRSA), are typically skin infections of buttocks, genitals or perineum in men who have sex with men.

Penicillin-resistant *Streptococcus pneumoniae* (PRSP) treatment is generally with a 3rd generation cephalosporin, or vancomycin.

Stenotrophomonas (Pseudomonas) maltophilia ('steno') infection is with an aerobic, non-fermentative, Gram-negative bacterium of low virulence found in aquatic environments. It frequently colonizes fluids in hospitals (e.g. irrigation solutions, intravenous fluids) and is found in patient secretions (e.g. secretions, urine, exudates). *Stenotrophomonas maltophilia* is susceptible to trimethoprim–sulfamethoxazole, meropenem, minocycline, quinolones and colistin/polymyxin B.

Vancomycin-resistant Enterococci (VRE) are often present in the normal intestinal flora and female genital tract, as well as in the environment. Most infections occur in hospitals acquired from other people or contaminated food or water. Most VRE infections can be treated with antibiotics other than vancomycin.

Vancomycin-intermediate *Staphylococcus aureus* (VISA) and vancomycin-resistant *Staphylococcus aureus* (VRSA) infections are seen usually in people with underlying health conditions (e.g. diabetes, chronic kidney disease), devices (e.g. catheters), previous infections with MRSA, and recent exposure to vancomycin and other antimicrobials. Quinupristin–dalfopristin, linezolid, tetracycline, trimethoprim–sulfamethoxazole (TMP-SMX), tigecycline and daptomycin, have been used for treatment of VISA.

Surgical wound infections (surgical site infections; SSIs)
Aetiopathogenesis

SSIs usually arise from the patient's own flora or from healthcare workers or articles brought into the operative field. Factors promoting infection include preoperative removal of hair, especially when there is skin abrasion, inadequate skin preparation with bactericidal solution, poor surgical technique, lengthy operations (>2 h), intraoperative contamination, prolonged stay in hospital, hypothermia, trauma, non-viable tissue in the wound, haematoma, foreign material (including drains and sutures), dead space, pre-existing sepsis (local or distant), immunocompromised or malnourished host, hypovolaemia, poor tissue perfusion, or obesity, and delayed prophylaxis with, or incorrect choice of, antibiotics.

The usual pathogens on skin are Gram-positive aerobic cocci (mainly staphylococci), but anaerobes and Gram-negative aerobes may be involved. Gram-negative aerobes may be a problem in patients who have been hospitalized or treated with radiotherapy. Most infections are transient with few untoward sequelae but some can cause serious, recurrent, disseminated or persistent lesions – especially in immunocompromised persons, such as neutropenic patients, those with organ transplants, and in HIV/AIDS.

Clinical presentation

Classic features are heat (*calor*), swelling (*tumour*), pain (*dolor*) and loss of function (*functio laesi*).

Diagnosis

On clinical grounds, supported by smears, culture, testing for immune responses (serology) and, increasingly, by examining for nucleic acids.

Treatment

Open the wound, evacuating pus and cleansing the wound – inspecting deeper tissues for integrity and for deep space infection or source. Often also antibiotics. The choice depends on the known or probable infecting microorganism, and factors such as severity of SSI, patient's age, hepatic and renal function, allergies and other medication(s). First choices are flucloxacillin in the absence of allergy if staphylococci or streptococci are implicated; metronidazole or clindamycin for anaerobic infections; cefuroxime for Gram-negative organisms; amoxicillin or co-amoxiclav for enterococcal infection.

Central line-associated bloodstream infections (CLABSI)

CLABSI is one of the most deadly and costly hospital-associated infections. Microorganisms implicated can be any of hundreds of common commensals (i.e., diphtheroids, *Bacillus* spp., *Propionibacterium* spp., coagulase-negative staphylococci [including *S. epidermidis*], viridans group streptococci, *Aerococcus* spp., and *Micrococcus* spp.). CLABSI can involve central lines (catheters) placed in great blood vessels.

The following devices are *not* considered central lines:

- Extracorporeal membrane oxygenation (ECMO)
- Femoral arterial catheters
- Haemodialysis reliable outflow (HeRO) dialysis catheters
- Intra-aortic balloon pump (IABP) devices.

To prevent CLABSI, healthcare providers should always:

- Select a vein where the catheter can be safely inserted and the infection risk is small.
- Clean hands with an alcohol-based hand rub before inserting the catheter.
- Wear mask, cap, sterile gown, and sterile gloves. The patient will be covered with a sterile sheet.
- Clean the patient's skin with an antiseptic cleanser before inserting the catheter.
- Clean their hands, wear gloves, and clean the catheter opening with an antiseptic solution before using the catheter to draw blood or give medications. Healthcare providers should also clean their hands and wear gloves when changing the bandage that covers the area where the catheter enters the skin.
- Remove the catheter as soon as it is no longer needed.
- Carefully handle medications and fluids that are given through the catheter.

Bites and puncture wounds

Bites

Dogs and cats cause most large animal bites in the UK. Dog bites may cause severe tissue injury to tissues as well as infections. Cat bites are more frequently (approximately 50%) infected.

Animal bite infections are usually bacterial – typically polymicrobial (staphylococci and anaerobes). Tetanus must be considered but is rarely transmitted by bites. Bites from non-immunized domestic animals and wild animals may carry the risk of rabies, which is more common in raccoons, skunks, bats and foxes than in cats and dogs. Rabbits, squirrels and other rodents rarely carry rabies. Cat scratch disease (CSD) is caused by a bacterium *Bartonella henselae* usually by being bitten or scratched by a cat (about 40% of cats carry *B. henselae* at some time in their lives but show no signs). Patients develop lymphadenopathy, especially around the head, neck, and axilla, and may develop fever, headache, fatigue, and anorexia.

Human bites are more likely to cause infections than are animal bites, since the oral flora contains many potentially pathogenic aerobic and anaerobic bacteria, among which are *Staphylococcus*, *Streptococcus*, *Clostridia* (and other anaerobes), and fusiform species. Tetanus is rarely a concern unless the wound is also contaminated by soil. Bites from humans may also carry the risk of blood-borne virus infections (BBV, e.g. haemorrhagic fevers, hepatitis B or C, or HIV): consideration of post-exposure prophylaxis (PEP) may then be important (see below).

Treatment of bites may include debridement, and antimicrobial coverage for staphylococci (co-amoxiclav) and anaerobes, and consideration of the possibilities of tetanus, rabies, and BBV. Any human bite could be from abuse and therefore should be assessed, preferably by a forensic clinician.

Puncture wounds

A puncture wound is caused by an object piercing the skin and creating a small hole. Some punctures can be very deep and do not often result in obvious excessive bleeding; they tend to close fairly quickly spontaneously. A puncture wound from a cause such as stepping on a nail can become infected. Treatment may be necessary to prevent tetanus or other infections. Most healthy people without signs of infection do not require antibiotics, but these may be given to people with diabetes, peripheral vascular disease, contaminated wounds or deep wounds to the foot.

Tetanus is a non-communicable infection caused by wound contamination with *Clostridium tetani* spores with mortality up to 60%. The spores are ubiquitous in soil or dust, particularly where there is faecal contamination, as on agricultural land. Tetanus is most likely to follow contaminated deep wounds, such as puncture wounds, especially if there is tissue necrosis, but it may also follow trivial wounds, or even bites or burns. Most cases of tetanus in the developed countries are seen in those who were never immunized, or in those whose immunity has declined – hence the risk is greatest in older people. The incubation period is between 4 and 21 days, commonly about 10 days.

Clostridium tetani produces a neurotoxin (tetanospasmin) responsible for violent muscular spasms: trismus (lockjaw) due to masseteric spasm the single most common early sign. Facial spasm produces a so-called sardonic smile (risus sardonicus) where the eyebrows are raised with eyes closed and the lips are drawn back over clenched teeth. Spinal muscle spasm produces arching of the back (opisthotonos), while laryngeal spasm can lead to asphyxiation. Autonomic dysfunction can cause cardiac arrhythmias and fluctuations in BP. Death may follow within 10 days of the onset of tetanus, usually from asphyxia, autonomic dysfunction or bronchopneumonia.

Patients who have contaminated wounds, such as those associated with road traffic or riding accidents, are at greatest risk from tetanus. Wounds that are considered tetanus-prone include any wound or burn sustained more than 6 h before surgical treatment of the injury, or that shows a significant degree of devitalized tissue; a puncture wound; contact with manure or soil; or clinical sepsis. Management of wounds where tetanus is likely includes anti-tetanus immunoglobulin (give early as it is ineffective after the toxin has become bound to nervous tissue) – human anti-tetanus immunoglobulin (ATG; Humotet, 500 units or more), antibiotics and active immunization with tetanus toxoid, but it is not good practice to give toxoid after every minor injury, as severe allergic reactions can occasionally follow.

Prophylaxis is active immunization tetanus in childhood; the duration of immunity is not known but current practice is to boost it every 10 years. Groups at highest risk (e.g. farm workers) should be given boosters every 5 years.

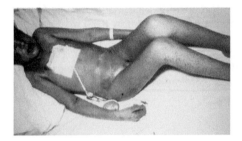

Figure 7.7 Tetanus. Reprinted from Porter SR, Scully C, Welsby P, Gleeson M (1999) Medicine and Surgery for Dentistry: Colour Guide. Churchill Livingstone. With permission from Elsevier.

Herpes viruses

Herpes simplex viruses (HSV)
Definition and aetiopathogenesis
Type 1 HSV (HSV-1) typically causes primary infection with acute stomatitis. HSV-2 typically causes anogenital infections but may cause oral or oropharyngeal infections. HSV thereafter remains latent in the sensory ganglia but may be reactivated by systemic infections, sunlight, trauma, stress, menstruation or immune incompetence.

Clinical presentations
Primary oral infection with HSV, usually HSV-1, typically causes acute gingivostomatitis, ulcers, fever, cervical lymph node enlargement and irritability, but may cause primary pharyngeal or anogenital infection (almost always caused by oral–genital contact with an infected person). Oral herpes is common in young children, sometimes misdiagnosed as 'teething', or may be subclinical, and resolves in 10 days. HSV-2 infection usually causes anogenital blisters which break, leaving tender ulcers that may take 2–4 weeks to heal. It is almost always contracted sexually and may affect the mouth or oro-pharynx. Women should avoid contracting HSV-2 during pregnancy because a first episode risks transmission to the newborn, with potentially fatal foetal outcomes. If a woman has active genital herpes at parturition, a Caesarean delivery is therefore usually performed. Primary herpes infections

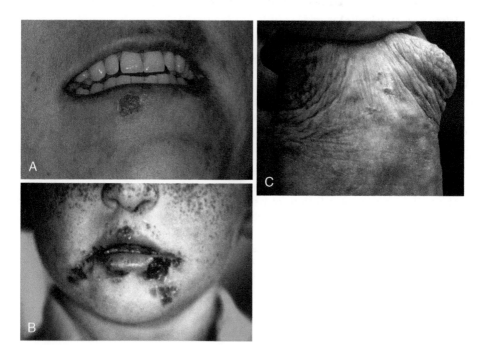

Figure 7.8 Herpes simplex viruses. **(A)** Herpes labialis (cold sore) on woman's lip; **(B)** Herpes labialis on immunocompromised child lips/around mouth; **(C)** Genital herpes.

are limited to the area but, in immunosuppressed or eczematous patients, may spread locally or disseminated infection may result.

Secondary infections (recurrences) may cause blistering at mucocutaneous junctions.

Diagnosis

Clinical but PCR or immunostaining can help.

Treatment

Antivirals (e.g. aciclovir) are effective against primary HSV or recurrent infections. Labial recurrences respond well to penciclovir or aciclovir creams or to hydrocolloid patches. Systemic aciclovir, famciclovir or others are essential to control primary infections or recurrences in immunocompromised patients. Treatment in primary infections is supplemented with adequate fluids, antipyretics and analgesics and good hygiene.

Dental considerations

Oral manifestations may include:

- Primary herpetic gingivostomatitis: painful ulcers, fever, cervical lymphadenopathy and irritability.
- Recurrent herpes labialis: painful vesicles typically on lip, that burst, ulcerate, then scab.
- Facial palsy.
- Erythema multiforme.

Herpes varicella zoster virus (VZV: Human herpesvirus 3)

Chickenpox (Varicella)

Definition

A highly contagious disease caused by the herpes varicella-zoster virus (VZV).

Aetiopathogenesis

Primary varicella infection spreads by droplets. During viraemia, VZV enters epidermal cells, causing a typical rash; enters sensory nerves travelling via retrograde axonal transport to neuronal cell bodies in sensory dorsal root ganglia, to become latent there.

Clinical presentation

Typically in children below age of 10 years, fever, malaise and a centripetal (mainly on trunk and face) rash which passes through macular, papular, vesicular and pustular stages before scabbing. There are about 3–5 crops of lesions. Patients are infectious from 1 to 2 days before the rash, until it scabs and dries. There may be mucosal ulcers.

Infants, adolescents, adults and immune-compromised persons are at risk for complications, such as disseminated or haemorrhagic varicella. Adults, especially those who are pregnant or who smoke, are at risk from fulminating varicella pneumonia. There is also a risk to the foetus and neonate if the mother contracts chickenpox in the first 20 weeks of pregnancy (congenital varicella syndrome – microcephaly, cataracts, growth retardation and limb hypoplasia) with a high mortality. Later in pregnancy, chickenpox may result in zoster in an otherwise healthy infant. Chickenpox around delivery time may cause severe or fatal infection of the neonate.

Diagnosis

Clinical usually (see also Herpes zoster).

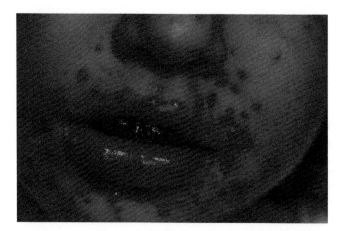

Figure 7.9 Chickenpox.

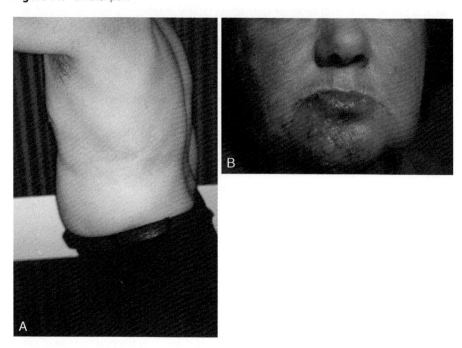

Figure 7.10 (A and B) Herpes zoster.

Treatment

Varicella-zoster immunoglobulin, or aciclovir, valaciclovir or famciclovir, may be indicated for pregnant or immunocompromised non-immune persons.

Prevention

Immunization of children against VZV can prevent or modify varicella if used within 3 days, and possibly up to 5 days of exposure, and reduces the risk of zoster later. If a person susceptible to VZV infection has close exposure to a person with zoster, post-exposure prophylaxis with varicella vaccine can be helpful: this is now also offered to older patients.

Dental considerations

Oral manifestations; mouth ulcers. Chickenpox is very contagious.

Herpes zoster (shingles)

Most (98%) of the adult population have non-infectious VZV latent within dorsal root ganglia but, if reactivated, as in immunocompromised (e.g. as a result of HIV/AIDS or a neoplasm, particularly a lymphoma) or older people, it can lead to shingles, when VZV migrates through axons to the skin, spreads from cell to cell, and penetrates the epidermis, causing pain, followed by a rash. Approximately 50% of persons aged 85 years or more will have experienced zoster.

Clinical presentation

Zoster is a painful, unilateral vesicular rash across closely overlapping dermatomes of the involved sensory nerve roots, usually of the chest or face. Zoster presents typically with a prodrome of headache, photophobia, and malaise. The rash is initially erythematous and maculopapular, but progresses to coalescing clusters of clear vesicles over several days and then evolves through pustular, ulcer, and crust stages over 7–10 days, with complete healing within 2-4 weeks. Trigeminal ophthalmic zoster may cause facial rash and pain and ulcerate the cornea. Zoster of the maxillary or mandibular divisions of the trigeminal nerve may cause facial rash and pain (sometimes simulating toothache) and ipsilateral oral ulceration.

Zoster is usually most severe in older adults and post-herpetic neuralgia (PHN), a persistent pain after resolution of the rash ranging from any duration after rash resolution to from >30 days to >6 months after rash onset is a common consequence of zoster in older people. PHN varies from mild to excruciating in severity, constant, intermittent, or triggered by trivial stimuli.

Diagnosis

Clinical. VZV can be identified by tissue culture, direct fluorescent antibody (DFA) staining or polymerase chain reaction (PCR) of a scraping.

Treatment

Aciclovir, famciclovir, and valacyclovir are treatments for zoster. Intravenous antivirals are needed in immunodeficient patients, particularly in those with HIV/AIDS, for whom zoster can be life-threatening.

The pain of PHN may not respond well to analgesics, but may respond to tricyclic antidepressants, carbamazepine or capsaicin, local heat; a cold spray; or transcutaneous electric nerve stimulation (TENS).

Dental considerations

Oral manifestations; unilateral pain and mouth ulcers in trigeminal zoster.

HIV/AIDS

Definitions

Infection with human immunodeficiency virus (HIV), a retrovirus, causes HIV disease which may be symptomless but, over time, ultimately damages CD4+ T lymphocytes, producing symptoms mainly from infections and/or neoplasms and the acquired immune deficiency syndrome (AIDS) (Table 7.5).

Table 7.5 AIDS-defining illnesses

Fungi
Candidosis
Pneumocystis carinii (jiroveci) pneumonia
Cryptococcus
Histoplasmosis
Others
Viruses
Herpes simplex
Herpes zoster
Epstein–Barr virus
Cytomegalovirus
Human herpes virus-8 (HHV-8)
Human papillomaviruses (HPV)
Molluscum contagiosum
Parasites
Toxoplasmosis
Leishmaniasis
Bacteria
Mycobacteria
Tuberculosis
Atypical mycobacterioses
Tumours
Kaposi sarcoma (HHV-8)
Lymphoma (EBV)
Cervical carcinoma (HPV)

Table 7.6 HIV/AIDS stages

CDC stage*				
1	**2**	**3**	**4a**	**4b–d**
Primary seroconversion illness	Asymptomatic	Persistent generalized lymphadenopathy (PGL)	AIDS-related complex (ARC)	AIDS: infections or tumours are AIDS indicator illnesses

*CDC, Centers for Disease Control, and Prevention Atlanta, Georgia, USA.

Aetiopathogenesis

There are two main viruses: HIV-1 (most common) and HIV-2. Both infect cells with CD4 surface receptors, mainly T-helper lymphocytes and brain glial cells; they then replicate within them and damage them. Body fluids such as semen may contain HIV as may saliva, breast milk and blood. HIV transmission is mainly sexual: most new cases are via heterosexual intercourse. HIV can also be transmitted by infected blood or blood products, including plasma, or tissues. HIV transmission by contaminated needles and syringes is an important route in injecting drug users. Cross-placental transfer is not uncommon. Transmission by needlestick ('sharps') injury is an occasional risk for healthcare workers.

There is no reliable evidence for HIV transmission by normal social contact or by biting insects.

Clinical presentations and classification

The incubation is weeks or months. CDC stages are:

A – asymptomatic, acute infection or persistent generalized lymphadenopathy.
B – symptomatic, not A or C conditions.
C – AIDS-defining illnesses.
CD4 T-cells categories include:
1. >500 × 10^6/L.
2. 200–500 × 10^6/L.
3. <200 × 10^6/L.

Early HIV infection may be symptomless or there may be glandular fever-like illness or persistent generalized lymphadenopathy (PGL). HIV antibodies develop and appear in the serum within 6 weeks to 6 months from infection (seroconversion).There is usually then a long asymptomatic period, but the risk of development of severe immunodeficiency, and symptoms of disease, increase with time, as the HIV damages CD4 helper cells in the immune and nervous systems lead to a lymphopenia and a fall in the ratio of CD4 to suppressor (CD8) lymphocytes. HIV damage to CD4+ lymphocytes leads to a profound cell-mediated immune defect, and *HIV disease*, symptomatic with infections and sometimes other features. HIV/AIDS common manifestations are infections, neoplasms, neurological and autoimmune disorders. Infections with viruses, mycobacteria, fungi and parasites, particularly *Pneumocystis carinii* (*jiroveci*) pneumonia and mucosal candidosis, are common. Loss of weight and wasting ('slim disease') is common. Without treatment, all eventually develop AIDS and die prematurely.

AIDS develops within 5 years in about 20%. AIDS is a lethal infection, defined as HIV infection plus one or more AIDS-defining illnesses and a CD4 T lymphocyte count <200 × 10^6/L.

Table 7.7 The more common oral manifestations of HIV infection

Condition	Features	Diagnosis	Management*
Candidosis	White removable lesions or red lesions	Clinical plus investigations; smear, culture, rinse, or biopsy	Antifungals
Hairy leukoplakia	White non-removable lesions almost invariably bilaterally on the tongue	Clinical plus investigations; cytology; EBV-DNA studies or biopsy	None usually
Periodontal disease	Linear gingival erythema, necrotizing gingivitis or periodontitis. Rarely leads to gangrenous stomatitis-cancrum oris or noma	Clinical	Oral hygiene, plaque removal, chlorhexidine, metronidazole
Herpesvirus ulcers	Chronic ulcers anywhere but often on tongue, hard palate or gingivae. Zoster increased by HAART	Clinical plus investigations; cytology, EM, DNA studies or biopsy	Antivirals
Aphthous-like ulcers	Recurrent ulcers anywhere but especially on mobile mucosae	Clinical plus investigations; possibly biopsy	Corticosteroids or thalidomide or granulocyte colony stimulating factor
Papillomavirus infections	Warty lesions, increased by HAART	Clinical plus investigations; DNA studies possibly biopsy	Excise or remove with heat, laser, or cryoprobe, imiquimod or podophyllin
Salivary gland disease	Xerostomia and sometimes salivary gland enlargement	Clinical plus investigations; sialometry, possibly biopsy	Salivary substitutes and/or pilocarpine or cevimeline
Kaposi's sarcoma	Purple macules leading to nodules, seen mainly in the palate	Clinical plus investigations; biopsy	Chemotherapy, usually vinblastine, or laser or radiation
Lymphomas	Lump or ulcer in fauces or gingivae	Clinical plus investigations; biopsy	Chemotherapy or radiation or both
Neurological	Dementia		
Autoimmune	Purpura		

*HAART (highly active antiretroviral treatment) reduces many manifestations.

Candidosis is universal especially in HIV subtype B strain CRF19 infection, but other infections in HIV/AIDS depend also upon their environmental exposure; thus for example, TB is particularly common in people from Africa and in urban IV drug-users in USA; leishmaniasis is common in persons from around the Mediterranean; mycoses such as penicillosis are seen mainly in northern Thailand.

Neoplasms may include virally related Kaposi sarcoma, lymphomas, or carcinomas (Table 7.5).

HIV-infected persons may also be at risk from viral hepatitis and other SSI.

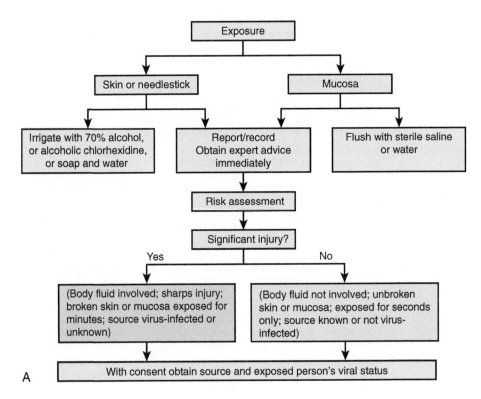

Figure 7.11 Needlestick injuries – PEP (continued below).

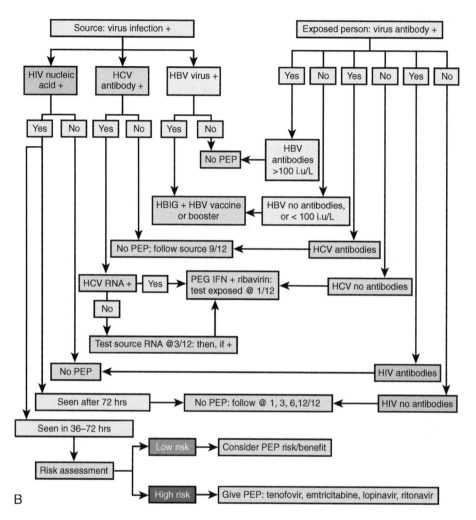

B

Figure 7.11, cont'd (from Samaranayake L, Scully C. Needlestick and occupational exposure to infections: a compendium of current guidelines. Br Dent J. 2013 Aug;215(4):163-6)

Diagnosis

Clinical plus blood tests:

- Lymphopenia.
- CD4 counts – low.
- CD4/CD8 ratio – reduced from a normal of about 2, to about 0.5 in AIDS.
- 'AIDS test' – HIV antibodies (usually ELISA [enzyme linked immunosorbent assay] or agglutination screening tests and a supplemental [confirmatory] test such as western immunoblotting).
- PCR can clarify indeterminate western blot results, is sensitive and detects HIV in seronegative HIV-infected persons.
- HIV viral load is also assayed.

It is important to apply at least two methodologically different assays; repeat the test 2–3 months later; and treat test results and diagnosis with confidentiality.

Prevention

Pre-exposure prophylaxis (PrEP) using safe sex practices plus tenofovir and emtricitabine is highly effective.

Treatment

No effective treatment exists for the underlying immune defect. Anti-retroviral drugs are effective though costly and often associated with resistance and/or adverse reactions. Immune reconstitution inflammatory syndrome (IRIS) may follow anti-retroviral therapy (ART) and can include exacerbation of some lesions such as tuberculosis, *Mycobacterium avium* complex (MAC), zoster, HPV, cytomegalovirus, cryptococcosus and Kaposi sarcoma. Specific antiretroviral drug groups include nucleoside analogues, protease inhibitors and non-nucleoside reverse-transcriptase inhibitors (Table 7.8). Some combinations – (ART; Active Retroviral Therapy) – show an especially increased antiviral activity.

Patients are monitored by CD4 counts and viral load since these correlate well with clinical progress; at CD4 counts <200/microlitre, patients are at high risk of *Pneumocystis carinii (jiroveci)* infection, and at counts below 100/microlitre, CMV, TB and *Mycobacterium avium-intracellulare* infections are risks.

Current PEP (Post-exposure prophylaxis); Figure 7.11 for BBV in UK consists of:

- HIV: tenovir, emtricitabine, lopinavir, ritonavir.
- HBV: hepatitis immunoglobulin plus HBV vaccine or booster.
- HCV: Interferon plus ribavirin.

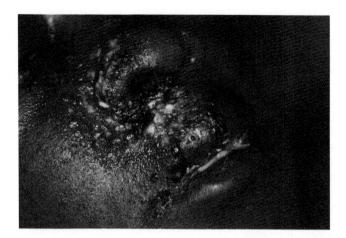

Figure 7.12 Skin lesions in maxillary Herpes zoster in HIV +ve patient (Courtesy of Dr D Malamos, Athens).

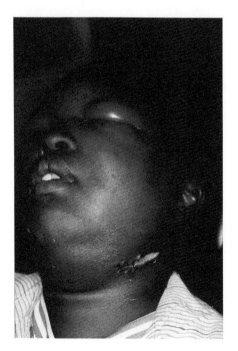

Figure 7.13 Osteomyelitis in HIV +ve patient.

Dental considerations

Oral manifestations may include: candidosis – the most common lesion, followed by hairy leukoplakia, Kaposi sarcoma, aphthous-like ulcers, herpes simplex, necrotizing ulcerative gingivitis, non-Hodgkin lymphoma, and xerostomia. Challenges in HIV/AIDS healthcare may include:

- Infections; HIV; other blood-borne viruses; sexually shared infections; tuberculosis; herpesviruses; candidosis; postoperative infections. Every effort must be made to avoid needlestick (sharps) injuries to anyone – as these could transmit HIV, hepatitis viruses, or other infections. In the event of such an injury, speed is of the essence, and where appropriate, counselling and post-exposure prophylaxis (PEP) given (Fig. 7.11).
- Bleeding (there is often thrombocytopenia). Local infiltrations or intraligamentary injections may be warranted as deep block injections can result in complications.
- In patients with advanced HIV/AIDS there can be delayed wound healing.
- Drug interactions or adverse effects of ART, chemotherapy or anti-infective agents.
- Prescribe sugar-free medication, if possible.

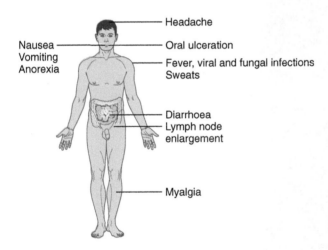

Figure 7.14 HIV/AIDS.

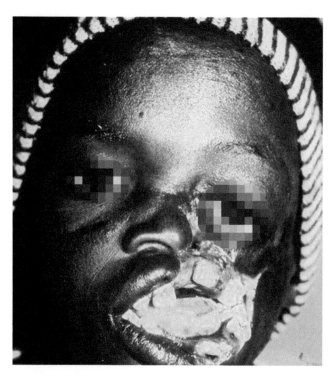

Figure. 7.15 Cancrum oris.

Table 7.8	Anti-retroviral agents	
Reverse transcriptase inhibitors	Nucleoside analogues (NRTIs)	Abacavir (ABC) Didanosine (ddI) Lamivudine (3TC) Stavudine (d4T) Zalcitabine (ddC) Zidovudine (AZT)
	Non-nucleoside	Adefovir (ADV) Delavirdine (DLV) Efavirenz (EFV)
	Nucleotide analogues (NNRTIs)	Nevirapine (NVP) Tenofovir (TFV)
Protease inhibitors	(PIs)	Amprenavir (APV) Atazanavir (ATV) Darunavir (DRV) Fosamprenavir (FPV) Indinavir (IDV) Lopinavir (LPV) Nelfinavir (NFV) Ritonavir (RTV) Saquinavir (SQV) Tipravanir (TPV)
Entry inhibitors	Integrase inhibitors	Raltegravir (RAL)
	Fusion inhibitors	Enfuvirtide (ENF, T-20)
	CCR 5 antagonists	Maraviroc (MVC)

Human papilloma viruses (HPVs)

Definition
Ubiquitous DNA viruses.

Aetiopathogenesis
Viral transmission via close contact.

Clinical presentation and classification
Over 100 HPV types are recognized. They are transmissible and mostly cause:
- Benign warts and other epithelial lesions, of skin and mucosae, including mouth and genitals.
  - *Skin* warts (verruca vulgaris) are common, especially in children, and spread mainly in wet environments such as changing rooms.
  - *Genital* warts (condylomata acuminata) may be found on the penis, vulva or vagina or perianally, or may be unseen in the urethral meatus or cervix.
  - *Oral* warts and papillomas. Heck disease (multi-focal epithelial hyperplasia) is an unusual condition, caused by HPV-13 and 32), mainly in ethnic groups such as Inuits and American Indians.
- Malignant disease: *oncogenic* or *high risk* HPVs – for example HPV-16, 18 and 33 are associated with cervical, ano-genital or oro-pharyngeal carcinomas.

Diagnosis
Clinical +/– biopsy.

Treatment
Local surgery or podophyllum resin has been the usual treatment for non-malignant HPV-related lesions. Immune stimulators such as interferon-alpha and imiquimod are now available.

HPV vaccines protect against some oncogenic and low-risk HPV types. There are two vaccines; both safe and usually given as a 3-shot series.

Cervarix: protects against HPV 16 and 18; recommended for females from 10 to 25 years of age.

Gardasil: protects against HPV 6, 11, 16 and 18; recommended for 11- and 12-year-old girls, and females 13 to 26-year-old and 9- to 26-year-old males.

Dental considerations
Oral manifestations: painless, soft, exophytic, cauliflower-like, lumps. Some HPV (e.g. HPV-16) are also associated with oropharyngeal carcinoma.

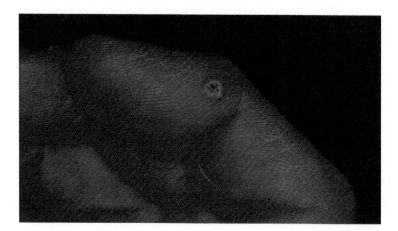

Figure 7.16 HPV – common wart.

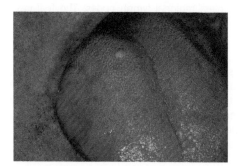

Figure 7.17 Papilloma on tongue.

Syphilis

Definition
Infection by *Treponema pallidum*.

Aetiopathogenesis
A bacterium transmitted by direct contact with syphilis lesions. An SSI, it can be transmitted via vaginal, anal, or oral sexual contact. Incidence is rising – over 80% of cases are in men who have sex with men (MSM). Infected pregnant women can pass it to their foetus.

Clinical presentation and classification
The average time between infection and appearance of first symptoms is 21 days (range 10–90 days).

Primary syphilis
Over 80% of cases are in MSM. *T. pallidum* causes a chancre (primary or Hunterian chancre), a small, firm, pink and typically single macule (usually on glans penis or vulva). Chancres occasionally involve the lips or tongue. The chancre changes to a papule and ulcerates to form a painless round ulcer with raised margin and indurated base. Untreated chancres are highly infectious, associated with enlarged painless regional lymph nodes. The features resolve clinically with or without treatment in 3–8 weeks, but if not adequately treated progress to the secondary stage.

Secondary syphilis
Follows primary stage after 6–8 weeks and is the great mimic. Rashes (characteristically symmetrically distributed coppery maculopapules on the palms and soles), and/or sores in the mouth, vagina, or anus mark this stage but features may be non-specific, with malaise, weight loss, fever, headache, hair loss, and generalized painless lymph node enlargement with unusual enlargement of epitrochlear nodes. Large, raised, grey or white lesions (condylomas) may develop in warm, moist areas such as the mouth, axilla or groin. Mucosal lesions are highly infectious. The features resolve clinically with or without treatment, but unless treated, it will progress to latent and possibly late stages.

Latent and late stages
The person, although infected, may exhibit no signs or symptoms. About 15% of untreated people develop late stage syphilis, up to 10–30 years after infection. Syphilis damages brain, nerves, eyes, heart, blood vessels, liver, bones, and joints and can result in death. The main feature is a localized non-infectious granuloma (termed gumma), varying in size from a pinhead to several centimetres which breaks down to form a deep punched-out ulcer. Skin gummas heal with depressed shiny scars (tissue-paper scars). Bone gummas may affect the long bones (especially the tibia – 'sabre tibia') or skull, producing lytic lesions and periostitis with new bone formation. Mucosal gummas may destroy bone, particularly the palate or involve the tongue. Features may also include muscle incoordination, paralysis, numbness, blindness, and dementia. Cardiovascular syphilis (aortitis, coronary arterial stenosis or aortic aneurysms) affects about 10% of patients. Meningovascular neurosyphilis also affects about 10%. Early symptoms vary, but late effects may be lesions of the IInd, IIIrd and VIIIth cranial nerves, or hydrocephalus and the pupils are also unequal and unresponsive to light (Argyll Robertson pupils). Paretic neurosyphilis begins insidiously with subtle mental disturbance going on to severe personality changes, complete dementia and widespread paralyses (general paresis of the insane; GPI). Tabes dorsalis (locomotor

ataxia) is characterized by atrophy of lumbar posterior nerve roots and sometimes the optic nerves, and characterized by sudden attacks of lightning-like pain and paraesthesiae of leg or trunk, with loss of normal pain sensation and of deep proprioceptive reflexes. These latter cause a tabetic gait in which the feet are slapped on the ground as a result of loss of sense of their position, and the neuropathic joints then become disorganized (Charcot joints).

Syphilis associated with HIV
May take an atypical, accelerated course with rapid progress to the tertiary stage; gummata may develop while the secondary stage is still active (lues maligna). The antibody response is atypical and unpredictable.

Congenital syphilis
A pregnant woman with syphilis can, after the fifth month, pass infection to her foetus with resultant low birth weight, premature delivery or stillbirth, or learning disability, deafness, blindness, frontal bossing, saddle nose and Hutchinson's teeth – screwdriver-shaped incisors. Affected children are highly infectious until about 2 years of age.

Diagnosis

Primary syphilis
Microscopy of lesional exudate (Darkfield microscopy) and serology. Biopsy may be suggestive, and diagnostic if specific antibodies are used. Serology is required but often negative at this stage. Non-specific (reaginic) serological tests, useful for screening such, include the Venereal Disease Research Laboratory (VDRL), rapid plasma reagin (RPR) card test, automated reagin test (ART) and toluidine red-treated serum test (TRUST). Treponemal enzyme immunoassays (EIAs) are an appropriate alternative but another treponemal assay such as TPHA (*T. pallidum* haemagglutination test) is confirmatory. The VDRL test appears positive towards the end of primary syphilis and usually becomes negative 1–2 years after treatment but remains positive in untreated secondary or tertiary syphilis. False-positive VDRL results may be seen after immunizations, in autoimmune disease and in some other infections (treponematoses, HIV, viral pneumonia, tuberculosis, malaria or leptospirosis). Specific serological tests such as fluorescent treponemal antibody absorbed (FTA-Abs) test, TPHA and the treponemal immobilization (TPI) test overcome the problem of false-positive VDRL results, but cannot differentiate syphilis from other treponematoses. The FTA-Abs is probably best reserved for specimens giving discrepant results. Specific tests become positive during primary and remain positive through untreated secondary or tertiary syphilis but, in contrast to VDRL, remain positive even in treated syphilis. *T. pallidum* Polymerase Chain Reaction (Tp-PCR) aids early diagnosis since it may be reactive before conventional serological tests are.

Secondary syphilis
Lesions examined for *T. pallidum* as above and blood taken for serological examination.

Tertiary syphilis
Diagnosis is confirmed by serology.

Treatment

Early syphilis
Benzathine penicillin G single dose is first-line therapy, with azithromycin single dose as a second-line alternative.

Late syphilis

Benzathine penicillin G three weekly doses is first-line therapy (except for neurosyphilis: procaine penicillin G with concomitant oral probenecid remains first-line therapy).

Azithromycin-resistant *T. pallidum* have appeared.

Dental considerations

Oral manifestations:

- *Primary:* Oral chancres.
- *Secondary:* condylomas, "snailtrack" ulcers, mucous patches, fever, malaise, rash and generalized lymphadenopathy.
- *Tertiary:* gumma.
- *Congenital:* Peg-shaped incisors (Hutchinson incisors) or multiple, supernumerary cusps on molars (mulberry molars), a high-arched palate and perioral rhagades (fissures).

Tuberculosis (TB)

Definition

An infectious chronic disease, caused by *Mycobacterium tuberculosis* (M.tb), an acid-fast non-motile aerobic rod bacterium.

Aetiopathogenesis

Humans are the only reservoir for the most common agent *M. tuberculosis.* Uncommon bacteria which together comprise the *M. tuberculosis* complex are *M. bovis, M. africanum, M. microti, M. caprae, M. pinnipedii, M. canetti* and *M. mungi.* TB is a major global health problem: one-third of the world's population is infected, most coming from resource deprived areas. TB incidence is rising, through worsening social deprivation, diabetes, homelessness, immigration, intravenous drug abuse and HIV/AIDS. In immunocompromised people, in prisons, or institutions the organism is frequently multi-drug resistant (MDR).

TB is characterized by granulomas – aggregates of immune cells (macrophages, foamy epithelioid cells and multinucleated giant Langerhans cells surrounded by lymphocytes) which concentrate the immune response of CD4 T cells, chemokines which bind to CCR2 receptor, TNF (tumour necrosis factor), IFNγ (Interferon gamma), IL-2 (Interleukin), lympho-toxin A, CD8 T cells and γδ T cells which localize and contain M.tb to the area.

Clinical presentation and classification

Primary TB infection mainly spreads to lungs by droplets usually transmitted by infected sputum. In normal persons inhaled mycobacteria may cause lesions subpleurally and in the regional lymph nodes (primary complex). Infection is usually localized, asymptomatic and subclinical (latent TB), though bacteria remain viable.

Acute active TB (fever, night sweats, cough, anorexia, weight loss and weakness) can follow massive infections, mainly when body defences are impaired, and may disseminate in the blood to produce miliary TB (lesions in lungs, genitourinary tract, bone, joint, eyes or elsewhere).

Latent TB infection (LTBI) means that *M. tuberculosis* is present, but no TB disease and people cannot spread the infection. However, reactivation may occur – usually only after many years and if the patient becomes immune-incompetent (e.g. diabetes, HIV, corticosteroids, cancer) and then causes post-primary TB.

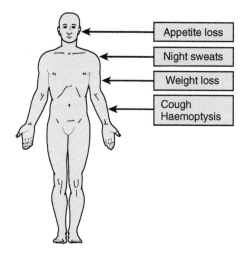

Figure 7.18 Tuberculosis.

Post-primary TB may be pulmonary, or can spread widely (e.g. to meninges, bone, renal tract, etc.) – in these cases there are organ-specific symptoms.

Diagnosis

Clinical, confirmed by:

- Tuberculin skin testing (tuberculin, Mantoux or Heaf test). A positive result means that a person has been infected but does not necessarily have active TB.
- Chest radiography.
- Smears and culture are cheap and quick, but of low sensitivity and culture takes 4–8 weeks but gives definitive diagnosis. PCR has accelerated the diagnosis and speciation of mycobacteria.
- The mycobacteria growth indicator tube (MGIT) system gives results as early as 3–14 days.
- Blood assay for *M.tb* (BAMT) may be positive by interferon-gamma release assay (IGRA). A positive test result suggests *M.tb* infection; a negative result suggests it unlikely.
- Histology of infected organs or tissues.

Prophylaxis

Immunization using BCG (Bacille Calmette–Guérin) gives some protection but is not highly reliable.

Treatment

Antibiotic chemotherapy is indicated for people ill with TB, those infected but not sick, or who are close contacts to infectious TB cases. Treatment starts with three antibiotics in combination to avoid the emergence of resistance, and must be given for at least 6 months (9 months in the immunocompromised). Initial therapy is daily isoniazid + rifampicin + pyrazimamide or ethambutol for 2 months. Continuation therapy of TB is with daily isoniazid + rifampicin for a further 4 months.

Drug-resistant TB is increasingly common, especially in HIV/AIDS, where it can be multi-drug resistant (MDR-TB).

Patients with HIV disease who have MDR-TB have been effectively treated with capreomycin. Extended drug resistance (XDR-TB) is increasing, but new agents such as bedaquiline and spectinamides are now appearing.

Atypical mycobacteria include *M. avium, M. intracellulare (M. avium-intracellulare complex: MAC), M. kansasii, M. scrofulaceum, M. fortuitum, M. marinum, M. ulcerans, M. chelonae* and *M. xenopi,* widely distributed in water, soil, animals and man. Infections with such non-tuberculous mycobacteria (NTM – also known as MOTT – mycobacteria other than TB) are believed to emanate from environmental exposure.

Dental considerations

Oral manifestations of TB may include:

- Mucosal ulceration
- Osteomyelitis
- Scrofula (infection of cervical and submandibular lymph nodes).

Defer elective care in patients with clinically active TB and positive sputum cultures.

Avoid NSAIDs if patient is taking fluoroquinolones (second-line antituberculosis drugs) as they may cause adverse CNS effects. Avoid aspirin with streptomycin, amikacin, kanamycin, and capreomycin.

Various other relevant infections

Some viral infections can only be managed symptomatically but rarely have systemic complications. Enteroviruses such as Coxsackie viruses can cause mouth ulcers in hand, foot and mouth disease, or herpangina. Mumps virus causes sialadenitis with painful swelling of salivary glands; routine vaccination in childhood should prevent this.

Further reading

<www.cdc.gov/hicpac/mdro/mdro_toc.html>
<www.cdc.gov/hicpac/BSI/BSI-guidelines-2011.html> <www.cdc.gov/hicpac/cauti/002_cauti_toc.html>.

8 Chemical dependence (drug addiction or substance abuse)

Chemical dependence

Definition

Chemical self-administration in a manner that deviates from the cultural norm. Drugs are abused experimentally, for recreation, in special circumstances or compulsively. In compulsive drug abuse or addiction the individual takes the drug without any medical indication, despite adverse effects and social consequences, due to their intense dependence. Chemicals used produce CNS stimulation, depression or hallucinations, or distort perception, thinking or judgement.

People who inject drugs (PWID) may have, and pose to healthcare workers and others, issues with blood-borne, sexually shared and other infections.

Clinical presentation

Findings that may suggest drug addiction include:

- Personality change – moods, anxiety, depression, impulsive behaviour, suicidal thoughts or gestures, or deteriorating interpersonal relations.
- Progressive deterioration in appearance/hygiene.
- Unreliability in keeping appointments, meeting deadlines, and at work.
- Work absenteeism, disappearances, improbable excuses, frequent or long trips to toilet.

Care should also be taken with any person who:

- makes a self-diagnosis and requests a specific drug, especially a psychoactive agent;
- appears to have a dramatic but unexpected complaint such as neuralgia;
- has subjective symptoms but no objective evidence of any physical disorder;
- has no interest in the diagnosis or investigation results, or refuses a second opinion;
- firmly rejects treatments that exclude psychoactive drugs.

Common signs may include (alphabetical):

- Bruxism (amphetamines or ecstasy).
- Drug-associated diseases.
- Dubious personal appearance and hygiene.
- Hyperpyrexia (with ecstasy).
- Needle tracks or abscesses.
- Pigmentation.
- Psychoses (with marijuana).
- Pupils dilated (cocaine/crack) or constricted (opioids).
- Sniffing (cocaine).
- Tachycardia (amphetamines).
- Viral hepatitis, HIV and other blood-borne agents.

Main dental considerations

(*See also generic guidance under main dental considerations on page 63 top, and also Section 2).

In addition to patients, drugs are sometimes abused by some medical and dental staff and students, mostly for 'recreational' puposes. Alcohol and tobacco are the substances abused most frequently by patients, followed by opiates (mainly hydrocodone and oxycodone), and nitrous oxide. Other substances abused include marijuana; opiates (e.g. morphine, fentanyl, meperidine, hydromorphone and oxycodone); minor opiates such as hydrocodone and codeine; 'legal highs' and anxiolytics such as alprazolam and diazepam.

Drug abuse may be associated with dental issues:

- *Rampant caries* seen in opioid abuse, stimulant abuse ('meth mouth'), cocaine, ecstasy and barbiturate abuse may be predisposed by:
  - Drug-induced hyposalivation.
  - Poor oral hygiene
  - Consumption of large amounts of carbonated sugary drinks.
  - Methadone if in a sugar syrup form.
- *Periodontal diseases:*
  - Addicts tend to have poor oral hygiene, and many also smoke tobacco – another periodontal disease risk factor.
- *Tooth surface loss* and masseteric hypertrophy may be caused by:
  - Bruxism, and clenching (mainly with opioids and stimulants)
  - Hyposalivation
  - Erosive (acidic) drinks
  - Regurgitation, bulimia and vomiting (mainly in alcoholism).
- *Candida infection* is commonly due to:
  - Dry mouth
  - Compromised immunity
  - Poor dental appliance hygiene.
- *Potentially malignant and malignant lesions* (particularly in alcohol, tobacco, betel and marijuana use).

Elective care may be carried out 24 hours after use of a stimulant drug (e.g., cocaine) or after marijuana/mescaline use. Dental management issues in addicts may include (alphabetical):

- acute anxiety, dysphoria, and paranoid thoughts
- behavioural problems
- compliance with treatment may be poor
- immune defects
- liver damage causing bleeding tendency and impaired drug metabolism
- malnourishment
- viral hepatitis (C and/or B), HIV or other infections.

NSAIDs are best for pain control. Pain management may be challenging for several reasons:

- anxiety
- resistance to local anaesthetics
- general anaesthesia or sedation can trigger a relapse.

If methadone has been prescribed, it should be maintained during treatment. Local anaesthesia with epinephrine may prolong the acute tachycardia already induced by cannabis.

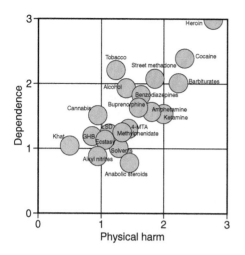

Figure 8.1 Drug dependency chart showing extent of dependency and physical harm (heroin worst).

Alcohol use

Alcohol depresses the CNS, releasing inhibitions, impairing capacity to reason, and interfering with the cerebellum (causing ataxia and motor incoordination) and then higher centres (causing unconsciousness).

Acute effects are mainly on judgment, concentration and coordination (Table 8.1). Social difficulties and conflicts are common. Mortality is high, mainly from road traffic accidents and assaults. After a large alcoholic binge, suppression of protective reflexes can cause vomit inhalation, asphyxia and death.

Later effects of chronic alcohol abuse may also include cardiomyopathy, liver disease (fatty liver, alcoholic hepatitis, cirrhosis), malnutrition, peripheral neuropathy, amnesia and confabulation (in Wernicke and Korsakoff CNS syndromes), cerebellar degeneration, or dementia. Prolonged abuse also can also cause anaemia, immune defects, gastritis, peptic ulcer, pancreatitis, hypertension and cardiomyopathy.

Diagnosis

From history and clinical features; blood tests – FBC (macrocytosis without anaemia) and/or raised levels of alcohol, gamma glutamyl transpeptidase (GGT) or carbohydrate deficient transferrin (CDT; the most specific marker).

Treatment

Counselling and a high-protein, high-calorie and low-sodium diet (+/– vitamin supplementation), cognitive therapy and possibly naltrexone or acamprosate.

Table 8.1 Acute effects of alcohol use

Blood alcohol level in mg/dL					
<100	100–200	200–300	300–400	400–500	>500
Dry and decent	Delighted and devilish	Delinquent and disgusting	Dizzy and delirious	Dazed and dejected	Dead drunk

Main dental considerations

(*See also generic guidance under main dental considerations on page 63 top, and also Section 2).

The most common oral effect of alcoholism is neglect, leading to caries and periodontal disease, and there is sometimes tooth surface loss also from dental erosion from regurgitation and/or attrition from bruxism. Wound healing may also be impaired and alcoholism may be a common factor in patients with osteomyelitis following jaw fractures. Alcohol may be a cause of leukoplakia and other potentially malignant disorders. There may be folate deficiency or other anaemia causing glossitis and sometimes angular stomatitis or recurrent aphthae. A rare manifestation is bilateral painless parotid swelling (sialosis).

Many alcoholics present no dental management problems, though there may be issues related to informed consent, or bleeding (if there is liver damage) but challenges may also include erratic attendance for dental treatment and aggressive behaviour. Alcoholics are best given an early morning appointment, when they are least likely to be under the influence. Liver cirrhosis delays drug metabolism and may cause a bleeding tendency. Alcohol can interact with warfarin, paracetamol/acetaminophen and benzodiazepines. Sedatives (including benzodiazepines and antihistamines) or hypnotics generally have an additive effect with alcohol, although these interactions are not entirely predictable. GA is best avoided, especially if patients have pre-medicated themselves with alcohol, because of increased risk of vomiting and inhalation of vomit. Alcoholics are especially prone to aspiration lung abscess. Aspirin and NSAIDs should be avoided: they are more likely in the alcoholic patient to cause gastric erosions and precipitate bleeding. The hepatotoxic effects of acetaminophen (paracetamol) are enhanced, though it is probably the safest analgesic. Heavy drinkers, however, become tolerant not only of alcohol but also of other sedatives.

Alcohol-containing mouthwashes, should be avoided in patients given metronidazole within the last 48 h. Metronidazole inhibits the liver breakdown of acetaldehyde, which accumulates to cause vasodilatation, nausea, vomiting, sweating, headache and palpitations similar to the Antabuse reaction.

Amphetamine use

Amphetamines stimulate alpha- and beta-adrenergic receptors and thus the CNS and peripheral nervous systems and are used orally usually for their euphoriant effect, to stave off fatigue, and for slimming.

Acute amphetamine toxicity causes aggression, dilated pupils, dry mouth, hallucinations, tachycardia, talkativeness, and tachypnoea, leading to seizures, hyperpyrexia, arrhythmias and collapse. High doses of amphetamines can cause mood swings, and psychoses – including hallucinations and paranoia and can cause respiratory failure and death.

Chronic amphetamine toxicity causes high BP, sleeplessness, restlessness, hyperactivity, loss of appetite and weight, tremor, and repetitive movements.

Amphetamines have no true withdrawal syndrome and, in this respect, differ from opioids or barbiturates.

Main dental considerations

(*See also generic guidance under main dental considerations on page 63 top, and also Section 2).

Bruxism and picking at the face, and dry mouth.

Cocaine and crack use

Cocaine is a powerfully addictive drug with profound almost immediate effects by potentiating catecholamines and interfering with dopamine reabsorption. The major routes of use of cocaine (including the hydrochloride and free-base or crack cocaine) are snorting (via nose), injecting or smoking. 'Crack' is the street name for cocaine processed with ammonia or sodium bicarbonate (baking soda) and water and heated to remove the

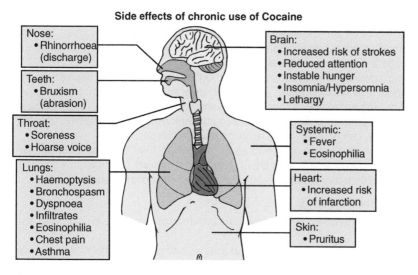

Side effects of chronic use of Cocaine

Nose:
- Rhinorrhoea (discharge)

Teeth:
- Bruxism (abrasion)

Throat:
- Soreness
- Hoarse voice

Lungs:
- Haemoptysis
- Bronchospasm
- Dyspnoea
- Infiltrates
- Eosinophilia
- Chest pain
- Asthma

Brain:
- Increased risk of strokes
- Reduced attention
- Instable hunger
- Insomnia/Hypersomnia
- Lethargy

Systemic:
- Fever
- Eosinophilia

Heart:
- Increased risk of infarction

Skin:
- Pruritus

Figure 8.2 Adverse effects of chronic use of cocaine.

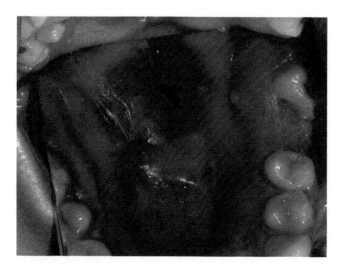

Figure 8.3 Oro-antral fistula – in cocaine abuse. (Courtesy of Professor JV Bagan, Valencia, Spain.)

hydrochloride to make a free base for smoking. The term 'crack' refers to crackling sounds heard when it is smoked (heated). Crack smoking can produce aggressive paranoid behaviour.

Cocaine euphoric effects appear in <5 minutes and include hyperstimulation, reduced fatigue, and heightened mental clarity. Physical effects mimic catecholamines, with constricted peripheral blood vessels, dilated pupils, and raised temperature, pulse rate, and BP. The cocaine addict has aptly been described as a 'sexed-up extrovert with dilated pupils'.

Cocaine misuse may induce angina, coronary spasm, arrhythmias, myocardial infarction, Sniffing is common. cerebrovascular accidents, convulsions, respiratory depression and death. Large doses of cocaine cause paranoia, visual hallucinations (snowlights) and tactile hallucinations. The latter are typically of insects crawling over the skin (formication, 'cocaine bugs'). Prolonged cocaine snorting can result in ulceration of the nasal mucous membrane and can damage and collapse the nasal septum.

On stopping cocaine, symptoms proceed through a crash phase of depression and craving for sleep, a withdrawal phase of lack of energy and then an extinction phase of recurrence of craving evoked by various external stimuli but of lesser intensity. Depression, fatigue and bradycardia may be seen. Behavioural interventions, particularly cognitive behavioural therapy, can be effective in reducing cocaine misuse.

Some use cocaine plus heroin intravenously ('speedballing'), which is especially dangerous. When people mix cocaine and alcohol consumption the liver manufactures cocaethylene, that intensifies euphoric effects, and raises the risk of sudden death.

Main dental considerations

(*See also generic guidance under main dental considerations on page 63 top, and also Section 2).

Oral use of cocaine temporarily numbs lips and tongue, and can cause gingival or mucosal erosions, dry mouth and bruxism or dental erosion. Caries and periodontal disease, especially acute necrotizing gingivitis, are more frequent. Snorting cocaine predisposes to palatal ulceration, sphenoidal sinusitis, and occasionally brain abscess. Cocaine may precipitate cluster headaches. Children born to cocaine-using mothers are more prone to have ankyloglossia. Injected cocaine brings the risk from blood-borne infections. It is important to avoid epinephrine-containing LA in persons using cocaine until at least 2 h have elapsed, because of enhanced sympathomimetic action and subsequent arrhythmias, acute hypertension or cardiac failure. Therefore, it is best to defer dental treatment until 6 h after the last use of cocaine.

Ecstasy (MDMA: methylene-dioxy methamphetamine) use

Ecstasy (MDMA) is, a synthetic, psychoactive with sympathomimetic properties, with both stimulant (amphetamine-like) and hallucinogenic (LSD-like) properties. Ecstasy affects dopamine-containing neurones that use serotonin to communicate.

Ecstasy is usually taken by mouth, and effects appear after 20–60 minutes and resemble other amphetamines, with euphoria and appetite suppression – but it is more potently hallucinogenic. Users face risks similar to those with amphetamines and cocaine, which are not dose-related. Ecstasy can produce psychiatric sequelae such as agitation or paranoia; neurological effects such as ataxia and seizures; cardiovascular such as tachycardia, arrhythmias or infarction; renal or hepatic failure, or other effects. Psychological difficulties include confusion, depression, sleep problems, drug craving, severe anxiety, and paranoia – and can extend weeks after taking MDMA. Physical symptoms may include muscle tension, involuntary teeth clenching, nausea, blurred vision, rapid eye movement, faintness, and chills or sweating. Raised heart rate and BP, are special risks for people with circulatory or heart disease. Also, there is evidence that people who develop an acneiform rash after using MDMA may be risking severe adverse effects, including liver damage. After long-term use of ecstasy, tolerance develops but there is no physical dependence or withdrawal symptoms.

Main dental considerations

(*See also generic guidance under main dental considerations on page 63 top, and also Section 2).
Bruxism and 'Meth mouth' – a term used to describe the oral neglect and disease seen.

Lysergic acid diethylamide (LSD) use

LSD ('acid') is usually sold as tiny squares of paper with pictures on them, but can be found as a liquid, pellets or squares like gelatin. LSD is taken orally, licked off paper or in a gelatine or liquid that can be put in the mouth or eyes. LSD is not considered an addictive drug since it does not produce compulsive drug-seeking behaviour as do cocaine, amphetamine, heroin, alcohol, and nicotine. Most LSD users voluntarily limit or cease use over time.

LSD however, is a major hallucinogen producing, within 30 to 90 minutes, several different emotions simultaneously or which swing rapidly. There is often lability of mood, panic ('bad trip') and delusions of magical powers, such as being able to fly. The user's sense of time and self changes. If taken in a large dose, LSD produces delusions and visual hallucinations. Synaesthesia, the overflow from one sense to another when, for example, colours are heard, is common. The effects of LSD are unpredictable but prolonged, often to about 12 hours, depending on the amount taken; the user's personality, mood, and expectations; and the surroundings in which the drug is used. Many LSD users experience flashbacks, recurrence of certain aspects of a person's experience, without the user having taken the drug again. A flashback comes suddenly, often without warning, and may come within a few days or more than a year after LSD use. LSD users may experience severe, terrifying thoughts and feelings, and despair, and fatal accidents have occurred during LSD intoxication.

LSD physical effects are similar to those of catecholamines and include dilated pupils, raised body temperature, heart rate and BP, sweating, loss of appetite, sleeplessness, dry mouth, and tremors.

Main dental considerations

(*See also generic guidance under main dental considerations on page 63 top, and also Section 2).
Oral manifestations may include a metallic taste and dryness.

Inhalant use

Inhalants are breathable chemical vapours that have psychoactive effects. Inhalants include:

- Gases (aerosol propellants, butane, propane and medical anaesthetic gases (e.g. nitrous oxide, halothane, ether, chloroform).
- Nitrites (cyclohexyl, amyl and butyl nitrite).
- Solvents (paint thinners, degreasers, petrol, glues, etc.).

Inhalant misuse is increasingly common and has led to many deaths of children and young adults. Inhalants can directly induce hypoxia, cardiac arrhythmias, liver damage, neurological damage, delusions and sudden death. Problems are most common with fluorocarbons and butane-type gas misuse. Deliberately inhaling from an attached paper or plastic bag or in a closed area greatly increases the chances of suffocation.

Solvent misuse signs include slurred speech, euphoria, anorexia and a circumoral rash (glue sniffers). Jaundice may be seen and the pulse may be irregular. Chronic solvent misuse can impair memory and concentration and occasionally causes permanent brain, liver or kidney damage. Specific chemicals may also have additional side-effects:

- Benzene (gasoline/petrol) – bone marrow damage.
- Hexane (glues, gasoline/petrol) and nitrous oxide (whipping cream, gas cylinders) – peripheral neuropathies or limb spasms. Nitrous oxide induces impaired consciousness with a sense of dissociation and often of exhilaration (laughing gas). Addiction, an occupational hazard of anaesthetists and dental staff, can interfere with vitamin B_{12} metabolism and cause neuropathy. Deaths from nitrous oxide abuse are rare.
- Organic nitrites ('poppers', 'bold,' and 'rush') and methylene chloride (varnish removers, paint thinners) – hypoxia.
- Petrol/gasoline – respiratory damage, anaemia, lead poisoning and cranial nerve palsies.
- Toluene (paint sprays, glues, dewaxers) and trichloroethylene (cleaning fluids, correction fluids) and chlorinated hydrocarbons (correction fluids, dry-cleaning fluids) – CNS, liver and kidney damage, hearing loss.

Main dental considerations

(*See also generic guidance under main dental considerations on page 63 top, and also Section 2).

Glue-sniffer's rash may be seen circumorally. A syndrome of learning impairment, scaphocephaly (long narrow head), prominent malar bones and hypotonia (fetal gasoline/petrol syndrome) has been seen in children of mothers who inhaled petrol in pregnancy.

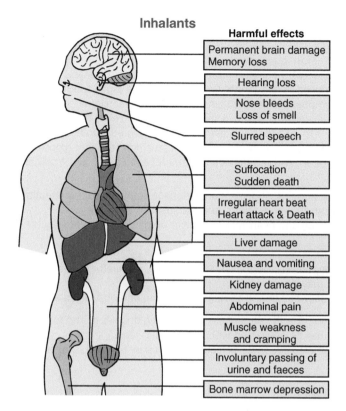

Inhalants

Harmful effects

- Permanent brain damage Memory loss
- Hearing loss
- Nose bleeds Loss of smell
- Slurred speech
- Suffocation Sudden death
- Irregular heart beat Heart attack & Death
- Liver damage
- Nausea and vomiting
- Kidney damage
- Abdominal pain
- Muscle weakness and cramping
- Involuntary passing of urine and faeces
- Bone marrow depression

Figure 8.4 Inhalant use. Adapted from www.inspirationsyouth.com/inhalants-abuse/ with kind permission from Inspirations for Youth and Families, LLC.

Marijuana use

Marijuana (cannabis) – the most commonly used illicit drug in the developed world (apart from alcohol and tobacco), originates from the hemp plant (Cannabis sativa or Cannabis indica). Usually smoked as a cigarette (joint, nail), or in a pipe (bong), it is also smoked in blunts (cigars emptied of tobacco and refilled with marijuana, often with another drug). As a more concentrated, resinous form, marijuana is called hashish and, as a sticky black liquid, hash oil. The main active chemical is THC (delta-9-tetrahydrocannabinol); this binds to brain receptors which influence pleasure, memory, thought, concentration, sensory and time perception, and coordinated movement. Adverse effects of cannabis can include:

- Behavioural problems and poor visual perception, language comprehension, attention, and memory in babies born to women who used marijuana in pregnancy.
- Cardiovascular – increased BP and heart rate and lower oxygen-carrying capacity of blood.
- Immune impairment.
- Psychological – depression, anxiety, personality disturbances, impaired attention, memory, and learning. It may precipitate schizophrenia.
- Respiratory – infections, daily cough and sputum production, and obstructed airways.

Marijuana fortunately does not directly cause death but smoking doubles it, and triples the risk of lung cancers, and it may be associated with some oral cancers.

Marijuana use is also promoted for some perceived health benefits, and is legalized in some countries.

Main dental considerations

(*See also generic guidance under main dental considerations on page 63 top, and also Section 2).

There is a tendency to a dry mouth and increased cravings for certain foods ('the munchies'), hyposalivation, increased *Candida* carriage, white lesions and cancer. There are no specific aspects of marijuana addiction that influence dental management.

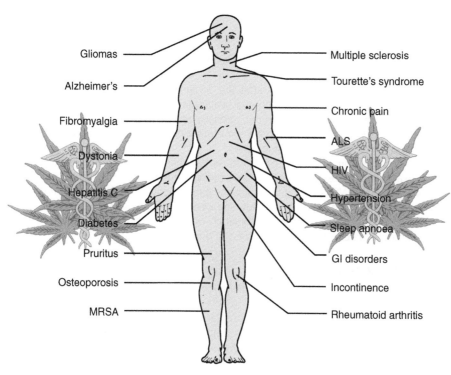

Figure 8.5 Potential therapeutic use of medical marijuana. Adapted from: http://visual.ly/
herbal-benefits-medical-marijuana. MRSA = methicillin-resistant Staph. aureus;
ALS = amyotrophic lateral sclerosis.

Nicotine use

Nicotine is absorbed readily from tobacco smoke in the lungs, and is one of the most heavily used addictive drugs.

Nicotine binds to a CNS receptor, raises the dopamine level (like cocaine, heroin, and marijuana), as well as opioids and glucose, activating the nucleus accumbens. Nicotine also causes a discharge of adrenaline from the adrenals, which stimulates the CNS.

Nicotine addiction results in withdrawal symptoms when a person tries to stop smoking, with excessive anger, hostility, and aggression.

Pharmacological combined with psychological treatments produce some of the highest long-term abstinence rates. Treatments include hypnotherapy, electronic cigarettes, nicotine replacement therapy (NRT – transdermal nicotine patch, nicotine nasal spray, nicotine gum, nicotine lozenge, sublingual nicotine tablet, and nicotine inhaler) – and bupropion, vareni-cline, clonidine or nortriptyline. The combination of an opiate antagonist mecamylamine with the nicotine patch has increased successful quit rates.

Main dental considerations

(*See also generic guidance under main dental considerations on page 63 top, and also Section 2).

Smoking tobacco may cause smokers keratosis, leukoplakia, erythroplakia, and oral cancer. Smoking also predisposes to pigmentary incompetence, and extrinsic staining of teeth, periodontal disease, implant failure, dry socket, candidosis and xerostomia. Difficulties in dental management of tobacco users may include associated chronic obstructive pulmonary disease, ischaemic heart disease, alcoholism or peptic ulcer. Smokers metabolize some other drugs more rapidly and require, for example, higher doses of benzodiazepines than do non-smokers.

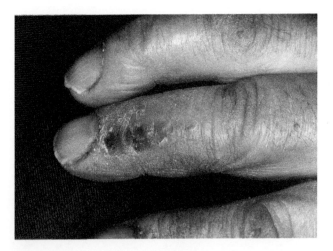

Figure 8.6 Nicotine use – stained fingers.

Opioid and heroin use

Opioids, and synthetic compounds such as methadone, dipipanone, dihydrocodeine and pethidine are widely used medically to provide potent analgesia. Opioids such as morphine and heroin derived from the opium poppy act by mimicking brain peptides – enkephalins and endorphins. The addictive dependence of heroin (diacetyl morphine) is due to conversion to morphine. Morphine binds to opioid receptor molecules in the brain area that controls pain and reward. Codeine is metabolised to by cytochrome p450 to morphine products. Oxycodone is a semi-syhthetic opioid in common use.

The brainstem, which controls automatic processes critical for life, such as respiration, BP, and arousal, also has opioid receptors and most heroin or morphine related deaths are caused by respiratory depression. Opioid misuse can be orally, sometimes smoked or sniffed as snuff, subcutaneously (skin popping), or intravenously. Heroin is a highly addictive opioid, processed from morphine, and differs from other opioids mainly in the difficulty in overcoming addiction. Heroin can be injected or sniffed, smoked from a tin-foil ('chasing the dragon').

Heroin misuse short-term effects appear soon after a single dose, with a surge of euphoria ('rush') accompanied by a warm flushing of the skin, dry mouth, and heavy extremities – probably due to histamine release. Following initial euphoria, which can last up to 4 hours, the heroin user goes 'on the nod,' an alternately wakeful and drowsy state as mental functioning becomes clouded due to CNS depression.

Common signs of abuse are:

- Pin-point pupils
- Needle tracks or abscesses
- Lymphadenopathy.

Opioid misuse leads to tolerance at an early stage, and physical dependence and addiction after some months. As a respiratory depressant, use predisposes also to pneumonia, lung abscesses and fibrosis. Heroin misuse is also associated with collapsed veins, infective endocarditis, abscesses, cellulitis, orthostatic hypotension, constipation, and neglect of health, diet and hygiene, and other conditions, including fatal overdose, spontaneous abortion, and infectious diseases, such as HIV/AIDS and hepatitis. 'Street' heroin contains only about 10% heroin: many additives do not readily dissolve and can result in infection or infarction in lungs, liver, kidneys, or brain.

Opioid withdrawal is unpleasant – though usually not dangerous, early features including lacrimation, rhinorrhoea, sweating and persistent yawning. After about 12 hours the addict enters a phase of restless tossing sleep (yen) when there is pupil dilatation, tremor, gooseflesh (cold turkey), anorexia, nausea, vomiting, muscle spasms and pain, orgasms, diarrhoea and abdominal pains. Pulse rate and BP also rise. Once the main features have subsided, there may be weakness and insomnia for several weeks or months.

Medical supervision and the use of opioid agonists such as oral methadone and levo-alpha-acetylmethadol (LAAM), or antagonists such as naltrexone, or lofexidine are used in the management of opioid dependence.

Main dental considerations

(*See also generic guidance under main dental considerations on page 63 top, and also Section 2).

There is often oral neglect, advanced periodontal disease and caries. If a patient is intoxicated, defer elective care. In the established addict, non-narcotic analgesics may be ineffective in controlling dental pain, so that large doses of opioids may have to be given. Pentazocine, being a narcotic antagonist, should not be used as it may precipitate withdrawal. Codeine is best avoided. Simulation of pain is a common manoeuvre to obtain analgesics. Prescription pads may be stolen or drug cabinets raided. Dental drugs that may attract the opiate addict include pethidine, codeine, pentazocine and dextropropoxyphene (in co-proxamol). Opioids may enhance the sedation of conscious sedation agents and GA. This patient population may miss appointments or call at weekends looking for prescription pain medications.

New psychoactive substances (NPS)

The United Nations Office of Drugs and Crime indicate that 540 different drugs can be classified as NPS (mainly 'legal highs'). Typically there are no quality controls for NPS and they are marketed as non-drug products with innocuous names and labelled 'not for human consumption' to minimize legal scrutiny. They are cheap, easy to obtain (often via the internet), and are not detectable by standard toxicology tests. Adverse effects of NPS include agitation, panic attacks, hallucinations, psychosis, violent behaviours, tachycardia, hyperthermia and seizures – and possible death. Targeted treatments or receptor antagonists cannot be given, since the precise substances ingested by a particular patient are usually unclear, and so treatment is mostly supportive, with benzodiazepines to reduce cardiovascular stimulation and agitation, and whole body cooling to treat hyperthermia (http://www.dana.org/Cerebrum/2016/The_Changing_Face_of_Recreational_Drug_Use/#sthash.EUS3kVq9.dpuf. Accessed 2016 March 22).

Legal highs are substances not covered by misuse of drugs laws. Sold under names like 'Clockwork Orange', 'Bliss', 'Mary Jane', users can never be certain what they are taking or what effects might be. Reduced inhibitions, drowsiness, excited or paranoid states, coma, seizures and death are possible. Some drugs marketed as legal highs actually contain some illegal ingredients.

Main dental considerations
(*See also generic guidance under main dental considerations on page 63 top, and also Section 2).
Mouth dryness and 'foaming at the mouth' have been reported.

Therapeutic modalities

Adverse drug reactions

Main dental considerations

(*See also generic guidance under main dental considerations on page 63 top, and also Section 2).

Adverse drug reactions (ADR) are responses to a medicinal product which are noxious and unintended. Drugs used in dentistry, and oral healthcare products may lead to such reactions.

Drug interactions are also possible and it is also important to bear in mind that over the counter (OTC) and herbal preparations, foods and other substances can also sometimes interact by affecting drug absorption or efficacy, or causing other interactions. An ADR may be a known side-effect or it may be previously unrecognized. The Yellow Card Scheme of the Medicines and Healthcare Products Regulatory Agency (MHRA) relies on reporting of suspected ADRs:

- Type A (augmented) reactions result from an exaggeration of a drug's normal pharmacological actions, such as respiratory depression with opioids or bleeding with warfarin.
- Type B (bizarre) reactions are novel responses such as anaphylaxis or rashes with antibiotics.
- Type C, or 'continuing' reactions, persist for a relatively long time such as drug/medication-induced osteonecrosis of the jaw (MRONJ), most common with bisphosphonates.
- Type D, or 'delayed' reactions, become evident only sometime after the use of a medicine (e.g. leukopenia, which can occur up to 6 weeks after a dose of lomustine).
- Type E, or 'end-of-use' reactions, are associated with the withdrawal of a drug – such as insomnia, anxiety and perceptual disturbances following benzodiazepine withdrawal.

Drug allergies

Any suggestion of a previous ADR or allergy, and particularly any adverse reaction during anaesthesia or imaging, must be taken seriously. Drug allergy or hypersensitivity often results from interactions between a drug and the immune system, mediated by IgE.

Identifiable risk factors for ADRs include:

- Advancing age
- Concurrent illnesses
- Female gender
- Previous hypersensitivity to related drugs.

Furthermore, patients with allergy to one drug, and patients with Sjögren syndrome or HIV disease may be particularly liable to ADRs.

Drug hypersensitivity is usually a diagnosis made on the basis of a rash or anaphylaxis. Laboratory testing may help, with skin testing. Treatment includes discontinuing the offending agent, symptomatic treatment, and patient education.

Anaesthetics and related agents

Local anaesthetic (LA) agents such as lidocaine with epinephrine/adrenaline are remarkably safe. However, the use of excessive amounts can be dangerous. The allergy risks with amide LAs, such as articaine, lidocaine, mepivacaine or prilocaine, are lower than with amines. The most sensitizing component of LA solutions has been the preservative: initially, methylparabens was used (now rarely used). There may be allergies to sulphite antioxidants or to latex in the LA cartridge diaphragm or bung. Methaemoglobinemia has been reported with all strengths of benzocaine gels and liquids, especially in young children. Therefore, benzocaine products should not be used on children under the age of two years.

Halothane may be a cause of hypersensitivity and 'halothane hepatitis'.

Intravenous anaesthetic agents can cause anaphylactic-type reactions, from hypersensitivity or by direct histamine release. Tachycardia, vascular collapse and skin reactions (flushing, oedema or urticaria) are the most frequent, but reactions can range from minor symptoms to bronchospasm and a sharp fall in BP. Treatment is as for anaphylaxis.

Muscle relaxants, particularly suxamethonium, thealcuronine, and tubocurarine are sometimes implicated in anaphylactoid reactions.

Analgesics

Non-steroidal anti-inflammatory drugs (NSAIDs) may, rarely, induce allergic reactions. Aspirin reactions, in relation to the scale of use, are almost negligible. Aspirin-induced asthma is rare, seen mainly in patients with nasal polyps ('triad asthma' – asthma, nasal polyps and aspirin sensitivity). Aspirin also readily causes platelet dysfunction, and it should also not be given to children, or to patients taking oral hypoglycaemics, valproic acid or carbonic anhydrase inhibitors. NSAIDs should not be taken by patients taking anticoagulants, alcohol or high-dose methotrexate. They should also be avoided in older or renally impaired patients taking digoxin, and avoided over the long term in those taking other NSAIDs.

Acetaminophen/paracetamol when given in large, or repeated doses, can cause severe liver damage, but may be given in the short term to any patient with a healthy liver. It should not be given to heavy alcohol drinkers or to persons who have recently stopped alcohol after chronic intake.

Codeine, as it is converted to morphine, is contraindicated in children who are having surgery.

Opioids should not be given to heavy alcohol drinkers.

BNF

In Confidence

YellowCard It's easiest to report online at www.yellowcard.gov.uk

MHRA

COMMISSION ON HUMAN MEDICINES (CHM)

SUSPECTED ADVERSE DRUG REACTIONS

If you suspect an adverse reaction may be related to one or more drugs/vaccines/complementary remedies, please complete this Yellow Card. See 'Adverse reactions to drugs' section in BNF or www.yellowcard.gov.uk for guidance. Do not be put off reporting because some details are not known.

PATIENT DETAILS Patient Initials:______ Sex: M / F Ethnicity:______ Weight if known (kg):______

Age (at time of reaction):______ Identification number (e.g. Your Practice or Hospital Ref):______

SUSPECTED DRUG(S)/VACCINE(S)

Drug/Vaccine (Brand if known)	Batch	Route	Dosage	Date started	Date stopped	Prescribed for

SUSPECTED REACTION(S) Please describe the reaction(s) and any treatment given:

Outcome
- Recovered
- Recovering
- Continuing
- Other

Date reaction(s) started:______ Date reaction(s) stopped:______

Do you consider the reactions to be serious? Yes / No

If yes, please indicate why the reaction is considered to be serious (please tick all that apply):

- Patient died due to reaction
- Life threatening
- Congenital abnormality
- Involved or prolonged inpatient hospitalisation
- Involved persistent or significant disability or incapacity
- Medically significant; please give details:______

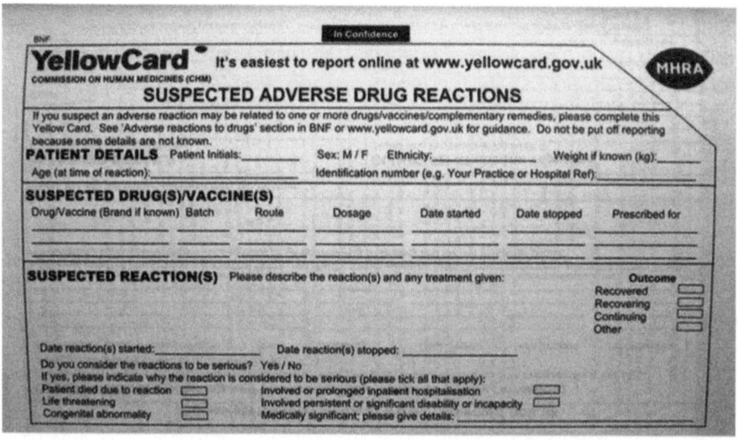

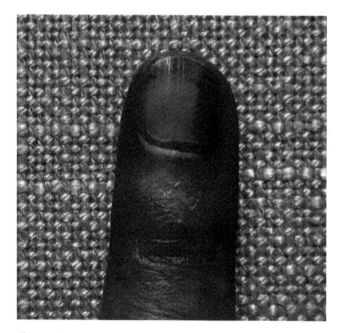

Figure 9.1 Adverse drug reactions – yellow card reporting.

Figure 9.2 Nail discolouration from chemotherapy.

Antibiotics

Allergies and anaphylaxis to antibiotics is a real possibility. Hypersensitivity reactions to beta-lactams (in penicillin and cephalosporins) are the most common reactions and more likely to follow parenteral than oral administration. Patients allergic to penicillin usually react to any other penicillin, except aztreonam. Patients with penicillin allergy should avoid carbapenems, and use caution with cephalosporins. A patient should of course be lying down when any injections are given, as fainting after injections is common and may be confused with anaphylaxis.

There are potential life-threatening interactions of some antimicrobials (erythromycin, clarithromycin, metronidazole, ketoconazole and itraconazole) with a host of other drugs whose metabolism is impaired by them. Antibiotics may also enhance the effects of warfarin via suppression of gut bacteria that produce vitamin K. Commonly employed antibiotics rarely impair the effectiveness of oral contraceptive agents.

Radiocontrast media (RCM) reactions

Intravascular iodinated RCM agents are based on a tri-iodinated benzene ring and can cause adverse reactions, which can be:

- Anaphylactoid.
- Nonanaphylactoid.
- Chemotoxic – organ-specific:
  - cardiovascular toxicity;
  - nephrotoxicity;
  - neurotoxicity.
- Vasovagal.

RCM usually act by directly releasing histamine from mast cells, rather than an allergic response. High-osmolar contrast media (HOCM) are the worst but have largely been superceded by less toxic non-ionic compounds – low-osmolar contrast media (LOCM).

People at higher risk for reactions to RCM include those:

- with past reactions to RCM;
- with asthma;
- with history of allergies;
- with history of heart disease;
- with history of kidney disease;
- taking beta-blockers;
- who are female;
- who are older.

Reactions to RCM are relatively quite common – 5 to 8% of people receiving an IV dye. Most reactions are mild, a feeling of warmth, nausea and vomiting, last only briefly and require no treatment. Moderate reactions, including severe vomiting, hives (urticaria) and swelling, occur in 1% of people receiving RCM, and may require treatment. Severe, life-threatening reactions, including anaphylaxis, occur in 0.1% of people receiving RCM and occasionally are fatal. Delayed contrast reactions can occur anywhere from 3 hours to 7 days following the administration of RCM.

Iodine and iodides are also present in some antiseptics such as povidone-iodine, and can provoke dangerous reactions. Povidone-iodine is a commonly used antibacterial agent also used in other products such as foods, drugs (e.g. antihistamines, diuretics and analgesics), hair products and toothpastes. Allergic contact reactions to povidone-iodine preparations are rare, and do not necessarily indicate reactivity to RCM.

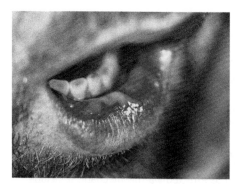

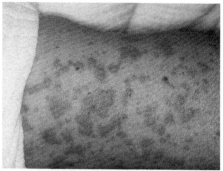

Figure 9.3 Adverse drug reactions – erythema multiforme lip lesions.

Figure 9.4 Adverse drug reactions – penicillin rash on arm.

Monoclonal antibodies and other biologics (see below)

Immunomodulator agents (see below)

Drug-induced hypersensitivity syndromes

Drug-induced hypersensitivity syndrome (DIHS) is a glandular fever-like syndrome (fever, rash, cervical lymphadenopathy, raised leukocyte count with atypical lymphocytes, and liver dysfunction) following use of certain drugs – especially anticonvulsants, isoniazid and sulphonamides. Many cases seem to be associated with reactivation of human herpesvirus 6 (HHV-6) or other herpesviruses.

Anticonvulsant hypersensitivity syndrome (AHS) is a potentially fatal drug-induced, multi-organ syndrome of urticaria, purpura, erythema multiforme, and exfoliative dermatitis reported with carbamazepine, phenytoin, phenobarbitone and lamotrigine with an ethnic predisposition, especially an association with HLA-B*1502 in some Asian patients.

Drug interactions

Drug absorption and activities can be impaired by other drugs or foods:

Antacids can cause early release of drugs from enteric-coated capsules, and can reduce absorption of antimicrobials.

Citrus fruit acids may cause some medications to dissolve prematurely in the stomach rather than the intestine and therefore, taking drugs with acid fruit juices (and carbonated sodas) is usually not recommended. Citrus juice, however, improves the absorption of iron.

Cranberry juice (*Vaccinium macrocarpon*) may enhance warfarin.

Garlic supplements appear to enhance anticoagulants.

Grapefruit, fresh, canned or frozen, or grapefruit juice, or drinks that contain grapefruit juice, can affect the metabolism of several drugs by cytochrome p450 (CYP450)
– typically enhancing their activity. Sour orange juice (e.g. Seville oranges), lime juice,

pomelos and tangelos (a grapefruit hybrid) possibly also have this effect. Some fruits and juices, including cranberry, Goji berry, and apple, contain other active moieties that can affect different P450 isoforms and transporters and interact with different drugs. These effects appear to last for at least 3 days. CYP3A4 is involved in the metabolism of around 50% of drugs, so a wide variety of drugs can be affected by the consumption of grapefruit juice and its furanocoumarins. Impaired metabolism of various cardiac drugs after ingestion of grapefruit juice has led to an increase in QT interval and torsades de pointes. Statins are also affected – leading to rhabdomyolysis.

A second mechanism involves the inhibition by grapefruit due to flavonoids such as naringin and hesperidin. The effect is reduced bioavailability of the drug and a decreased efficacy lasting about 4 hours. Drugs affected via this mechanism include aliskiren, celiprolol, ciprofloxacin, fexofenadine, and talinolol.

Finally, grapefruit juice constituents, including flavonoids, have also been implicated in activating P-glycoprotein, an intestinal-wall drug efflux mechanism.

The main problem with grapefruit is with drugs that act on the CNS (benzodiazepines, buspirone, carbamazepine, pimozide, quetiapine). Anticoagulants, antiarrhythmics, calcium channel blockers, cytotoxics, immunosuppressants (ciclosporin, tacrolimus, sirolimus) and statins (atorvastatin, simvastatin) are the other main problems.

Most other citrus fruits, such as lemons, sweet oranges and tangerines, are considered safe in this respect.

Medications such as itraconazole, ketoconazole, ciclosporin, diltiazem and erythromycin may inhibit both intestinal CYNA4 and hepatic CYP3A4.

Metoclopramide enhances absorption of aspirin and acetaminophen/paracetamol.

Minerals may influence drug absorption. Iron, magnesium and aluminium in drugs can impair tetracycline absorption. Aluminium can impair absorption of azole antifungals. Iron can reduce absorption of quinolones (e.g. ciprofloxacin). Calcium in dairy foods and in supplements chelates tetracyclines.

Phytates in chapattis bind calcium and impair its absorption.

Pomegranate may inhibit cytochrome p450 and increase the effects and adverse effects of codeine, carbamazepine, diclofenac, midazolam and tramadol, and other drugs.

Vitamin K in foods (e.g. liver, cabbage, spinach, cauliflower, green tea and broccoli), in contrast, can substantially reduce the effectiveness of warfarin.

Anti-thrombotic agents

Main dental considerations

(*See also generic guidance under main dental considerations on page 63 top, and also Section 2).

Anti-thrombotic agents are used for treatment of a thrombus – such as DVTs, PEs and other thromboses – to prevent them enlarging (Section 5), or to prevent thrombosis in people at risk, such as those who have:

- atrial fibrillation
- blood disorders, e.g. inherited thrombophilia, antiphospholipid syndrome.
- endocarditis
- mechanical heart valve
- mitral stenosis
- hip or knee replacements recently.

The two main classes of anti-thrombotic drugs are anticoagulants and antiplatelet drugs.
Anticoagulants slow clotting, thereby reducing fibrin formation and preventing clots from forming and growing. They include:
- Heparins;
- Vitamin K antagonists (VKAs – such as warfarin/coumarins);
- Newer oral anticoagulants (NOACs – such as dabigatran).
Antiplatelet agents such as aspirin or clopidogrel, prevent platelets from clumping and clots forming and growing.

All anti-thrombotic agents also produce a bleeding tendency and may cause postoperative bleeding. Dental preventive care is especially important in order to minimize the need for surgical intervention. In general, these agents should be stopped only where the risk of postoperative bleeding is high (e.g. major surgery) or where the consequences of even minor bleeding are significant (e.g. retinal and intracranial surgery) though, for other minor surgery, drug dose reductions are rarely needed and indeed may put the patient at risk from thromboses which can be lethal. This should be discussed with the patient, who also must be warned of the risk of intra- and postoperative bleeding and intra-/extraoral bruising.

Anticoagulants

Heparins

Heparin is a natural sulphated glycosaminoglycan, abundant in mast cells. Heparin blocks the conversion of fibrinogen to fibrin, acts on factors IX–XII and inhibits thrombin-induced platelet activation. Heparin acts by potentiating anti-thrombin III which inhibits the activation of clotting factors II, IX, X and XI prolongs the APTT. Use for more than 5 days can induce thrombocytopenia. Heparin is used subcutaneously or intravenously for acute thrombo-embolic episodes and to prevent DVT and PE (Section 5).

Heparin is available as standard (unfractionated [UFH] – which has an immediate effect on blood clotting which is usually lost within 6 hours of stopping it), or low molecular weight (LMWH) heparins. Unfractionated heparin (UFH) is given via intravenous infusion, with the dose titrated according to the APTT. The half-life of UFH is 1 hour, making it useful where rapid normalisation of anticoagulation is required e.g: before surgery.

LMWHs (ardeparin, certoparin, dalteparin, danaparoid, enoxaparin, nadroparin, reviparin, tinzaparin) interact with factor Xa and are given once daily to reduce DVT as they

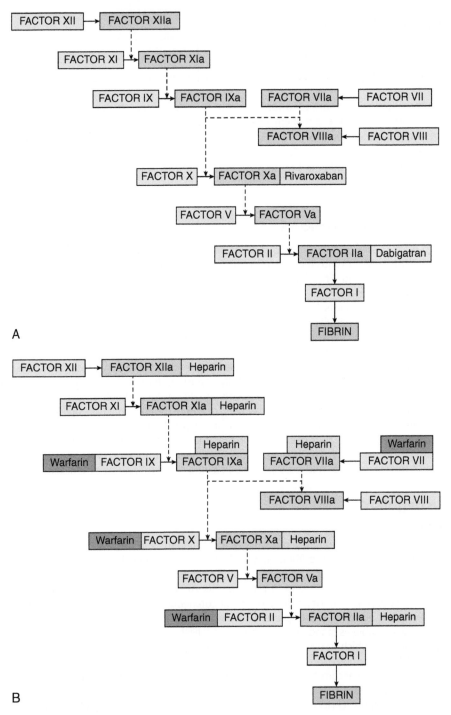

Figure 9.5 Blood coagulation cascade showing sites of action of: **(A)** NOACS; **(B)** heparin/warfarin.

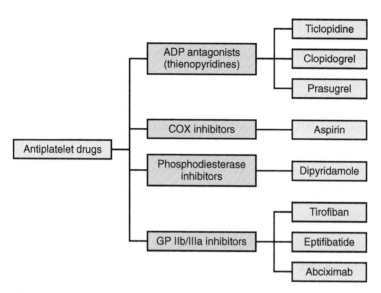

Figure 9.6 Anti-platelet drugs.

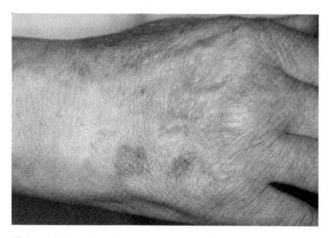

Figure. 9.7 Bruising secondary to warfarin.

have longer action. The APTT is normal; a Factor Xa assay can be used to monitor the anticoagulant effect of LMWH, but is not routinely required. Heparin anticoagulation can be reversed by withdrawal, or by protamine sulphate.

Vitamin K antagonists (VKAs)

Warfarin

VKAs include coumarins (e.g. warfarin). They reduce liver synthesis of several coagulation factors, especially factors II (prothrombin), VII, IX and X and proteins C, S and Z. Warfarin effects begin after 8–12 hours, are maximal at 36 hours, but persist 72 hours. Warfarin is commonly used for patients who have had cardiac surgery, organ transplants, or thromboses. The prothrombin time (PT) and activated partial thromboplastin times (APTT) are prolonged as is the International Normalised Ratio (INR) – the PT ratio (patient's PT/control PT) that would have been obtained if an international reference thromboplastin reagent had been used. In a person with a PT within the normal range, the INR is approximately 1. An INR above 1 indicates that clotting will take longer than normal. An INR of 2 to 3 is the usual therapeutic range for DVT, and an INR of up to 3.5 is required for patients with prosthetic heart valves.

The management of surgical patients on anticoagulants should consider the type of procedure and INR value. Stopping warfarin preoperatively is not necessarily the best policy since it does not significantly reduce bleeding but, in contrast, may cause hypercoagulability and rebound thrombosis which has damaged prosthetic cardiac valves and even caused deaths. Therefore, unless serious bleeding is anticipated, warfarin should be continued.

Warfarin can be reversed in emergency situations, by vitamin K, fresh-frozen plasma, prothrombin complex concentrate, or recombinant factor VIIa.

Newer oral anticoagulants (NOACs)

Novel oral anticoagulants (NOACs), such as direct thrombin inhibitors (DTI) *(gatrans)* and anti-Xa (xabans), target the single coagulation enzymes thrombin (dabigatran) or factor Xa (apixaban, rivaroxaban, and edoxaban). In contrast to warfarin, NOACs have minimal food and drug interactions. Moreover, compared with warfarin, NOACs do not require monitoring and have less thrombotic events and lower rates of major bleeding events. NOACs are thus poised to replace VKAs for many patients with atrial fibrillation and may have a role after acute coronary syndromes.

Dabigatran and rivaroxaban are both quickly absorbed and have short half-lives compared to warfarin so, in the event of excessive anticoagulant activity, discontinuing the drug is usually sufficient. They have no antidotes. There is no need for routine coagulation monitoring in the same way as warfarin using the prothrombin time or INR.

Concomitant administration of potent inducers of P-glycoprotein (P-gp:efflux membrane transporters), such as rifampicin, St. John's wort, carbamazepine, and phenytoin which can decrease dabigatran plasma concentrations should be avoided. Rivaroxaban is metabolized via CYP3A4 and CYP2J2 and is a substrate of P-gp, and is not recommended in patients receiving strong inhibitors of both CYP3A4 and P-gp, such as azole-antimycotics and HIV protease inhibitors (PIs). The known drug interaction profiles of both dabigatran and rivaroxaban as regards antimicrobials and analgesics are less restrictive than with warfarin. It may be better to confine analgesic use to paracetamol since NSAIDs have antiplatelet effects. Dabigatran and rivaroxaban have no antidotes. If reversal is essential, haemodialysis has been recommended, coagulation factor concentrates may be effective, and idarucizumab, an antibody fragment which binds it, can reverse dabigatran.

No preoperative blood testing, INR monitoring or dose adjustment is needed for NOACs but, in any patients with another clotting defect, recently placed stent, liver or kidney functional impairment, alcohol problems and in patients under treatment with cytotoxic agents, caution is advised. Table 9.1 compares VKAs and NOACs.

Antiplatelets

Platelets are critical in haemostasis: damaged endothelium activates platelets which then adhere and aggregate. Their release of thromboxane A2 and adenosine diphosphate (ADP) amplifies and propagates the process by stimulating surrounding platelets. Production of

Table 9.1 VKAs and NOACs

	Warfarin	Dabigatran	Rivaroxaban
Targets	Factors II, VII, IX and X; proteins C & S	Thrombin	Factor Xa
Effective half-life	20–60 h (mean ~40 h)	Adult 12–17 h; Old people 14–17 h (normal renal function)	Young 5–9 h; Old people 11–13 h
Food and other effects on absorption	Food may delay absorption rate	Acidic environment needed. Absorption reduced by proton pump inhibitors and antacids	Food increases rate and extent of absorption by 25–35%
Need for routine monitoring of coagulation	Yes (PT/INR)	No	No
Antidote/reversal agent available	Yes (vitamin K)	Idarucizumab	Andexanet
Drug and food interactions: increased anticoagulation	**Antifungals:** miconazole, ketoconazole, fluconazole (lesser degree: itraconazole) **Antibiotics:** erythromycin, clarithromycin, (metronidazole possibly) azithromycin, tetracycline, doxycycline, cephalosporins, levofloxacin **Analgesics:** NSAIDs, (antiplatelet agents: aspirin, clopidogrel), ibuprofen, diclofenac, paracetamol (prolonged regular use) **Food/herbs:** cranberry juice, St John's wort, alcohol, many dietary supplements	**Antifungals:** ketoconazole, itraconazole **Antibiotics:** erythromycin, clarithromycin **Analgesics:** NSAIDs, (antiplatelet agents: aspirin, clopidogrel), ketorolac (diclofenac appears not to interact) **Food/herbs:** alfalfa, anise, bilberry	**Antifungals:** ketoconazole, itraconazole (miconazole if renal function impaired) **Analgesics:** NSAIDs, (antiplatelet agents: aspirin, clopidogrel) **Food/herbs:** grapefruit juice, alfalfa, anise, bilberry
Drug and food interactions giving decreased anticoagulation	Green leafy vegetables (vitamin K), vitamin E	Dexamethasone Carbamazepine Rifampicin St John's wort	Phenytoin Rifampicin St John's wort

thrombin via the coagulation cascade is also accelerated, stabilizing the thrombus by the conversion of fibrinogen to fibrin.

Antiplatelet drugs act by inhibiting platelet aggregation and thrombus formation and are most effective for arterial clots (composed largely of platelets). There is no suitable test available to assess the increased risk of bleeding in patients taking antiplatelet medications. The different classes of antiplatelets act at different points:

- **Aspirin** – a non-selective, irreversible inhibitor of cyclo-oxygenase (COX) – catalyses thromboxane and prostaglandin production and reduces thromboxane A2.
- **Clopidogrel** – an ADP receptor antagonist, inhibits ADP from binding to platelet receptors, preventing up-regulation of glycoprotein (GP) IIb/IIIa receptor, blocking amplification of platelet aggregation. Importantly, it is routinely used in treatment of acute coronary syndromes (ACS) and post-percutaneous coronary intervention (PCI) stenting (in conjunction with aspirin). Clopidogrel is used alone in those who cannot tolerate aspirin.
- **Prasugrel** – a prodrug from the same family as clopidogrel – is more efficient at platelet inhibition. Prasugrel is used in combination with aspirin in ACS patients undergoing PCI (Section 5) when:
  - immediate PCI is necessary for ST segment elevation myocardial infarction (STEMI); or
  - stent thromboses during treatment with clopidogrel; or
  - diabetic patients.
- **Dipyridamole** – acts by inhibiting platelet adenosine uptake and reducing ADP-induced aggregation.
- **Glycoprotein IIb/IIIa antagonists** – inhibit the final common pathway of platelet aggregation where fibrinogen binds to GP IIb/IIIa receptor. The monoclonal antibody abciximab was the original but can be used once only, as inhibitors form. Newer agents include eptifibatide and tirofiban. GP IIb/IIIa antagonists can cause severe bleeding, most often from the site of femoral puncture for percutaneous transluminal coronary angioplasty (PTCA).
- **Vorapaxar** – a protease-activated receptor (PAR) antagonist.

Main dental considerations of anti-thrombotic agents

(*See also generic guidance under main dental considerations on page 63 top, and also Section 2).

All dental professionals encounter patients who experience prolonged bleeding following operative procedures. Often causal is a dental extraction. Saliva contains fibrinolytic agents which may aggravate the situation. In most cases the cause is local and bleeding can be managed using simple local haemostatic measures such as applying pressure to the wound with sterile pads (moistened with water, normal saline or 5% tranexamic acid solution), absorbable oxidized cellulose sponges, suturing, and also giving postoperative instructions verbally and in writing.

Surgery should ideally be planned and done:

- At the beginning of the day – this allows more time to deal with immediate re-bleeding problems.
- Early in the week – this allows for delayed re-bleeding episodes occurring after 24–48 hours to be dealt with during the working week.

Avoid intramuscular injections. Regional LA block or floor of mouth injections may present a hazard, as they can result in excessive bleeding into fascial spaces. Direct mucosal LA infiltrations, intraligamentary or intrapapillary injections can usually be performed safely. Routine dental care, such as supragingival scaling, non-surgical endodontics, removable and fixed prosthodontics and direct restorative root planing procedures, can usually be performed without additional concern. Usually, antithrombotic therapy should not be stopped before dental procedures such as biopsy, implant placement, periodontal surgery, endodontic surgery and dentoalveolar surgery (1–3 teeth). Use haemostatic agents (e.g. Gelfoam) as required.

If there is concern, consult the patient's physician. If maxillofacial surgery is needed, refer the patient to a hospital setting. Antimicrobials may affect anticoagulation states, and increased monitoring will be required until 3–4 days post-treatment: avoid beta-lactam antibiotics, ciprofloxacin, doxycycline, erythromycin, metronidazole, quinolones, and tetracyclines; and azoles (e.g. fluconazole, ketoconazole, miconazole). Avoid NSAIDs in patients taking ANY antithrombotic. Tramadol and paracetamol can enhance warfarin.

Heparins

For uncomplicated forceps extraction of 1–3 teeth, there is usually no need to interfere with heparin or LMWH anticoagulation. Before more advanced surgery in a heparin-treated patient, medical advice should be sought. Where heparin has been stopped, any surgery can safely be carried out after 6–8 h. In renal dialysis patients, or patients having cardiopulmonary bypass or other extracorporeal circulation with heparinization, surgery is best carried out on the day after dialysis. LMWH may have little effect on post-operative bleeding, despite their longer activity (up to 24 h). However, the advice of the haematologist should be sought before surgery.

Warfarin and VKAs

Surgery is the main oral healthcare hazard to the patient on warfarin and thus the possibility of alternatives, e.g. endodontics, should always be considered. The INR is used as a guideline to care and should be checked on the day of operation or, if that is not possible, within 24 hours prior to surgery. Anticoagulant treatment should not be altered without the agreement of the clinician in charge, and stopping it preoperatively is rarely the best policy, since it does not necessarily significantly reduce bleeding but, in contrast, may cause hypercoagulability and rebound thrombosis – which has damaged prosthetic cardiac valves and even caused thrombotic deaths in dental patients. Hospital or specialist referral is indicated in the presence of:

- INR >4.0;
- need for more than a simple surgical procedure;
- presence of additional bleeding risk factors or logistical difficulties; or
- drug interactions with warfarin especially, azoles, erythromycin and metronidazole (Table 9.1). http://www.bcshguidelines.com/pdf/WarfarinandOralSurgery26407.pdf http://www.npsa.nhs.uk/nrls/alerts-and-directives/alerts/anticoagulant/

Novel oral anticoagulants (NOACs)

NOACs include dabigatran etexilate and rivaroxaban both of which are quickly absorbed and have short half-lives so, in the event of excessive anticoagulant activity, discontinuing the drug is usually sufficient. Most dental situations such as removal of a small number of teeth would be comparable to treating a patient with an INR ≤ 4, relying on local haemostatic measures.

NOAC therapy can be recommenced 4 hours after a surgical procedure.

Antiplatelet drugs

There is no evidence that continuing antiplatelet monotherapy causes major bleeding problems during or after minor surgery such as dental extractions. Antiplatelet agents when prescribed as primary thrombus prevention may be safely withdrawn 7 days before surgery, but any decision to stop antiplatelet therapy used for secondary prevention, must balance the risk of thrombosis and ischaemia with bleeding. The risk of bleeding is greater with aspirin–clopidogrel or prasugrel–aspirin combinations, but these patients are generally already at a higher risk of thromboembolic events; therefore advice from a specialist should be sought before considering withholding treatment, or the patient may need to be referred to a hospital setting for the procedure. Patients who should *not* have their medications stopped or altered prior to dental surgical procedures in primary care include those taking:

- aspirin (low-dose);
- clopidogrel;
- dipyridamole.

Consensus is that for dentoalveolar surgical procedures, antiplatelet medications should not be stopped or doses altered, but that local haemostatic measures be used to control bleeding. Patients taking antiplatelet medication with the following medical problems however, should not be treated in primary care without medical advice – or should be referred to a dental hospital or hospital based dental clinic:

- liver impairment and/or alcoholism;
- renal failure;
- thrombocytopenia, haemophilia or other disorder of haemostasis;
- those currently receiving a course of cytotoxic medication.

Patients requiring major surgery should usually be treated in a secondary care setting.

Other parenteral agents

Other parenteral agents influencing haemostasis include *heparinoids* such as danaparoid; *hirudins* such as lepirudin and desirudin. The physician should be consulted before any major surgical procedure but dentoalveolar surgery is usually uncomplicated.

Biological therapies

Biopharmaceuticals (biologics or biologicals) are any medicinal product manufactured in or extracted from a biological source, which can include materials ranging from blood to stem cells and vaccines but is usually used for gene-based and cellular biologics, often generated by DNA recombinant biotechnology. Biologics include:

- Small molecules.
- Biologics nearly identical to key signalling proteins such as erythropoeitin, colony stimulating factors, growth hormone or biosynthetic human insulin.
- Monoclonal antibodies; 'custom-designed' using hybridoma or other technology to counteract or block a given substance, or target a cell type.
- Receptor constructs or 'fusion proteins'; based on a natural receptor giving specificity, linked to the immunoglobulin frame, which gives stability.

Biologics are often used to target immunocytes or their products and thus specific steps in pro-inflammatory pathways, or are used in cancer therapy. Biologics often target T lymphocytes, B cells, granulocytes, antigen-presenting cells (APCs; dendritic cells [DCs], macrophages) or other immunocytes and mediators (cytokines, chemokines, growth factors, complement components).

Biologics include a number of human (suffix mab), humanized (suffix: zumab) or chimeric (mouse–human) (suffix: ximab) monoclonal antibodies or variant fusion proteins (suffix: cept). They are expensive, and must be given by injection or infusion.

As the number of biologics increases exponentially, reports of ADRs are also increasing; they have an inherent risk for infusion reactions, cytokine storms, fatigue, arthralgias, immunosuppression, autoimmunity, potential malignancy and other disorders. Despite these serious potential adverse effects, biologics are generally considered safe.

The three main broad classes of biologicals used currently are tumour necrosis factor-alpha (TNF-α) inhibitors, lymphocyte modulators and interleukin inhibitors.

TNF-α inhibitors (anti-TNFs)

TNF-α, a key proinflammatory cytokine, is central in the pathogenesis of immunologically driven disease acting via pathways to promote increased leukocyte activation and recruitment to sites of tissue inflammation. TNF-α inhibitors (e.g. infliximab, etanercept, and adalimumab), the most common biologics, blocking TNF effects upon target inflammatory cells.

Injection and infusion site reactions are the most common adverse effects from TNF-α blockers. However, the most important safety problem is an increased risk of infections including upper respiratory tract infections, opportunistic infections and reactivation of tuberculosis. Fungal infections are also increased. Viral infections may also be seen. A further important safety problem related to many biologic agents is an increased risk of neoplasms.

Skin reactions have been reported with all TNF-α blockers. Aplastic anaemia and/or pancytopenia may complicate treatment with etanercept or adalimumab. Autoimmune diseases, including systemic (lupus erythematosus, vasculitis, sarcoidosis, antiphospholipid syndrome and inflammatory myopathies) and organ-specific (interstitial lung disease, uveitis, optic neuritis, peripheral neuropathies, multiple sclerosis, psoriasis, inflammatory bowel disease and autoimmune hepatitis) disorders have been reported. Demyelinating diseases or flare-ups of existing demyelinating diseases can occur with TNF-α antagonists.

Lymphocyte modulators and interleukin inhibitors

Lymphocyte modulators act on specific CD antigens and are either T-cell modulators (e.g. alefacept – a chimeric fusion protein targeting CD^{2+} on memory T and natural killer (NK) cells, so blocking the LFA-3/CD2 interaction in antigen presentation and also inducing T

Table 9.2 Detail of targets and effects of biologics

mAb/fusion protein	Common names	Targets*	Applications
Abatacept	Orencia	CD80 & CD86	Transplant rejection, rheumatoid arthritis
Abciximab	ReoPro	gpII/IIIa	Coronary interventions
Adalimumab	Humira	TNF alpha	Crohn's; rheumatoid arthritis, psoriasis
Alefacept	Amevive	CD2	Psoriasis
Alemtuzumab	Campath	CD52	Chronic lymphoid leukaemia, rheumatoid
Anakinra	Kineret	IL-1R	Rheumatoid arthritis
Basiliximab	Simulect	IL-2R	Transplant rejection
Belatacept	Nulojix	CD80 & CD86	Transplant rejection
Bevacizumab	Avastin	VEGF	Cancers (various)
Bortezomib	Velcade	Proteasome	Multiple myeloma
Canakinumab	Ilarts	IL-1 beta	Juvenile arthritis
Catumaxomab	Removab	Epithelial cell adhesion molecule	Cancers
Certolizumab	Cimzia	TNF alpha	Crohn's; rheumatoid arthritis, psoriasis
Cetuximab	Erbitux	EGFR	Head and neck cancer
Daclizumab	Zenapax	IL-2R	Transplant rejection
Denileukin diftitox	Ontak	IL-2R	Lymphoma
Denosumab	Prolia	RANKL	Osteoporosis
Eculizumab	Soliris	C5	Paroxysmal nocturnal haemoglobinuria
Etanercept	Enbrel	TNF alpha	Crohn's; rheumatoid, psoriasis, sarcoid
Gemtuzumab	Mylotarg	CD33	Acute myeloid leukaemia
Golimumab	Simponi	TNF alpha	Crohn's; rheumatoid arthritis, psoriasis
Ibritumomab	Zevalin	CD20	NHL
Infliximab	Remicade	TNF alpha	Crohn's; rheumatoid arthritis, psoriasis, sarcoid
Muromonab	Orthoclone OKT3	CD3	Transplant rejection
Natalizumab	Tysabri	Integrin receptor antagonist	Multiple sclerosis, Crohn's
Omalizumab	Xolair	IgE	Asthma
Palivizumab	Synagis	Respiratory syncytial virus	Respiratory syncytial virus
Panitumumab	Vectibix	EGFR	Cancers

Table 9.2 Detail of targets and effects of biologics—cont'd

mAb/fusion protein	Common names	Targets*	Applications
Ranibizumab	Lucentis	VEGF	Age-related macular degeneration
Raxibacumab	ACthrax	*Bacillus anthracis*	Anthrax
Rilonacept	Arcalyst	IL-1	Autoinflammatory disease
Rituximab	Rituxan or Mabthera	CD20	NHL, rheumatoid arthritis
Tocilizumab	Actmera	IL-6R	Rheumatoid arthritis
Tositumomab	Bexxar	CD20	NHL
Trastuzumab	Herceptin	ErbB2 (Her 2)	Breast cancer
Ustekinumab	Stelara	IL-12 & IL-23	Psoriasis

*See text.

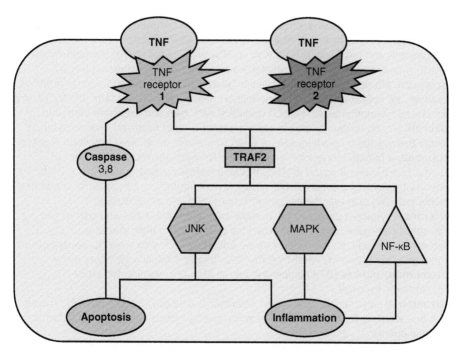

Figure. 9.8 Tumour Necrosis Factor (TNF) roles in inflammation. Downstream signalling pathways of TNF leading to cell death by apoptosis, or to inflammation and survival. Inflammatory mediators: TRAF = TNFR-associated factor; JNK = Jun N-terminal kinase; MAPK = mitogen-activated protein kinases; NF-κB = nuclear factor-κB. (After Georgakopoulou E, Scully C 2015 Biological agents; what they are, how they can affect oral health and how they can modulate oral health care. British Dental Journal 26;218(12):671-7)

cell apoptosis); or B-cell modulators (e.g. rituximab – targets CD20, on mature B cells, so depleting them). Rituximab can have serious adverse effects including cutaneous eruptions, infections (some fatal), and tumour lysis syndrome (TLS).

Interleukin inhibitors are a group of immunosuppressive agents which include anakinra, basiliximab, briakinumab, canakinumab, daclizumab, mepolizumab, rilonacept, secukinumab, tocilizumab, and ustekinumab. Interleukin inhibitors have a broad spectrum of clinical uses depending on the interleukin they target. For example, anti-IL6 agent tocilizumab is used for rheumatoid arthritis (RA), anti-IL12 and -IL23 agent ustekinumab is used for psoriasis. Basiliximab is a chimeric anti-interleukin-2 receptor monoclonal antibody which is used to prevent acute renal transplantation rejection. The most usual undesirable effects of basiliximab in adult patients are constipation, infections, pain, nausea, peripheral oedema, hypertension, anaemia, headache, hyperkalaemia, hypercholesterolaemia, raised serum creatinine, and hypophosphataemia.

Daclizumab is another anti-interleukin-2 receptor antibody used to prevent acute transplant rejection and appears to share a similar safety profile with basiliximab.

Other biologicals

Anticoagulant and anti neo-vascularization agents include:

Abciximab, the Fab section of the chimeric human-murine monoclonal antibody 7E3 which binds to the platelet receptor glycoprotein IIb/IIIa and inhibits blood clot formation. The main adverse effects are bleeding and thrombocytopenia.

Bevacizumab is a vascular endothelial growth factor (VEGF) inhibitor which blocks angiogenesis and has been labelled with an FDA warning for arterial thromboembolic events, hypertension, reversible posterior leukoencephalopathy syndrome (RPLS), proteinuria, infusion reactions, and ovarian failure. The most common adverse reactions, however, are epistaxis, headache, hypertension, rhinitis, proteinuria, taste alterations, dry skin, rectal haemorrhage, lacrimation disorders, back pain and exfoliative dermatitis.

Cetuximab, an anti-epidermal growth factor receptor used in head and neck or colorectal cancer therapy, has a common adverse effect of a severe generalized acneiform eruption.

Denosumab, a human monoclonal antibody which targets the receptor activator of nuclear factor-kappa B ligand (RANKL) blocking RANKL binding to RANK, and inhibiting osteoclast growth and action, hence reducing bone resorption, can cause severe adverse events including skin exanthemas and infections, and jaw osteonecrosis.

Interferons – cytokines produced by immune cells and fibroblasts – and part of the non-specific immune response, are used for various therapeutic purposes. Recombinant products of interferons have adverse effects which are flu-like symptoms and psychiatric disorders, while they may also trigger immunologic phenomena.

Panitumumab, another EGFR competitor, has an FDA box warning for severe dermatologic toxicities.

Pertuzumab, a recombinant humanized monoclonal antibody directed at HER2, has an FDA box warning for fetal toxicity: common adverse effects are febrile neutropenia and leukopenia.

Trastuzumab, a humanized monoclonal antibody targeting HER-2/neu has severe adverse effects, which include congestive heart failure while there are cases of patients who have developed leukaemia.

Main dental considerations

(*See also generic guidance under main dental considerations on page 63 top, and also Section 2).

Consider the possible drug sequelae (e.g. bleeding tendency, immunosuppression, delayed healing).

Chemotherapy (CTx)

Chemotherapy drugs are used especially in:

- lymphoproliferative disease (leukaemias/lymphomas) treatments;
- cancer control; and
- conditioning for bone marrow (HSCT) transplantation.

These agents are many, and they act mainly by interaction with cancer cell DNA or RNA and are used singly or in combinations (Box 9.1).

Various hormones (ethinyloestradiol, megestrol medroxyprogesterone, or norethisterone) or drugs for prostate cancers (diethylstilbestrol, fosfestrol) are also used to control tumours such as breast cancer. Hormone antagonists are used in some tumours, such as breast (tamoxifen, toremifene, aminoglutethimide, anastrozole, letrozole, exemestane, trilostane, goserelin) and prostate cancers (buserelin, goserelin, leuprorelin, triptorelin, cyproterone acetate, flutamide, bicalutamide).

Box 9.1   Classification of chemotherapy drugs

Alkylating agents
Alkane sulfonates, e.g. busulfan
Cyclophosphamide
Nitrogen mustard-based agents (mechorethamine)
Nitrosoureas, e.g. carmustine
L-phenylalanine mustard-based agents (mephalan)

Antimetabolites
Cytosine arabinose (e.g. cytarabine)
Fluoropyrimidines (e.g. 5FU [fluorouracil], capecitabine)
Gemcitabine
Methotrexate

Antimicrotubule agents
Taxanes (paclitaxel, docetaxel)
Vinca alkaloids (vinblastine, vinorelbine)

Antitumour antibiotics
Actinomycin D
Anthracyclines (daunorubicin, doxorubicin)
Bleomycin
Camptothecines (irinotecan, topotecan)
Mitomycin C
Podofylotoxines (etoposide, teniposide)

Platinum co-ordination complex agents
Carboplatin
Cisplatin
Oxaliplatin

Others
Monoclonal antibodies, signalling inhibitors.

Antibodies linked to toxins or radionuclides can kill cells. Monoclonal antibodies can block cancer cell growth or effects. Gene therapy is being developed to replace damaged tumour suppressor genes, or otherwise influence cell activity.

The type of CTx prescribed by the oncologist depends on many factors, often including:

- cancer type
- cancer size
- cancer location
- patient's other cancer treatments.
- patient's age and other medical conditions
- adverse effects of CTx.

Some agents doses must be tailored depending on host genetic patterns and enzyme activities (Table 9.3). Chemotherapy is typically given intravenously, sometimes via a 'port' or central venous line. Drugs used must be handled with gloves, with care, especially by women as they are teratogenic.

Most cytotoxic agents cause complications by killing other rapidly dividing cells, particularly if treatment is prolonged or in high dosage, especially causing:

- Alopecia.
- Bone marrow suppression (causing a bleeding tendency and liability to infections) and hyperuricaemia.
- Constipation or diarrhoea.
- Fatigue.
- Mucositis.
- Nausea and vomiting.
- Neuropathies.
- Reproductive function suppression.
- Skin reactions.

Table 9.3 Tailored chemotherapy

DME	Enzyme	Drugs affected	Actions
CYP2D6	Cytochrome P450 (CYP2D6)	Tamoxifen (nolvadex), Codeine, SSRIs	Care with doses
CYP2B6	Cytochrome P450 (CYP2B6)	Cyclophosphamide (cytoxan) ifofsamide, protease inhibitors	Care with doses
DPD	Dihydropyrimidine	5-FU capecitabine (xeloda)	Genetic screen
G6PD	Glucose 6 phosphate dehydrogenase	Rasburicase (elitek)	Contraindicated
MTHFR	Methylene tetrahydrofolate reductase	Methotrexate (rheumatrex)	Care with doses
TMPT	Thiopurine methyl transferase	6-mercaptopurine, azathioprine	Dose reduction
UGT1A1	Uridine diphosphate glucuronyl transferase	Irinotecan (camptosar), nilotinib (tasigna)	Care with doses

DME = drug metabolising enzyme.

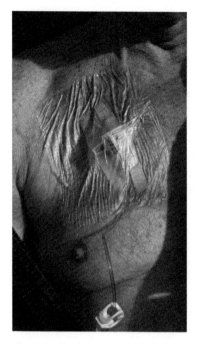

Figure 9.9 Chemotherapy – cannula in chest for Hickman line.

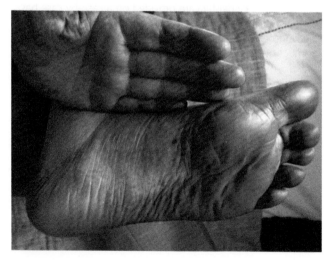

Figure 9.10 Palmar-plantar erythrodysesthesia (PPE; hand–foot syndrome) from chemotherapy.

Some toxicities are related to genetic enzyme defects such as dihydropyrimidine dehydro-genase (DPD deficiency) which may result in life-threatening toxicity after exposure to 5-FU or capecitabine.

See: www.macmillan.org.uk/Cancerinformation/Cancertreatment/Treatmenttypes/Chemo therapy/Chemotherapy.aspx

Central line-associated bloodstream infection (CLABSI)

This is serious and presents with fever, skin erythema and soreness around the line entry point (Section 7). Isolates may include *Staphylococcus aureus, Klebsiella pneumonia, E. coli, Pseudomonas aeruginosa* and *Candida* spp. – and resistance can be an issue.

Palmar plantar erythrodysaesthesia (PPE; or hand-foot syndrome)

This is a toxicity with specific chemotherapy that affect the palms of hands and soles of feet, with pain, swelling, numbness, tingling, redness or desquamation (Fig. 9.10).

Main dental considerations

(*See also generic guidance under main dental considerations on page 63 top, and also Section 2).

Oral manifestations may include:

- Mucositis
- Infections
- Dysgeusia
- Xerostomia and hyposalivation
- Bleeding
- Halitosis.

Advice on preventive care, oral hygiene and diet is important. Consider the possible drug sequelae (e.g. bleeding tendency, immunosuppression). Generally, elective care is deferred during active chemotherapy, with emergency dental care provided on a case-by-case basis after consultation with the oncologist. If surgery or other invasive procedures are required, allow at least 10–14 days of healing before re-initiation of chemotherapy. Provide topical anaesthetics for oral pain from mucositis. Avoid the use of NSAIDs.

Complementary and alternative medicine

In the resource-rich world, therapies that are not currently considered an integral part of *conventional* (allopathic) medical practice are termed *complementary* (when used in addition to), and *alternative* (when used instead of), conventional treatments. Such therapies (complementary and alternative medicine – or CAM) include, but are not limited to, acupuncture, chiropractic, specialized diets, faith healing, folk medicine, herbal (natural) medicine, homoeopathy, naturopathy, new age healing, massage and music therapy. However, there is only limited evidence of efficacy for many CAM therapies – though acupuncture for knee pain, insomnia, nausea or vomiting and back pain may have some benefit.

Many proven effective conventional drugs originated from plant sources. Examples include aspirin (from willow bark), digoxin (foxglove), morphine (opium poppy) and quinine (cinchona bark). However, other natural or herbal products may not be safe, and research into safety and efficacy of most has been limited because of product variability, lack of controlled studies and few legal controls. Some herbal drugs do appear to be effective and fairly safe and there are reliable published data supporting a potential medicinal role for aloe vera, melatonin, saw palmetto, and St John's wort. Reliable published efficacy data are weaker for gingko biloba and alpha lipoic acid, but contradictory for valerian and echinacea.

There are potential drug interactions with some herbals and others (e.g. opioids, cocaine and peyote) are addictive; many are highly toxic (e.g. some Chinese weight loss herbs are nephrotoxic; and kava-kava [*Piper methysticum*] is hepatotoxic). Chamomile, licorice root, quassia, and red clover all contain coumarin derivatives, and other herbal products may impair platelet aggregation, thus prolonging bleeding while others pose a risk for cardiac patients.

In many cultures, traditional medicine is widely practised, particularly in Asian and African cultures. Traditional Chinese medicine (TCM) is typically delivered using acupuncture, herbs, and other methods such as cupping, dietary therapy, massage, mind–body therapy, and moxibustion (the burning of mugwort, a small herb). Acupuncture has the largest body of evidence and is considered safe if practised correctly. Some Chinese herbal remedies may be safe; others may not be.

Ayurvedic medicine (Ayurveda) originated in India and involves herbs, massage, and specialized diets. Some Ayurvedic products may be harmful (causing adverse effects or interacting with conventional medicines).

Main dental considerations

(*See also generic guidance under main dental considerations on page 63 top, and also Section 2).

There are few RCTs on acupuncture use for orofacial conditions. Any efficacy may be explained by possible release of endogenous opiates (beta-endorphin, enkephalin, endomorphin and dynorphin) during acupuncture.

There are weak data on the possible effects of aloe extracts, berries, chamomile, cocoa, coffee, grapes, honey/propolis, myrtle, polyphenols (stilbenes, flavonoids and proanthocyanidins) and tea on various oral diseases but no strong evidence. Herbals may influence dental treatment, especially with drug interactions as for example, when benzodiazepine sedation is used or if they produce a bleeding tendency. St John's wort (*Hypericum perforatum*; SJW) induces various drug-metabolizing enzymes (cytochrome P450 isoenzymes, CYP3A4, CYP2C9, CYP1A2, and the transport protein P-glycoprotein), which lowers blood levels and therapeutic effects of some drugs – notably anticoagulants, anticonvulsants, antidepressants and azole antifungals. It is important also to note that, when patients stop taking SJW, blood levels of interacting medicines may rise, resulting in toxicity. SJW should be stopped at least 5 days or more before surgery.

Graft versus host disease (GVHD)

Definition and classification

A severe complication following allogeneic haematopoietic cell transplantation (bone marrow transplantation) (HSCT or BMT).

Acute GVHD – a syndrome of dermatitis, hepatitis, and enteritis developing within 100 days of BMT.

Chronic GVHD – more diverse, developing after day 100.

Aetiopathogenesis

HSCT recipient's immune system is damaged by iatrogenic immunosuppression (chemotherapy with or without total-body irradiation [TBI]). Lymphocytes transferred to the host attack the host's tissues.

Clinical presentation

Acute GVHD manifests initially with a pruritic or painful lichenoid rash. Asymptomatic bilirubin, alanine amino-transferase (ALT), aspartate aminotransferase (AST), and alkaline phosphatase rises herald liver involvement. Gastrointestinal involvement affects the distal small bowel, and colon, resulting in diarrhoea, intestinal bleeding, cramping abdominal pain, and ileus.

Other findings include increased risk of infectious and non-infective pneumonia and sterile effusions, haemorrhagic cystitis, thrombocytopenia, and anaemia, and a haemolytic–uraemic syndrome (HUS: thrombotic microangiopathy).

Chronic GVHD manifestations may include also:

- Autoimmune phenomena – such as myasthenia gravis or polymyositis.
- Neuromuscular manifestations – weakness, neuropathic pain, and muscle cramps
- Ocular manifestations – burning, irritation, photophobia, from lack of tear secretion.
- Oral and gastrointestinal manifestations – dryness, dysphagia, and increasing pain.
- Pulmonary manifestations – obstructive lung disease with wheezing, dyspnoea, and chronic cough non-responsive to bronchodilator therapy.
- Skin lichenoid lesions or sclerodermatous thickening of the skin – sometimes causing contractures and limitation of joint mobility.

Thus it may mimic systemic progressive sclerosis, systemic lupus erythematosus, lichen planus, Sjögren syndrome, eosinophilic fasciitis, rheumatoid arthritis, or primary biliary cirrhosis.

Treatment

GVHD prophylaxis is ciclosporin or tacrolimus in combination with methotrexate and/or prednisone.

Acute GVHD is treated with methotrexate IV for up to 14 days. The grade of acute GVHD predicts outcome, with highest mortality rates in grade IV, or severe, GVHD.

Chronic GVHD is treated with oral prednisone alone or in combination with ciclosporin. Chronic GVHD mortality rates are higher in patients with extensive disease, progressive-type onset, thrombocytopenia, and HLA-non-identical marrow donors. The overall survival rate is 40%, but patients with progressive onset of chronic GVHD have only a 10% survival rate.

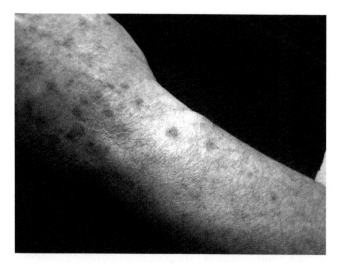

Figure 9.11 Graft versus host disease lichenoid rash.

Main dental considerations

(*See also generic guidance under main dental considerations on page 63 top, and also Section 2).

Oral manifestations may include mucositis, infections, dysgeusia, xerostomia and lichenoid lesions. Advice on preventive care, oral hygiene and diet is important. Consider the possible drug sequelae (e.g. immunosuppression). Mucositis affects the majority; provide topical anaesthetics. Generally, elective care is best deferred during acute GVHD, with emergency dental care provided on a case-by-case basis after consulting the physician.

Haemodialysis

Haemodialysis involves removal from the blood of excess levels of any solute such as potassium, phosphorus or sodium ions which otherwise can be dangerous and lead to:

- arrhythmias
- osteoporosis
- seizures (fits) and coma
- sudden death.

Haemodialysis involves solute diffusion across a semipermeable membrane, using countercurrent flow where a dialysate flows in the opposite direction to blood in an extra-corporeal circuit. Fluid removal is achieved by altering the dialysate hydrostatic pressure, causing free water and dissolved solutes such as urea, creatinine and electrolytes to cross the membrane along a gradient.

Haemodialysis is carried out at home or as an outpatient, for two to three, 3 to 6-hourly sessions per week. An arteriovenous fistula, Gortex or PTFE graft, or an indwelling tunnelled cuffed catheter is usually created to facilitate infusions. The patient is heparinized to keep infusion lines and dialysis machine tubing patent. 40–50 mL of blood are transferred through a needle at any one time to a dialyser or dialysis machine. The dialysis machine consists of a series of membranes, and the dialysate (a sterile solution of mineral ions). The membranes filter waste products, sodium, potassium and phosphates, into the dialysate fluid which is removed from the dialyser and 'clean' blood is passed back into the body through a second needle.

Diet plans for patients needing dialysis take into consideration avoiding eating foods high in:

- Salt:
  - bacon
  - cheese
  - ham
  - ready-to-eat meals (including ready-to-eat sandwiches)
  - smoked fish.
- Potassium:
  - baked potatoes
  - bananas
  - chocolate
  - oranges.
- Phosphorus.

and

- Baked beans.
- Bran cereals.
- Dairy products, such as cheese.
- Lentils.
- Sardines.
- Yoghurt.

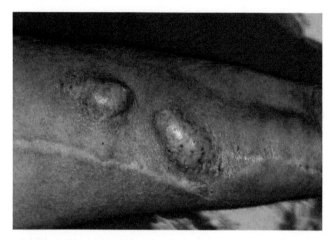

Figure 9.12 Haemodialysis – fistulae.

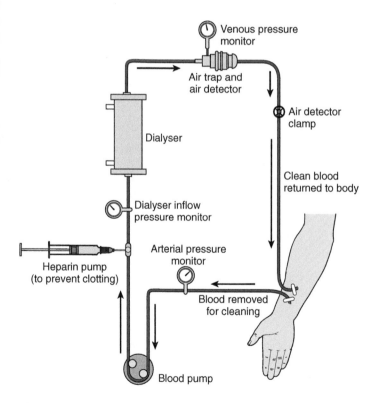

Figure 9.13 Haemodialysis.

Main dental considerations

(*See also generic guidance under main dental considerations on page 63 top, and also Section 2).

Oral manifestations of chronic kidney disease (CKD; Section 5) may include:

- Periodontal disease
- Infections
- Signs of secondary hyperparathyroidism (see Section 5):
  - loss of lamina dura
  - osteoporosis
  - central giant cell lesions.
- Dry mouth.
- Halitosis.
- Increased calculus.
- Metallic taste.

Infection control is of paramount importance, as infection with hepatitis viruses, HIV or other blood-borne agents, and tuberculosis, was common in the past. Consider other comorbid diseases. Patients on haemodialysis are severely compromised, and many require anticoagulation.

Defer elective dental treatment on day of dialysis. Appointments should be scheduled on day after dialysis. Lidocaine is the safest LA to use, followed by articaine and prilocaine. Midazolam is preferable to diazepam because of its lower associated risk of thrombophlebitis. Diazepam should be safe, except that it is long acting, requires renal dosing and has a risk of propylene glycol toxicity if given via IV (at high/prolonged dosage). It is not dialyzable. Never put a cannula (IV) into the arm with the shunt.

Antimicrobial use may be:

- *Usually safe (no dosage change required):* azithromycin, cloxacillin, doxycycline, flucloxacillin, fucidin, minocycline, rifampicin.
- *Fairly safe (change dosage only in severe CKD):* ampicillin, amoxicillin, benzylpenicillin, clindamycin, co-trimoxazole, erythromycin, ketoconazole, lincomycin, metronidazole, phenoxymethyl penicillin.
- *Less safe (dosage reduction in all patients):* aciclovir, cephalosporin, ciprofloxacin, fluconazole, levofloxacin, ofloxacin, sitafloxacin, and vancomycin.

Avoid (*do not use in any patients*): aminoglycosides, carbenicillin, cefadroxil, cefixime, cephalexin, cephalothin, gentamicin, imipenem, itraconazole, sulfonamides, tetracyclines, and valacyclovir.

Analgesics may be:

- Usually safe (no dosage change required): acetaminophen/paracetamol
- Fairly safe (dosage change only in patients with severe CKD): codeine
- Less safe (dosage reduction in all patients): NSAIDs.
- Avoid (*do not use in any patients*): dextropropoxyphene, meperidine, morphine, opioids, pethidine, tramadol.

Other drugs:

Diazepam and midazolam are usually safe (*no dosage change required*): but dosage reduction is needed in all patients given carbamazepine, gabapentin or lamotrigine.

Immunosuppressive treatment

Used to control immune reactions in diseases such as autoimmunity, in therapy of some cancers (e.g. haematological), and to prevent transplant rejection, immunosuppressive therapy may range from the use of total body irradiation (TBI) to destroy all lymphocytes and white cells before bone marrow transplantation (BMT [haematopoietic stem cell transplant or HSCT]); to potent immunosuppressive drugs which have less dramatic effects (traditionally the corticosteroids); to biologics (see above).

Many immunosuppressive regimens predominantly inhibit cell-mediated responses. Some 'steroid-sparing' drugs such as azathioprine, cyclophosphamide and chlorambucil are cytotoxic to a range of cells, including some immunocytes. Ciclosporin, tacrolimus or mycophenolate mofetil are more specific, and thalidomide and the newer 'biologics' target specific lymphocyte types or cytokines (see Biologicals, and Steroids).

Classification

Induction immunotherapy is not commonly used after transplantation, although the recent introduction of IL-2 receptor-blocking antibodies, daclizumab and basiliximab, may change this.

Maintenance immunosuppression is usually based on a corticosteroid, and/or calcineurin inhibitor (i.e. ciclosporin or tacrolimus), sirolimus, sometimes combined with antimetabolites (e.g., mycophenolate mofetil) or antiproliferative agents (e.g., rapamycin).

- Corticosteroids may decrease inflammation by reversing increased capillary permeability and suppressing PMN activity.
- Ciclosporin is a highly lipid-soluble drug metabolized by liver cytochrome P-450 enzymes (CYP3A4). Inhibitors of the cytochrome P-450 hepatic microsomal enzyme system increase or decrease its clearance.

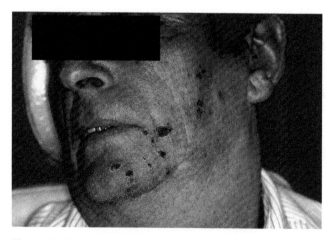

Figure 9.14 Herpes zoster (mandibular shingles).

- Tacrolimus is a macrolide antibiotic similar to ciclosporin which inhibits IL-2, interferon-gamma, and IL-3 production; transferrin and IL-2 receptor expression; and cytotoxic T generation. Tacrolimus is metabolized by the same cytochrome P-450 system as ciclosporin.
- Sirolimus is a non-calcineurin inhibiting immune-suppressant which inhibits lymphocyte proliferation.
- Azathioprine is a second-line immune-suppressive agent metabolized by the enzyme thiopurine methyl transferase (TPMT) to mercaptopurine which acts as purine analogue that interacts with DNA and inhibits lymphocyte cell division, and may cause myelo-suppression and hepatotoxicity. Testing TPMT activity is mandatory.
- Mycophenolate mofetil is a second-line immune-suppressive agent that may be used as an alternative to azathioprine in solid organ transplantation, acting via selective inhibition of T and B cell proliferation.

Complications

People on systemic immunosuppressive therapy may be liable to drug interactions and many of the challenges facing HIV-infected patients (Section 7), apart usually from the risk from HIV itself, notably a liability to:

- Drug interactions and toxicities:
  - Corticosteroid toxicities.
  - Azathioprine – myelosuppression.
  - Ciclosporin – gingival swelling (drug induced gingival overgrowth; DIGO), hepatotoxicity, hypertension, hypertrichosis, nephrotoxicity and tremor.
  - Tacrolimus – cardiomyopathy, hyperglycaemia, nephrotoxicity, neurotoxicity.
  - Sirolimus – hyperlipidaemia.
  - Rapamycin – cytopenia, hyperlipidaemia.
- Infections.
- Neoplasms, at least some of which are virally-related (Kaposi's sarcoma; HHV-8), lymphomas (EBV) and squamous cell carcinomas of the skin, anogenital region and the lip (HPV).
- Teratogenicity.

Main dental considerations

(*See also generic guidance under main dental considerations on page 63 top, and also Section 2).
Patients are immunocompromised and liable to infections – which should be handled with caution. Mammalian target of rapamycin (mTOR) inhibitors, rapalogs, (e.g. everolimus, ridaforolimus, temsirolimus) may cause mouth ulceration.

Implanted devices

Medical implants are devices or tissues that are placed inside the body or on the surface. Many implants are prostheses intended to replace missing body parts; others deliver medication, monitor body functions, or provide support to organs and tissues.

Some implants are made from skin, bone or other body tissues; others are made from materials such as metal, plastic, or ceramic.

Implants may be placed with intent to be permanent (e.g. stents, limbs, joints, cochlear, dental or aesthetic implants). Other implants can be removed once they are no longer needed (e.g. chemotherapy ports or bone screws). Some resorb over time (e.g. drug delivery systems). Implant types may include those listed in Box 9.2, and notes on some of the more common are given below.

Complications

The risks with implants, apart from failure, include mainly the surgical risks during placement or removal, infection, or reactions to implant materials.

Surgical risks invariably include some pain, swelling, and bruising. Infections mostly arise from skin bacterial contamination at the time of surgery.

Main dental considerations

(*See also generic guidance under main dental considerations on page 63 top, and also Section 2).

Comments on specific implants

Breast implants – devices implanted under the breast tissue or under the chest muscle to increase breast size (augmentation) or to rebuild breast tissue after mastectomy or other damage to the breast (reconstruction). There are two main types – saline-filled or silicone gel-filled. Breast implants are not lifetime devices; as many as 20% need removal within 10 years. There may be a low but increased risk of developing anaplastic large cell lymphoma (ALCL) in breast tissue around the implant.

Cardiac implantable electronic devices (CIEDs) (see Section 5). Cardiac pacemakers and implantable cardioverter defibrillators help correct abnormal heart rhythms.

 Pacemakers are small implanted electronic devices that stimulate the heart to beat, and 'pace' the rate when it is too slow (bradycardia). Modern pacemakers work mainly on demand, are rate-adaptive, bipolar, implanted in the right ventricle transvenously via the subclavian or cephalic vein, and typically located on or beneath the skin, on the left upper chest wall or within the pectoral muscle or in the abdominal wall.

 Implantable cardioverter defibrillators (ICDs) achieve cardioversion by a cardioverter device which administers countershocks through electrodes on chest or on or in the heart. They can correct ventricular fibrillation (VF).

Disruption and complications

External electromagnetic radiation interference (EMI) and CIEDs: High frequency EMI from various sources can interfere with the sensing function of pacemakers and of ICDs, and may induce fibrillation.

Pacemakers can be disrupted by MRI from static magnetic, alternating magnetic and radiofrequency (RF) fields (Table 9.4). This hazard to pacemakers is real and so MRI is contraindicated. Diagnostic radiation and ultrasound have no effect on pacemakers.

Box 9.2 Prostheses and implants

- Artificial limbs
- Auditory brainstem implants
- Blood vessel prostheses
- Bone nails, plates, screws
- Breast implants
- Cardiac implanted electronic devices (CIEDs)
- Cochlear implants
- Dental implants
- Drug implants
- Electrodes, implanted
- Embolic protection devices
- Vena cava filters
- Eye, artificial
- Fiducial markers (an object placed in the field of view of an imaging system which appears in the image produced, for use as a point of reference)
- Glaucoma drainage implants
- Heart valve prostheses
- Heart, artificial
- Heart-assist devices
- Internal fixators
- Joint prostheses:
  - Elbow prostheses
  - Hip prosthesis
  - Knee prostheses
  - Other joint prostheses
- Neurostimulators
- Larynx, artificial
- Lenses, intraocular
- Orbital implants
- Ossicular prostheses
- Penile prostheses
- Ports
- Septal occluder devices
- Stents
- Suburethral slings
- Suture anchors
- Testicular implants
- Tissue expansion devices
- Tissue scaffolds
- Urinary sphincter, artificial
- Visual prostheses.

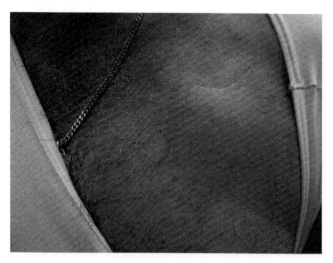

Figure 9.15 Pacemaker scar.

Table 9.4 Possible effects on cardiac pacemakers of equipment used in healthcare

May affect	Unlikely to affect
Diathermy	Electric toothbrushes
Electrosurgical units	Electronic tooth apex locators
Lithotripsy	Piezoelectric ultrasonic scalers
MRI	Sonic scalers
Radiotherapy	
Transcutaneous electric nerve stimulation (TENS)	
Ultrasonography	
Ultrasonic cleaning baths	

Pacemakers can also be disrupted by ionizing radiation, and some ultrasonic EMI. Modern bipolar pacemakers have titanium insulated interference-resistant circuitry, and thus the risk of EMI is very small and usually only if the devices are placed in close approximation to the pacemaker (Table 9.4). Digital mobile phones, and even television transmitters and faulty or badly earthed equipment may cause interference, but the risk is very small and only when used in close proximity to the device. Brief exposure of pacemakers to electromagnetic anti-theft or surveillance devices, as found in airports, shops, libraries and some teaching, clinical and other facilities, causes little, if any, dysfunction. Domestic appliances – even remote controls, CB radios, electric blankets, heating pads, shavers, kitchen appliances, and microwave ovens – are safe.

Implantable cardioverter defibrillators (ICDs) may activate without significant warning, potentially causing the patient to flinch, bite down, or perform other sudden movements that may result in injury to the patient or the clinician. Some patients with ICDs lose consciousness when the device is activated. This is less likely to occur with newer devices that initially emit low level electrical bursts followed by stronger shocks if cardioversion does not occur immediately.

An implanted ICD will not only trigger airport security alarms, but also the use of strong magnets over the device may adversely affect its function.

Digital mobile phones, and even television transmitters and faulty or badly earthed equipment may cause interference, but the risk is very small and only when used in close proximity to the device. Domestic appliances – even remote controls, CB radios, electric blankets, heating pads, shavers, kitchen appliances, and microwave ovens – are safe.

If an ICD shuts off, switch off all possible sources of interference and give CPR to the supine patient.

CIED infection. There is no scientific basis for the use of prophylactic antibiotics before routine invasive oral, gastrointestinal, or genito-urinary procedures to prevent CIED infection.

Endocarditis. Unless a cardiac valve lesion is also present, patients with permanent pacemakers or ICD do not need antibiotic cover to prevent endocarditis.

Cochlear implants – electronic hearing devices used to produce useful hearing for people with profound hearing loss due to nerve deafness. These implants usually consist of an externally worn microphone, sound processor and transmitter system plus an implanted receiver and electrode system, that receives signals from the external system and sends electrical currents to the inner ear. A magnet holds the external system in place next to the implanted internal system.

MRI imaging is contraindicated: even being close to an MRI imaging unit will be dangerous because it may dislodge the implant or demagnetize its internal magnet. A cochlear implant may also set off theft detection systems or other security systems.

Dental radiography, cone beam computed tomography, computed tomography, electric pulp testing, panoramic radiography and digital radiography are safe in patients with cochlear implants. However, the speech processor component should be turned off, removed and kept away from the room containing X-ray equipment while taking radiographs. External parts of the implant should be removed when ultrasound tooth cleaning or during MRI scans, gamma camera and radiotherapy with cobalt units/linear accelerators.

If bipolar electrosurgery is used, the tip of the cautery should be at least 3 cm away from the implant. Bipolar diathermy is contraindicated closer than 2 cm to the cochlear implant.

Some procedures that can irreversibly damage a cochlear implant and should not be used include transcutaneous electrical nerve stimulation (TENS), ultrasonic imaging and therapy, monopolar electrosurgery, monopolar diathermy, microwave diathermy, shortwave diathermy and ultrasound diathermy.

May be affected by mobile phone users or other radio transmitters, may have to be turned off during aircraft take-offs and landings and may interact with other computer systems. Static electricity may temporarily or permanently damage a cochlear implant.

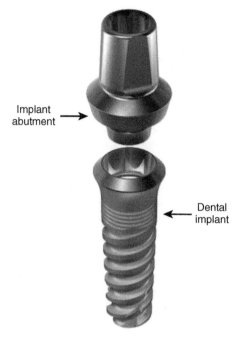

Implant
abutment →

← Dental
implant

Figure 9.16 Dental implant.

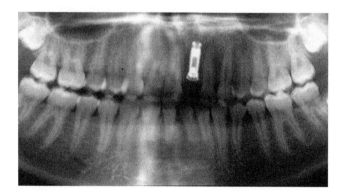

Figure 9.17 Implant in situ.

Neurostimulation devices – stimulate externally (e.g. tENS – Transcutaneous Electrical Nerve Stimulation) or implanted in the nervous system (IND – Implantable Neurostimulation Devices). The latter have increasing applications, mainly for tremors. Advice should be sought before use of ultrasonics or devices that may cause electromagnetic interference (e.g. MRI, diathermy). Simple radiography appears to be safe.

Metal-on-metal (MoM) hip implants – may be used for patients with hip joint deterioration who may benefit from total hip replacement or hip resurfacing. They may be 'metal-on-metal' implant in which the 'ball and socket' of the device are both metal or metal-on-metal resurfacing hip systems which consist of a trimmed femoral head capped with a metal covering and a metal acetabular component. All artificial hip implants carry risks including wear of the component material; MoM implants have unique additional risks since some of the implant metal ions (e.g. cobalt and chromium) can damage bone and/or tissue – sometimes referred to as an 'adverse local tissue reaction (ALTR)' or an 'adverse reaction to metal debris (ARMD).' Soft tissue damage may lead to pain, implant loosening, device failure, and the need for revision; some ions will enter the bloodstream so patients with MoM hip systems should be monitored for hypersensitivity (skin rash), cardiomyopathy, neurological or psychological status change, renal and thyroid function. However, there is not enough evidence to support the need for routine checking of blood metal ion levels or soft tissue imaging. See Section 5 for other comments.

Osseointegrated dental implants

A dental implant is a prosthetic replacement for a missing tooth. The root is the part of the tooth that is effectively replaced by an implant. There are three components – the implant itself (inserted directly into bone); abutment – the piece that connects the implant device to the third part – the overlying crown or denture. Metal implants are made usually of titanium, a metal that is biocompatible, strong, durable and fuses directly to bone – *osseointegration*. Zirconia might be used. Concern about titanium sensitivity or any adverse effects is controversial. MRI, though not contraindicated, may cause distortion artefacts around the implant. CT and cone beam CT are without problems.

Contraindications for dental implants may include:

• Cardiovascular events (MI; CVA) if recent, or valvular prosthesis surgery.
• Diabetes if poorly controlled.
• Immunosuppression.
• Inability to maintain high levels of dental plaque control (e.g. impaired manual dexterity or mental capacity).
• Intravenous bisphosphonate therapy.
• Radiotherapy to jaw bone.
• Smoking.
• Uncontrolled drug or alcohol use.
• Uncontrolled mental disorders.
• Untreated periodontal disease.

Phakic intraocular lenses

These are new devices, thin plastic or silicone lenses implanted permanently into the eye to correct myopia to correct eye refractive errors and reduce the need for glasses or contact lenses. Phakic refers to the fact that the lens is implanted into the eye without removing the natural lens.

Urogynaecologic surgical mesh implants

These are made from synthetic materials or processed and disinfected animal (pig [porcine] or cow [bovine]) intestine or skin. Non-absorbable mesh will remain in the body indefinitely and is considered a permanent implant, though it will degrade and lose strength over time. Animal-derived mesh is absorbable: there may be cultural issues in their use.

Surgical mesh can be used for urogynaecologic procedures, including repair of pelvic organ prolapse (POP) and stress urinary incontinence (SUI). It is not clear whether trans-vaginal POP repair with mesh is more effective than traditional non-mesh repair, nor how mini-slings for SUI compare with multi-incision slings with regard to safety and effectiveness. Mesh sling surgeries for SUI have similar effectiveness as non-mesh SUI surgeries, but mesh slings introduce a risk not present in traditional non-mesh surgery – erosion through the vagina (also called exposure, extrusion or protrusion).

Mucositis

Mucositis typically consists of erythema, ulceration and pain which appears after radiotherapy or chemotherapy. Mucositis significantly affects quality of life, is almost inevitable in radiotherapy where the field involves mucosae – and is particularly severe after chemoradiotherapy or total body irradiation (TBI).

Radiotherapy-induced mucositis can be reduced by:
- Improved radiation techniques.
- Lower radiation doses.
- Use of shielding.

Chemotherapy-induced mucositis may predict gastrointestinal toxicity and hepatic veno-occlusive disease and, with neutropenia, predisposes to septicaemia. There may be benefit in chemotherapy-induced mucositis from use of:
- Ice chips before giving 5-fluorouracil (5FU), methotrexate or melphalan.
- Folinic acid (as calcium folinate), levofolinic acid or disodium folinate before administration of methotrexate or 5FU.

Other approaches include use of:
- Anti-inflammatory medications.
- Biologic response modifiers (cytokines such as interleukin-1, interleukin-11, TGF-beta 3 or keratinocyte growth factor [Palifermin]).
- Colony-stimulating factors (CSF) – granulocyte macrophage (GM-CSF) and granulocyte (G-CSF).
- Cytoprotective agents (primarily free radical scavengers or antioxidants, such as amifostine, N-acetyl cysteine and vitamin E).
- Thalidomide – a TNF blocker and an angiogenesis-inhibiting drug.

Management of mucositis often necessitates use of:
- Analgesics – opioids, plus rinses or sprays (lidocaine or benzydamine).
- Improved hygiene.
- Prophylaxis for infectious complications.
- Special diets (Table 9.5) or tube feeding in oral mucositis.

Infections – are common and important and can become systemic. They are often termed mucosal barrier injury laboratory-confirmed bloodstream infections (MBI-LCBI).

Oral candidosis is common, caused by *Candida albicans* or, less often, other *Candida* species. Mucormycosis (phycomycosis) or aspergillosis are rare. Antifungals may be given prophylactically. Herpetic infections are common and may cause chronic skin or mucosal ulcers. Aciclovir or valaciclovir prophylactically lower the incidence of infections and mortality. Gram-negative oral infections due to *Pseudomonas*, *Klebsiella*, *Escherichia*, *Enterobacter*, *Serratia* or *Proteus* may develop and spread rapidly unless treated with, for example, gentamicin or carbenicillin.

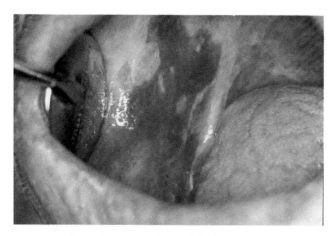

Figure 9.18 Mucositis. Reprinted from Scully C. et al. (2012) Pocketbook of oral disease. Churchill Livingstone Elsevier, with permission from Elsevier.

Table 9.5 Diet in oral mucositis

Typically acceptable diet	Foods to avoid	Lifestyle habits to avoid
Liquids Purees Ice Custards Non-acidic fruits (apple, banana, mango, melon, peach) Soft cheeses Eggs Smoothies	Rough food (chips, crisps, toast), spices, salt, acidic fruit (grapefruit, lemon, orange)	Smoking Alcohol

Palliative and end of life care

(See also Bedbound patients, Section 10.

The quality of life (QoL) is as important as, or more important than, its duration. Confidential compassionate communication with patient, partners, family and friends is crucial since many different persons are involved in the care, so that all are aware of the patient's psychological reactions, their understanding about their disease and:

- adverse effects of treatment
- prognosis.

Dignity and confidentiality are extremely important, and can too easily be lost in terminal disease.

Psychological health is crucial; patients may or may not know, or may not want to know, that they have terminal disease, and even if they are aware of it may not appreciate, or be willing to accept, the prognosis. Counselling is especially important and if appropriate should include family members and partners. Patients are subject to considerable distress and ~30% have anxiety or depression, which may even lead to suicide.

Pain control is of paramount importance. Potent analgesics, such as narcotics, sedatives or antidepressants, may be needed and are warranted in terminal disease. The World Health Organization (WHO) three-step analgesic ladder is a guideline for effective pain management. The essential concepts in the WHO approach are drug therapy:

- by the mouth;
- by the clock;
- by the ladder;
- for the individual and with attention to detail.

Adjuvant drugs to enhance analgesic efficacy, treat concurrent symptoms that exacerbate pain, and provide independent analgesic activity for specific types of pain may be used at any step.

- Step 1, for mild to moderate pain, involves the use of paracetamol/acetaminophen, aspirin, or another NSAID.
- Step 2, when pain persists or increases, advises that an opioid such as codeine or hydrocodone should be added (not substituted) to the regimen. When higher doses of opioid are necessary, the third step is used.
- Step 3, for pain that is still persistent, or moderate to severe, involves giving opioid and non-opioid analgesics separately, in order to avoid exceeding maximally recommended doses of paracetamol/acetaminophen or NSAID. Drugs such as codeine,

Table 9.6 Drugs for controlling severe pain

	Buccal	IV	PR	SC	Sublingual	Transdermal
Fentanyl	+					+
Hydromorphone		+	+	+		
Morphine		+	+	+	+	
Oxycodone		+				

I, intravenous. PR, per rectum. SC, subcutaneous.

or hydrocodone are used initially but may need to be replaced with more potent opioids (usually morphine, hydromorphone, methadone, fentanyl, or levorphanol) (Table 9.6). Morphine and diamorphine are the drugs of choice for severe pain. Phentazocine may be valuable in patients intolerant of, or allergic to, morphine. Pethidine has too short an action and the metabolite norpethidine can accumulate in renal failure and then cause convulsions. Buprenorphine is a partial agonist and should be avoided. Dextromoramide is only very short-acting but can be useful to 'cover' painful procedures. Carbamazepine or tricyclic antidepressants may relieve pain due to tumour infiltrating nerves. Transdermal fentanyl (skin patches) are increasingly used since they have an effect comparable with morphine and a duration of action of around 3 days.

Medications for persistent cancer-related pain should be administered on an around-the-clock basis, with additional 'as-needed' doses, because regularly scheduled dosing maintains a constant level of drug in the body and helps to prevent a recurrence of pain.

Patient-controlled analgesia (PCA), can be accomplished by mouth or subcutaneously, or epidurally, but is usually delivered via continuous systemic infusion, which allows patients to control the amount of analgesia they receive. Intravenous and subcutaneous PCA is contraindicated for sedated and confused patients.

Nutrition can be a problem, especially if there is dysphagia, when nasogastric (NG) intubation may be needed, but per-endoscopic gastrostomy (PEG) is a better long-term solution as it avoids the fear of choking and aspiration pneumonia.

The paraphernalia involved can be most disconcerting to the patient and others.

Box 9.3 Preferred practices for palliative and hospice care

- Provide palliative and hospice care by an interdisciplinary team of skilled palliative care professionals, including, for example, physicians, nurses, social workers, pharmacists, spiritual care counsellors, and others who collaborate with primary healthcare professional(s).
- Provide access to palliative and hospice care that is responsive to the patient and family 24 hours a day, 7 days a week.
- Provide continuing education to all healthcare professionals on the domains of palliative care and hospice care.
- Provide adequate training and clinical support to assure that professional staff is confident in their ability to provide palliative care for patients.
- Hospice care and specialized palliative care professionals should be appropriately trained, credentialled, and/or certified in their area of expertise.
- Formulate, utilize, and regularly review a timely care plan based on a comprehensive interdisciplinary assessment of the values, preferences, goals, and needs of the patient and family and, to the extent that existing privacy laws permit, ensure that the plan is broadly disseminated, both internally and externally, to all professionals involved in the patient's care.
- Ensure that upon transfer between healthcare settings, there is timely and thorough communication of the patient's goals, preferences, values, and clinical information so that continuity of care and seamless follow-up are assured.
- Healthcare professionals should present hospice as an option to all patients and families when death within a year would not be surprising and should reintroduce the hospice option as the patient declines.
- Patients and caregivers should be asked by palliative and hospice care programmes to assess physicians'/healthcare professionals' ability to discuss hospice as an option.
- Enable patients to make informed decisions about their care by educating them on the process of their disease, prognosis, and the benefits and burdens of potential interventions.
- Provide education and support to families and unlicensed caregivers based on the patient's individualized care plan to assure safe and appropriate care for the patient.
- Measure and document pain, dyspnoea, constipation, and other symptoms using available standardized scales.
- Assess and manage symptoms and side-effects in a timely, safe, and effective manner to a level that is acceptable to the patient and family.
- Measure and document anxiety, depression, delirium, behavioural disturbances, and other common psychological symptoms using available standardized scales.
- Manage anxiety, depression, delirium, behavioural disturbances, and other common psychological symptoms in a timely, safe, and effective manner to a level that is acceptable to the patient and family.
- Assess and manage the psychological reactions of patients and families (including stress, anticipatory grief, and coping) in a regular, ongoing fashion in order to address emotional and functional impairment and loss.

Box 9.3 Preferred practices for palliative and hospice care—cont'd

- Develop and offer a grief and bereavement care plan to provide services to patients and families prior to and for at least 13 months after the death of the patient.
- Conduct regular patient and family care conferences with physicians and other appropriate members of the interdisciplinary team to provide information, to discuss goals of care, disease prognosis, and advance care planning, and to offer support.
- Develop and implement a comprehensive social care plan that addresses the social, practical, and legal needs of the patient and caregivers, including but not limited to relationships, communication, existing social and cultural networks, decision making, work and school settings, finances, sexuality/intimacy, caregiver availability/ stress, and access to medicines and equipment.
- Develop and document a plan based on an assessment of religious, spiritual, and existential concerns using a structured instrument, and integrate the information obtained from the assessment into the palliative care plan.
- Provide information about the availability of spiritual care services, and make spiritual care available either through organizational spiritual care counselling or through the patient's own clergy relationships.
- Specialized palliative and hospice care teams should include spiritual care professionals appropriately trained and certified in palliative care.
- Specialized palliative and hospice spiritual care professionals should build partnerships with community clergy and provide education and counselling related to end of life care.
- Incorporate cultural assessment as a component of comprehensive palliative and hospice care assessment, including but not limited to locus of decision making, preferences regarding disclosure of information, truth telling and decision making, dietary preferences, language, family communication, desire for support measures such as palliative therapies and complementary and alternative medicine, perspectives on death, suffering, and grieving, and funeral/burial rituals.
- Provide professional interpreter services and culturally sensitive materials in the patient's and family's preferred language.
- Recognize and document the transition to the active dying phase, and communicate to the patient, family, and staff the expectation of imminent death.
- Educate the family on a timely basis regarding the signs and symptoms of imminent death in an age-appropriate, developmentally appropriate, and culturally appropriate manner.
- As part of the ongoing care planning process, routinely ascertain and document patient and family wishes about the care setting for the site of death, and fulfil patient and family preferences when possible.
- Provide adequate dosage of analgesics and sedatives as appropriate to achieve patient comfort during the active dying phase, and address concerns and fears about using narcotics and of analgesics hastening death.
- Treat the body after death with respect according to the cultural and religious practices of the family and in accordance with local law.

Continued

Box 9.3 Preferred practices for palliative and hospice care—cont'd

- Facilitate effective grieving by implementing in a timely manner a bereavement care plan after the patient's death, when the family remains the focus of care.
- Document the designated surrogate/decision maker in accordance with law for every patient in primary, acute, and long-term care and in palliative and hospice care.
- Document the patient/surrogate preferences for goals of care, treatment options, and setting of care at first assessment and at frequent intervals as conditions change.
- Convert the patient treatment goals into medical orders, and ensure that the information is transferable and applicable across care settings, including long-term care, emergency medical services, and hospital care.
- Make advance directives and surrogacy designations available across care settings, while protecting patient privacy and adherence to regulations, for example, by using Internet-based registries or electronic personal health records.
- Develop healthcare and community collaborations to promote advance care planning and the completion of advance directives for all individuals, for example, the Respecting Choices and Community Conversations on Compassionate Care programmes.
- Establish or have access to ethics committees or ethics consultation across care settings to address ethical conflicts at the end of life.
- For minors with decision-making capacity, document the child's views and preferences for medical care, including assent for treatment, and give them appropriate weight in decision making. Make appropriate professional staff members available to both the child and the adult decision maker for consultation and intervention when the child's wishes differ from those of the adult decision maker.
- **Dignitas** is a group, helping those with terminal illness and severe physical and mental illnesses to die, assisted by qualified doctors and nurses. www.dignitas.ch/?lang=en

(Adapted from National Quality Forum. A National Framework and Preferred Practices for Palliative and Hospice Care Quality. A Consensus Report. Available at www.qualityforum.org.)

Main dental considerations

(*See also generic guidance under main dental considerations on page 63 top, and also Section 2).

Preferred practices for palliative and hospice care are shown in Box 9.3.

Radiotherapy (RTx)

Internal or external beam radiotherapy (RTP, RXR or DXR) of various kinds are used to treat cancers (Table 9.7).

The type of RTx prescribed by a radiation oncologist depends on many factors, including the:

- cancer type
- cancer size
- cancer's location
- cancer proximity to radiation sensitive normal tissues
- body penetration the radiation needs to travel through
- patient's general health and medical history
- other types of cancer treatment used.

Several short-term complications can follow RTx but, with improved radiation techniques, and lower radiation doses or use of shielding, these complications can often be reduced. General short-term side-effects of radiotherapy, such as tiredness and skin reactions can accompany any RTx. The main side-effects of radiotherapy treatment include:

- Fatigue.
- Soreness and hair loss in the RTx beam path.

Table 9.7 Types of external beam radiotherapy used to treat cancer

Type	Source	Used for
Electron beam	Electrical	Superficial lesions
Low voltage	X-ray	Superficial lesions
Orthovoltage	X-ray	Skin lesions
Supervoltage	^{60}Cobalt	Deeper lesions
Megavoltage	Linear accelerator or betatron	Larger lesions

Table 9.8 Complications of RTx involving mouth/salivary glands

Week 1	Week 2+	Week 3+	Later
Nausea Vomiting	Mucositis Taste changes	Dry mouth	Infections Caries Pulp pain and necrosis Tooth hypersensitivity Trismus Osteoradionecrosis Craniofacial defects

There can also be short- and long-term side-effects of RTx related to particular parts of the body. For example, RTx affecting the:

- abdomen or pelvis can cause diarrhoea or pain;
- brain can cause nausea;
- chest can cause dysphagia, dyspnoea and weight loss;
- salivary glands can cause unpleasant effects, especially hyposalivation, weight loss and mucositis – usually transient.

Main dental considerations

(*See also generic guidance under main dental considerations on page 63 top, and also Section 2).

Mucositis dysphagia and oral soreness become maximal 2–4 weeks after RTx involving salivary glands but usually subside in a further 2–3 weeks. Symptomatic treatment is indicated.

Hyposalivation is almost invariable following radiotherapy of tumours of the mouth, naso-, and oro-pharynx, but can be reduced by:

- sparing at least one parotid gland;
- giving amifostine which is cytoprotective of acinar cells;
- drugs to stimulate salivation (e.g. pilocarpine or cevimeline).

Saliva substitutes (mouth wetting agents e.g. carboxymethylcellulose) may give symptomatic relief, as may salivary stimulants (e.g. sugar-free chewing gum).

Infections predisposed to by hyposalivation include caries, candidosis and ascending sialadenitis. Caries may be reduced by:

- control of dietary carbohydrates;
- fluoride and amorphous calcium phosphate applications;
- protecting salivary function as above.

Loss of taste (hypoguesia) follows RTx damage to the taste buds. If more than 6000 CGy have been given, loss of taste is usually permanent. In others, taste may start to recover within 2–4 months. Zinc sulphate supplementation may help.

Trismus (limitation of jaw opening) may follow endarteritis affecting masticatory muscles from replacement fibrosis. Jaw-opening exercises with tongue spatulas or wedges or use of Therabite, three times a day may help.

Osteonecrosis of the jaws – may arise from radiotherapy (osteoradionecrosis; ORN) or from certain drugs (osteonecrosis of the jaws; ONJ). ORN is a serious complication of radiotherapy, the risk being greatest in the mandible and when there is trauma/ surgery from 10 days before, to several years after; when the radiotherapy is internal, e.g. iridium 192 radiotherapy and >50–55 Gray (Gy) and is increased by:

- Chemotherapy
- Tobacco use
- Alcohol use
- Immune defects.

ORN typically results from dental extractions in the mandible after radiotherapy because of reduced bone vascularity following irradiation endarteritis and is heralded by pain and swelling. In severe cases the whole of the body of the mandible may be affected. ORN may be prevented by avoiding operations in patients who have irradiated jaw

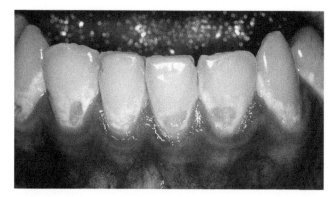

Figure 9.19 Caries due to dry mouth.

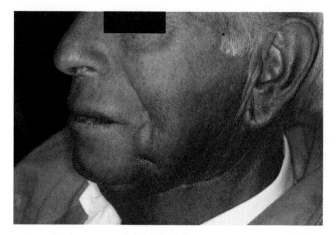

Figure 9.20 Radiotherapy effects on skin plus sinus from osteoradionecrosis in the mandible.

bones with endarteritis obliterans, and this is achieved best by leaving only those teeth which may be saved, and removing others with an interval of at least 2 weeks between extractions and starting radiotherapy. Hyperbaric oxygen (HBO) may help prevent ORN. Complete resolution can take 2 years or more despite intensive antimicrobial treatment. HBO and possibly surgical bone decortication may be required.

Craniofacial maldevelopment: craniofacial defects, tooth hypoplasia and retarded eruption can follow irradiation of developing teeth and growth centres. Children treated for neuroblastoma therefore, are at particularly high risk for abnormal dental development.

Most RTx can have a long-term increase in risk of second tumours.

Splenectomy

The spleen is essential for controlling erythrocyte quality, is the site of sequestration of effete erythrocytes and, if enlarged, sequesters platelets, and also has important functions in antibody production and the phagocytosis of opsonized microbes (or auto-antibody coated platelets). Two splenic opsonins, properdin and tuftsin, protect against bacteria such as pneumococci.

Aetiopathogenesis

Absence of a functional spleen may be due to:

- Congenital asplenia – uncommon.
- Acquired asplenia:
  - Splenectomy:
    - after serious splenic injuries in abdominal trauma or where the spleen is fragile as in infectious mononucleosis;
    - in haemolytic anaemias, hereditary spherocytosis, autoimmune haemolysis;
    - in idiopathic thrombocytopenic purpura treatment;
    - in some lymphomas.
  - Infarction in sickle cell disease (auto-splenectomy), and other disorders.

In the absence of a functional spleen there is a lifetime infection risk. Children are ten times more likely than adults to develop sepsis. The greatest risk is invariably by encapsulated bacteria: *Streptococcus pneumoniae* (pneumococcus) in particular, together with *Haemophilus influenzae* and *Neisseria meningitidis* (meningococcus).

Other infections may include *Escherichia coli*, tuberculosis, babesiosis, malaria, hepatitis C and (from dog bites) *Capnocytophaga canimorsus*.

Prophylaxis – oral phenoxymethylpenicillin is usually given for 2 years or until age 16 years, whichever is longer.

Main dental considerations

(*See also generic guidance under main dental considerations on page 63 top, and also Section 2).

All infections should be handled with special care and patients with asplenia, if acutely unwell, should promptly be given penicillin. Antimicrobial prophylaxis may be indicated for surgery.

Steroids (corticosteroids)

The adrenal glands secrete three main types of steroids: glucocorticoids, mineralocorticoids and sex hormones (see Section 5). Cortisol is the major glucocorticoid. It is involved in inflammatory responses, metabolic processes, vascular tonicity, and control of response to stress such as trauma, infection, GA or surgery. At such times there is normally an increased corticosteroid output related to the degree of stress but, in patients given exogenous steroids, the adrenals are suppressed and this response may not occur. Cortisol secretion is regulated via the hypothalamic-pituitary-adrenal (HPA) axis by a biological feedback involving adrenocorticotrophic hormone (ACTH).

Synthetic (cortisol-like) glucocorticoids are used frequently for immunosuppression, and occasionally to replace missing hormones (in Addison disease or after adrenalectomy) or to treat many diseases. Long-term systemic use of corticosteroids can cause many side-effects, often beginning soon after the start of treatment; they can cause significant morbidity or mortality, including:

- Adrenal suppression
- Cataracts
- Cushingoid weight gain – around the face (moon face) and upper back (buffalo hump) – and hirsutism
- Diabetes
- Growth retardation in children
- Hypertension

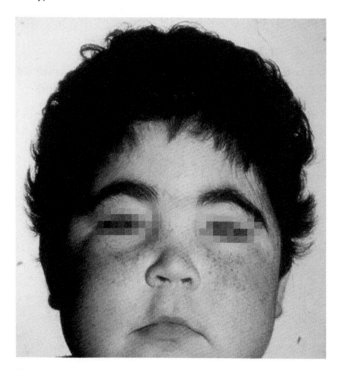

Figure 9.21 Steroid-induced 'moon face'.

- Infections
- Mood changes
- Muscle weakness
- Osteoporosis
- Perforated or bleeding peptic ulcers
- Tumours if given long-term
- Psychoses.

These complications may be reduced but not abolished if steroids are given on alternate days.

Patients on systemic steroids, in order to minimize the above effects are usually monitored for osteoporosis and BP, and also given ranitidine or proton pump inhibitors and calcium.

Main dental considerations

(*See also generic guidance under main dental considerations on page 63 top, and also Section 2).

Patients are immunocompromised; infections should be handled with caution. Conventional wisdom is that systemic corticosteroids suppress the hypothalamo-pituitary-adrenal (HPA) axis and thus the endogenous adrenal cortisol responses to stress become impaired. This can result in acute adrenal insufficiency (adrenal crisis – characterized by vomiting, headache and fever, with rapidly developing hypotension, collapse and possibly death). Before operation or GA, or during intercurrent illness or infection, or after trauma, these patients thus require an increase in corticosteroid dosage ('steroid cover').

Current guidance suggests 'steroid cover' may be indicated in these circumstances if:

- The patient is currently on daily systemic corticosteroids at doses above 10 mg prednisolone, or equivalent.
- Corticosteroids have been taken regularly during the previous 30 days.

Patients who have not received systemic steroids for more than 3 months are considered likely to have full recovery of HPA axis and require no perioperative supplementation. BP should be monitored.

Transplantation

Transplantation is a life-saving procedure for many patients with end-stage diseases, and is often the only viable treatment available. Organs, tissues, and cells transplanted include: kidneys, hearts, lungs, pancreas, liver, and small bowel; bone marrow, corneas, bones, and skin; and cells of muscle, bone, and pancreas. Transplant recipients selected are generally those with the following circumstances:

- Absence of other severe concomitant diseases.
- Ambulatory patient with rehabilitation potential.
- Limited life expectancy.
- Satisfactory emotional support system.
- Satisfactory psychosocial profile.
- Substantial limitation of daily activities.
- Untreatable end-stage disease.

Transplants donors can be living, sometimes from donors who are 'brain dead' (irreversible cessation of all brain and brainstem function), or transplants can be from cadaveric donors.

The major barrier to successful transplantation is rejection of the transplant and, except for transplants between identical twins, all transplant donors and recipients are immunologically incompatible. Transplant recipients thus undergo extensive immunological evaluation to avoid transplants at risk for antibody-mediated hyperacute rejection that includes; ABO blood group determination; Human leukocyte antigen (HLA) typing; serum screening for antibody to HLA phenotypes; and crossmatching.

Organ transplant success rates range from 50% to 90%. Rejection may be mild or severe but can lead to graft failure or patient death. Other complications from transplantation and associated medications may include:

- *Infections*: Patients are immunocompromised by virtue of drugs taken to prevent rejection. Infections may spread rapidly, may be opportunistic (involving micro-organisms that are normally commensal) and may be clinically silent or atypical. Infections are a serious threat and immunosuppression must then be reduced or stopped temporarily. Infections experienced depend on which microorganisms are in the environment and, to some extent, other treatments. Viral, fungal, mycobacterial and protozoal infections are a particular problem:
  - *Viral infections* account for substantial morbidity and mortality. Herpes simplex and zoster infections are common. Cytomegalovirus (CMV) infection is common. Epstein–Barr virus (EBV) may cause post-transplant lymphoproliferative disease (PTLD: see below).

Table 9.9 Donor cells used in HSCT

Donor	Comments
Autologous	Best for HSCT in non-malignant disease – no graft versus host disease (GVHD)
Sibling: syngeneic (identical twin)	No GVHD
Sibling (HLA-matched)	Minimal GVHD
Unrelated donor: HLA-matched	Some GVHD

- *Fungi* can cause severe local or invasive infections. *Candida* species (i.e., *Candida albicans, Candida tropicalis, Candida parapsilosis, Candida krusei*) are the most common. *Aspergillus niger, Aspergillus flavus,* or *Aspergillus fumigatus* may involve respiratory tract, skin, soft tissues, and CNS. *Cryptococcus neoformans* infections may cause pulmonary, CNS, and disseminated cutaneous disease. *Mucor* and *Rhizopus* infections (phycomycoses) are rare, but can produce destructive CNS or soft tissue infections that are difficult to eliminate.
- *Bacterial infections* must be treated aggressively. *Legionella* and *Pneumocystis* infections are more common. TB may reactivate.
- *Malignancies* (cancer of skin, lip, cervix, external genitalia, and perineum; Kaposi's sarcoma; post-transplant lymphoproliferative disease or lymphomas). These can be virally induced, such as HPV-associated carcinoma of the cervix, HHV-8 (KSHV) associated Kaposi's sarcoma, and EBV-associated post-transplant lymphoproliferative disease (PTLD) and lymphomas. PTLD is a heterogeneous group of tumours, ranging from benign B-cell hyperplasia to immunoblastic malignant lymphoma.
- *Graft dysfunction.*
- *Recurrent organ disease.*
- *Cardiac disease* (coronary heart disease or hypertension).
- *Endocrine problems*; adrenal suppression or diabetes mellitus.
- *Drug reactions.*
- *Graft versus host disease*, after bone marrow transplantation.

Bone marrow transplantation (BMT; Haematopoietic stem cell transplantation; HSCT)

The terms bone marrow transplant and stem cell transplant are interchangeable. HSCT is increasingly used in the treatment of aplastic anaemia, and haematological malignancies, and genetic defects. Bone marrow cells harvested from a donor are injected intravenously into a recipient. The donor cells are best harvested from an identical twin or a close relative who is also HLA – matched as much as possible to minimize graft rejection (Table 9.9). Most transplants are made between HLA-identical siblings, though other family members, or matched volunteers, may be used.

To reduce graft rejection patients must be profoundly immunosuppressed, often with cyclophosphamide (plus – in leukaemia – busulphan and total body irradiation [TBI] – to destroy malignant cells). An indwelling intravenous catheter (Hickman line) facilitates therapy. The donor marrow is mixed with heparin and infused intravenously to colonize the recipient marrow and, over the next 2–4 weeks, to produce blood cells.

Myeloablative treatment makes recipients extremely immune-incompetent, and they must be isolated from infection. Granulocytes, platelets or red cells, granulocyte colony stimulating factors, and antimicrobials may be needed until the marrow is functioning fully.

Heart transplantation

Selection of candidates is performed based on: ECG, echocardiogram and radionuclide scintillation studies. The donor heart usually comes from a brain-dead person as treatment for end-stage disease (cardiomyopathy, coronary artery disease, or valvular disease). All transplant recipients require life-long immunosuppression to prevent a T-cell, alloimmune rejection response, usually with ciclosporin, mycophenolate or azathioprine, corticosteroids and antithymocyte globulin, or tacrolimus.

The success of the transplantation is evaluated by means of: endomyocardial biopsies, ECG and coronary angiography. The 1-year survival is variable (20–80%), although post-operative mortality and morbidity are falling. Coronary artery stenosis develops in about 30% within a few years. Due to the absence of cardiac innervation, angina is rare and patients may experience 'silent' myocardial infarction or sudden death.

Liver transplantation

Surgical replacement is of a diseased liver with a healthy one or part of a normal liver from a living donor usually from a cadaveric or brain-dead donor. The 1-year survival after trans-plantation is around 80%. Recipients all require life-long T-cell immunosuppression. Recipients may be susceptible to recurrence of their original disease.

Lung transplantation

The lung for a transplant usually comes from a brain-dead organ donor. Recipients all require life-long immunosuppression to prevent a T-cell, rejection response (often a combination of ciclosporin, azathioprine, and glucocorticoids). Early graft failure following lung transplantation is diffuse alveolar damage (re-implantation oedema, reperfusion oedema, primary graft failure, or allograft dysfunction).

Pancreatic transplantation

The donor pancreas usually comes from a cadaver. About 85% of transplants are performed with a kidney transplant (a simultaneous pancreas–kidney [SPK] transplant), mostly in diabetic patients with renal failure. About 10% of cases are performed after a previously successful kidney transplant – a pancreas-after-kidney (PAK) transplant. An alternative new therapy that also may ameliorate diabetes is islet transplantation.

All transplant recipients require life-long immune-suppression to prevent a T-cell, alloimmune rejection response, using muromonab-CD3 – a mouse antihuman monospecific antibody against CD3 antigen on T lymphocytes; daclizumab – a humanized monoclonal antibody that blocks the interleukin-2 (IL-2) receptor on activated T cells; or basiliximab – a chimeric monoclonal antibody that blocks IL-2 receptor. The 1-year survival after pancreas transplantation is around 70%.

Renal transplantation

The donor kidney can be from cadaveric or living donors. Induction immunosuppression is a short course of intensive treatment with intravenous antilymphocyte antibodies (e.g. daclizumab and basiliximab). All recipients require life-long immunosuppression to prevent a T-cell, alloimmune rejection response, usually with a corticosteroid plus a steroid-sparing drug such as azathioprine or more commonly, ciclosporin or tacrolimus or sirolimus, or mycophenolate mofetil. Renal transplant survival can be as high as 90% at one year with an overall mortality of less than 5%, and about 70% survival at 5 years.

Main dental considerations in transplant patients

(*See also generic guidance under main dental considerations on page 63 top, and also Section 2).

Transplanted patients have been severely ill and remain immunocompromised, and often on medications such as anticoagulants or antihypertensive agents. Dental care should be done after consultation with the responsible physician/surgeon and patient, and elective care deferred until the patient is stabilized. Infection control and management are crucial.

Before transplantation

Where possible, active dental disease should be treated before transplantation:

- Eliminate oral infections.
- Extract unrestorable teeth.
- Educate patients about effective oral healthcare.

The timing of treatment, need for antibiotic prophylaxis, precautions to prevent excessive bleeding, and appropriate medication and dose should be considered. Some patients are only suitable for treatment in a hospital setting and factors that should be considered include:

- **Antibiotic prophylaxis.**
- **Infection:** active infections should be treated.
- **Excessive bleeding:** take precautions to limit bleeding.
- **Medication considerations:** transplantation patients are usually on multiple medications such as anticoagulants, beta-blockers, calcium channel blockers, diuretics, and others. Their adverse effects, and drug interactions must be considered.
- **Other medical problems:** Patients with end-stage organ failure may have comorbidities.

After organ transplantation

Treatment after organ transplantation requires consultation with the patient's physician. Except for emergency care, avoid dental treatment for at least 3 months following organ transplantation – when patients are at greatest risk for rejection and other serious complications.

Infection: Patients who have undergone organ transplant surgery are at increased risk for serious infection, especially immediately after surgery.

Medication considerations: Drugs that affect dental treatment include immunosuppressive agents that can cause gingival overgrowth, impaired healing, and infections and may interact with prescribed drugs. Anticoagulants may contribute to excessive bleeding, whereas a patient on steroids may be at risk for acute adrenal crisis. Several complications associated with marked immunosuppression manifest in the mouth, including candidiasis, herpes simplex/herpes zoster, hairy leukoplakia, aphthous-like ulcers, and infections. Progressive periodontal disease, delayed wound healing, and excessive bleeding may also become problems. Kaposi's sarcoma, lymphoma, and squamous cell carcinoma are among the oral malignancies that sometimes occur in organ transplant patients.

If organ rejection is occurring, only emergency dental care should be provided.

Further reading

www.npsa.nhs.uk/nrls/alerts-and-directives/alerts/anticoagulant/

http://circ.ahajournals.org/content/121/3/458.full

www.netce.com/coursecontent.php?courseid=844

10 Disability, vulnerability and impairment

Main dental considerations

(*See also generic guidance under main dental considerations on page 63 top, and also Section 2).

Oral manifestations may include dental caries and periodontal disease due to difficulties with oral hygiene practices. Treatment access has often been a barrier, but service providers in the UK are under a duty not to discriminate by refusing to provide good facilities or services or providing them at a lower standard or in a worse manner, or offering a service on worse terms than would be offered to other members of the public. Patients may have additional disabilities to consider, e.g. epilepsy, or defects of hearing, vision, speech, emotional disturbances or learning impairment. Advice on preventive care, oral hygiene and diet is especially important for patient and carers.

Bedbound patients

Bedbound people have the most severe degree of dependence, often with a weakness or a disability that makes it difficult for them to accomplish personal care routines and other activities of daily living (ADL), safely or independently. ADL include:

- Eating
- Bathing
- Dressing
- Toileting
- Transferring (walking)
- Continence

Aetiopathogenesis

Underlying causes may include neuropsychiatric disorders, osteoarthritis and cardiovascular illness but may be a physical disability, medical illness and/or mental health issue. Many are also people with ASA scores of III, IV and V (Section 2).

Clinical care

Common issues are constipation, uncontrolled bladder, skin breakdown (bedsores), muscle stiffening and gingivitis. Thromboses may arise, and respiratory and infectious complications are common. Many bedbound patients (such as those with a vascular catheter or urinary

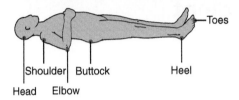

Figure 10.1 Points of pressure in bedbound patients – where pressure sores may arise.

catheter), are taking long-term antibiotics which may result in emergence of resistant bacteria. Prophylaxis to avoid the need for interventions is thus crucial.

- Encourage the person to do as much as possible themselves. If needed, raise the bed head to assist the patient with breathing, or at mealtimes, or when taking medications. If the patient has good upper body strength, a bed 'trapeze' lets them use arm strength to help with repositioning.
- Changing the patient's position frequently relieves pressure on backs, buttocks, heels and hips to help avoid bedsores. Check the skin twice daily – especially the back of the ears, buttocks, heels and back. Heel protectors provide protection. Avoid electric blankets or heating pads which may become warm enough to burn. Give a daily complete bed bath. Range-of-motion exercises help preserve joint and muscle function.
- Basic personal-care needs may include assisting feeding/eating, adequate bowel and bladder function and oral healthcare. Intimate hygiene care is important, when maintaining privacy for the client is crucial. Before a patient becomes totally incontinent, a bedpan may be offered on a regular basis for a woman or a girl who cannot get to the bathroom or a bedside commode, and a urinal may be used for males. If there is regular incontinence, special incontinence briefs to absorb fluids should be used and changed regularly, and incontinence pads should be placed beneath the person. Skin must be kept clean and dry, and if it becomes irritated or erythematous, should be cleansed with a wet soft cloth or disposable wet wipe, patted dry with clean soft towels, and a moisture barrier applied.
- Patients may need help with activities such as opening food or milk packages/cartons, to butter bread, cut up food or to eat. When assisting a dependent person with a meal, use a spoon, rather than a fork, offer small bites of food, give them enough time to chew and swallow each mouthful and offer small sips of drink frequently between bites; provide privacy. If eyesight is poor, they may need assistance to tell them where items are on the tray. Some people may not be able to feed themselves at all.

Main dental considerations

(*See also generic guidance under main dental considerations on page 63 top, and also Section 2).

Access for dental treatment is challenging, but equipment for domiciliary use is available and helpful.

Cerebral palsy (CP)

Definition
Abnormalities of motor control.

Aetiopathogenesis
Damage to a child's brain early in development by hypoxia, trauma, maternal infection or hyperbilirubinaemia. Risk factors include: breech presentation – when a fetus does not turn to the usual head-first position for birth, and low birth-weight babies.

Clinical presentation and classification
The most common congenital and irreversible physical handicap features are abnormalities of movement and posture. These may include delays in motor skill development, weakness in one or more limbs, abnormal walking gait with one foot or leg dragging, excessive drooling or difficulties in swallowing and poor control over hand and arm movement:

- **Spastic CP** – excessive muscle tone, contractures, pathological reflexes and hyperactive tendon reflexes. Limbs are affected differently in the different types:
  - Monoplegic; only one limb affected.
  - Paraplegic; lower extremities only.
  - Hemiplegic; one side upper/lower limbs.
  - Double hemiplegic; all, but arms mainly.
  - Diplegic; all limbs, mainly legs.
  - Quadriplegic; all limbs (tetraplegic).

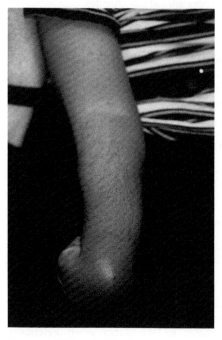
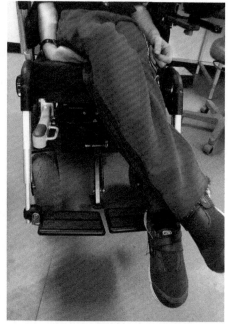

Figure 10.2 Cerebral palsy.   **Figure 10.3** Wheelchair for CP patient.

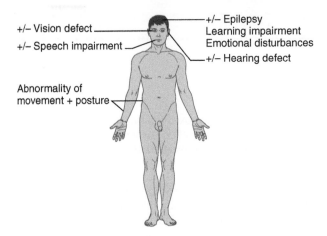

+/– Epilepsy
Learning impairment
Emotional disturbances
+/– Hearing defect

+/– Vision defect

+/– Speech impairment

Abnormality of
movement + posture

Figure 10.4 Cerebral palsy, possible features.

- **Athetoid CP** affects all limbs – smooth worm-like movements, exaggerated if patient is anxious.
- **Ataxic CP** – disturbance of balance.

Diagnosis
From signs and cerebral CT and MRI which may show anatomical changes.

Treatment
- Physical, occupational, speech therapy.
- Hearing and visual aids; joint surgery; possibly muscle relaxants and anticonvulsants; dietary advice.
- Life expectancy in CP has increased significantly, but respiratory infections are common, and aspiration pneumonia is a main danger.

Main dental considerations
(*See also generic guidance under main dental considerations on page 63 top, and also Section 2).
Oral manifestations may include:
- Bruxism and attrition.
- Spontaneous TMJ subluxation or dislocation.
- Drooling, and general poor control of oral structures and head posture.
- Delayed eruption of primary dentition.
- Enamel hypoplasia.
- Malocclusion.
- Papillary hyperplastic gingivitis.

Tilted back or supine positioning will often cause an apprehensive response. Manual support of head and jaw may be helpful. Anxiety tends to aggravate involuntary movements. Most drug therapies used are CNS depressants, so take caution when prescribing other CNS depressants (e.g., narcotics, muscle relaxants, anxiolytics).

Clefts

Definition

Clefts of the lip with or without cleft palate and cleft palate alone result from the failure of the first branchial arches to complete fusion processes and are the most common of all craniofacial anomalies.

Aetiopathogenesis

The primary palate will fuse laterally with the maxillary processes of the first branchial arch during the sixth and seventh week's gestation, forming the upper lip and alveolar bone. Impaired formation results in cleft lip (CL) which is clinically evident. Secondary palate development involves bilateral palatal shelves arising from the maxillary processes which fuse by the 10th week of gestation. Impaired formation results in cleft palate (CP), usually quickly recognized after birth, especially when associated with a cleft lip – but submucous cleft can be more difficult to diagnose.

Many but not all cases of clefting are inherited; a number of teratogens (environmental agents that can cause birth defects) have also been implicated, as well as defects in essential nutrients. Cleft lip/palate is more prevalent in lower socioeconomic groups. Environmental factors during the first trimester of pregnancy which may generate cleft palate, include maternal upper respiratory infection in the first trimester, smoking, obesity, diabetes, stress or exposure to various agents. Teratogens incriminated include isotretinoin (used to treat acne), which causes birth defects such as brain malformations, learning disability, heart problems, and facial abnormalities. Thalidomide given to pregnant mothers was, and anticonvulsants (phenytoin, valproic acid, lamotrigine, carbamazepine) and corticosteroids may be, associated with an increased incidence. Systemic corticosteroids have been reported to increase the risk (this is controversial) and there are also concerns about possible effects from topical steroids used in the first trimester. There has been concern but no real evidence about aspirin and diazepam as possible causes. Paternal smoking has also been implicated.

Clefting can occur independently or as part of a larger syndrome that may include the heart and other organs. The total incidence of facial clefting is between two and three per 1000 live births. A number of these fetuses do not develop to full-term. Facial clefts are associated with a syndrome in up to 15–60% of cases and are then termed syndromic clefts. More than 400 syndromes may include a facial cleft as one manifestation and cleft lip/palate (CLP) may be associated with many congenital syndromes.

Clinical presentation

The common clefts are cleft lip with or without cleft palate (CL ± P) and cleft palate only (CP). A unilateral CL occurs on one side of the upper lip. A bilateral cleft lip occurs on both sides of the upper lip. In its most severe form, the cleft may extend through the nose base. Cleft palate may be incomplete – or even submucous – involving only the uvula (bifid) and the muscular soft palate (velum). A complete cleft palate extends the entire length of the palate. Cleft palates can be unilateral or bilateral.

Affected infants with clefts have facial deformity and may have difficulty with feeding, breathing, speaking, and swallowing and are susceptible to respiratory infections. The neonate with a cleft palate is unable to suckle. Later, speech development is also impaired.

There may also be feeding difficulties and associated congenital defects such as dental, hearing and speech defects, or more serious anomalies – especially skeletal, cardiac, renal and central nervous system defects.

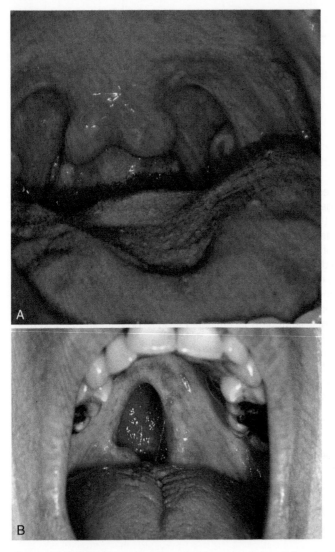

Figure 10.5 (A) Bifid uvula (often signifies submucous cleft palate). **(B)** Cleft palate.

Diagnosis

Clinical, imaging and pharyngeal function studies.

Treatment and main dental considerations

(*See also generic guidance under main dental considerations on page 63 top, and also Section 2).

A multidisciplinary cleft palate team includes: audiologists; maxillofacial, ear, nose and throat, and plastic surgeons; geneticists; neurosurgeons; nurses; dentists; paediatricians; social workers/psychologists; and speech and language pathologists.

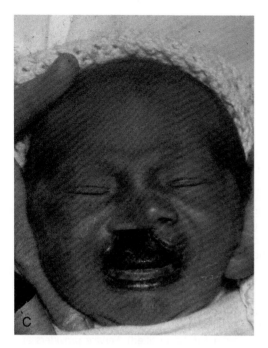

Figure 10.5, cont'd (C) Cleft lip and palate.

- Age – newborn to 12 months. Aesthetics is a major issue for parents, but treatment of the airway takes priority and may be managed with positioning but, in severe cases, may need tracheostomy. There can be significant difficulties in management of the airway for anaesthesia in children under the age of 5 years, particularly in young infants and in those with feeding difficulties, bilateral clefts and/or retrognathia. One of the problems for the child is feeding; a Rosti bottle with Gummi teat often helps.
- The timing of the initial cleft lip and palate repair is controversial. In general, when the lip alone is cleft, initial cosmetic repair is carried out at about 3–6 months of age, though earlier operations are becoming popular. Many repair cleft lip and palate within the first few days of life since, after repair, the appearance is dramatically improved, feeding difficulties are significantly minimized and speech develops better. If the palatal defect is too wide, it can be repaired 3 months later to allow for sufficient palatal growth. In any event, CP is now usually repaired before the child speaks, between 6 and 18 months, typically at 6–12 months of age.
- Age 1–5 years is when it is important to have good hearing and normal appearance to avoid low self-esteem and help speech develop. These children need a hearing assessment, and if it is impaired, ear ventilation tubes (grommets) may be indicated.
- Age 5–13 years is when orthodontists can help correct malocclusion and alveolar bone grafting may be needed. Speech, if poor despite the best efforts by the child and the speech pathologist, may be corrected with pharyngoplasty.
- Age 13–18 years is the time for final adjustments. Orthodontic and restorative care are usually indicated.

Disability and impairment

Definitions

An *impairment* is any loss or abnormality of psychological, physiological or anatomical structure or function. A *disability* is any restriction or lack (resulting from an impairment) of ability to perform an activity in the manner or within the range considered normal for a human being. A *handicap* is a disadvantage for a given individual, resulting from an impairment or a disability, which prevents the fulfilment of a role that is considered normal (depending on age, sex and social and cultural factors) for that individual. Disabilities may be classified in a variety of ways, as listed in Table 10.1.

Aetiopathogenesis

Developmental disabilities are caused by impairments that include intra-uterine infections, metabolic defects, fetal alcohol syndrome (FAS), chromosomal abnormalities, birth hypoxia, autism, cerebral palsy, and postnatal infections (e.g. meningitis or encephalitis). Acquired disabilities are caused by stroke, traumatic brain injury, spinal cord damage, multiple sclerosis, arthritis and Alzheimer disease.

Treatment

The main obstacle or barrier to healthcare had been access, but the Disability Discrimination Act 1995 (DDA) makes it unlawful to treat a person with disability less favourably for a reason related to that person's disability (unless it can be justified). Service providers are under a duty not to discriminate by refusing to provide good facilities or services or providing them at a lower standard or in a worse manner, or offering a service on worse terms than would be offered to other members of the public.

However, if the person with a disability poses a 'direct threat' (significant risk that cannot be eliminated using special procedures) to the health or safety of others, that person, e.g. an aggressive patient, may be refused access to the premises.

Main dental considerations

(*See generic guidance under main dental considerations on page 63 top, and also Section 2).

Table 10.1 Disability and impairment

Disabilities	Impairments
Physical	Mobility
	Respiratory
Mental	Emotional
	Social
Sensory	Hearing
	Visual
Cognitive	Learning
	Attention

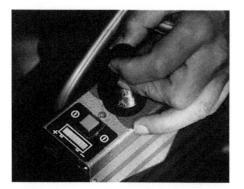

Figure 10.6 Motorized wheelchair control panel.

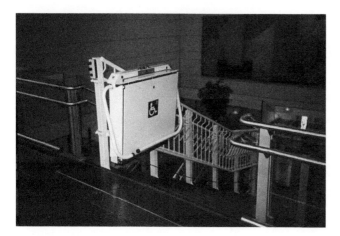

Figure 10.7 Staircase for disabled people.

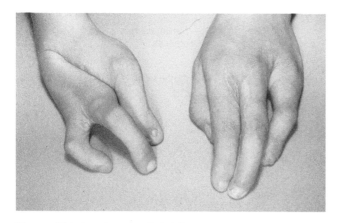

Figure 10.8 Hands-congenital deformities.

Down syndrome (DS)

Definition
The most common chromosomal disorder.

Aetiopathogenesis
An additional chromosome 21; three genetic variations (trisomy, mosaic trisomy, translocation trisomy).The likelihood of an extra copy of chromosome 21 increases dramatically as a woman ages.

Clinical presentation
DS affects many if not most organs. Characteristic features include:
- Neuropsychiatric disease:
  - Learning disability
  - Visual: cataracts
  - Hearing loss
  - Seizure disorders
  - Dementia, or memory loss and impaired judgment.

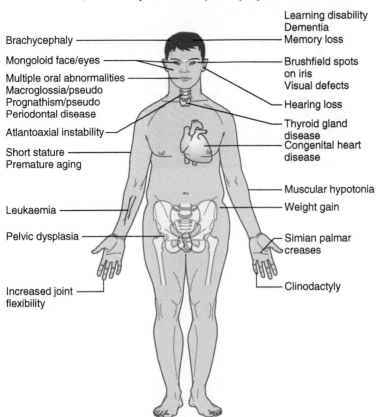

Figure 10.9 Down syndrome – features.

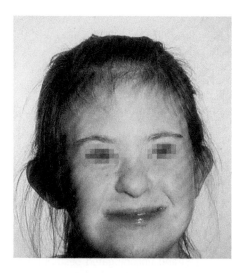

Figure 10.10 Down syndrome.

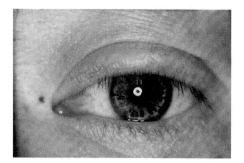

Figure 10.11 Down syndrome showing Brushfield spots in iris.

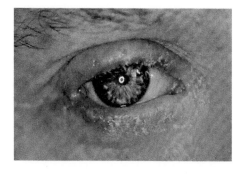

Figure 10.12 Blepharitis in Down syndrome.

- Physical changes:
  - Short stature, brachycephaly, mongoloid facies, Brushfield spots in the iris.
  - Muscular hypotonia, increased joint flexibility, pelvic dysplasia, atlantoaxial instability – can cause spinal cord compression if the neck is not handled considerately. Transient myelodysplasia, or defective development of the spinal cord. Clinodactyly (short fifth finger). Single palmar (simian) creases.
- Cardiac problems: Approximately 50% have atrial septal defect, or mitral valve prolapse.
- Malignant disease: leukaemia, retinoblastoma.
- Immune defects and infections.
- Endocrine: thyroid disease.
- Premature aging.

Diagnosis

Fetal screening tests include: nuchal translucency ultrasound scan, plus quadruple blood test (maternal serum alpha feto-protein [MSAFP; reduced in DS], beta chorionic gonado-tropin [beta hCG; raised in DS], inhibin-A [raised in DS] and unconjugated oestriol [uE3; reduced in DS]). Amniocentesis and chorionic villus sampling (CVS) may also be carried out, and percutaneous umbilical blood sampling (PUBS) for chromosomal karyotype.

Main dental considerations

(*See also generic guidance under main dental considerations on page 63 top, and also Section 2).
Tooth eruption is often irregular. Missing teeth are common. Morphological abnormalities, particularly teeth with short small crowns and roots are common. Anterior open bite, posterior cross-bite and other malocclusions are common. There is also a higher incidence of bifid uvula, cleft lip and cleft palate. The tongue may be large and fissured, the lips thick, dry and fissured. Severe early-onset periodontal disease may be due to poor oral hygiene, and impaired immunity. Most patients can be treated under LA with sedation if necessary. GA is best avoided, in view of other difficulties which may include cardiac defects, anaemia, possible atlantoaxial subluxation (care needed when extending neck) or respiratory disease.

Hearing impairment

Conductive hearing loss is due to middle or external ear disorders – when sounds that should be carried from the tympanic membrane to the inner ear are blocked by, for example foreign bodies, wax, fluid or infection, or abnormal bone growth.

Sensorineural hearing loss is due to defects of the cochlear nerve or its central connections, as in damage to the inner ear or auditory nerve (e.g. in birth defects, exposure to very loud noises [pop music, explosions, loud machinery, etc.], head injury, surgery, tumours, certain drugs, hypertension or stroke). Age-related changes include especially presbycusis – the most common hearing problems in older people are linked to inner ear changes.

Speech communications are easier for the hearing-impaired person if there is:

- Bright lighting.
- Little background noise.
- Speaker facing them directly, not wearing a face mask, not moving their head around, talking slowly, preferably one phrase at a time, at the optimal distance from the person (between 1 and 2 metres).

The sign language ('deaf') alphabet helps. Hearing aids available to help differ in design, size, amount of amplification, ease of handling, volume control, and special features. All include a microphone, an amplifier, and a receiver (miniature loudspeaker) to deliver the sound into the ear. Bone-anchored hearing aids are implantable devices which act by directly stimulating the inner ear. Hearing assistive devices are available for use with or without hearing aids.

People with a severe to profound hearing loss who cannot be helped with hearing aids may find cochlear implants of benefit.

Cochlear implants have external parts behind the ear (receiver), and internal (surgically implanted) electrodes which stimulate the auditory nerve directly, helping sensorineural hearing loss (see Implants; Section 9). However, people with cochlear implants are more likely to contract bacterial meningitis than those without. The US Centers for Disease Control (CDC) recommend that children with cochlear implants receive pneumococcal vaccination.

See http://thehearingfix.com/hearing-aid-reviews/

Main dental considerations

(*See also generic guidance under main dental considerations on page 63 top, and also Section 2).

Communication. Electromagnetic interference can be an issue with hearing aids.

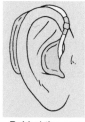
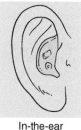
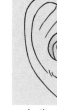

Behind-the-ear   In-the-ear   In-the-canal

Figure 10.13 Hearing aids.

Learning disability and impairment

Definition
Limitations in mental functioning (cognition) and in communicating, self-care or sociability.

Aetiopathogenesis
The result of brain damage, causes usually unknown but may include:
- *Birth* problems (e.g. during labour and birth).
- *Genetic* conditions (e.g. Down syndrome, fragile X syndrome [X chromosome changes]), etc.
- *Postnatal* problems (e.g. whooping cough, measles, meningitis, head trauma, extreme malnutrition or poisons like lead or mercury).
- *Pregnancy* problems (e.g. fetal alcohol syndrome or infections [e.g. rubella]).

Clinical presentation
Affected children often take longer to speak, walk, and take care of their personal needs such as dressing or eating, have trouble learning and may have trouble:
- remembering things
- seeing the consequences of their actions
- solving problems
- thinking logically
- understanding social rules
- understanding the need and how to pay for things.

Brain damage may also cause physical impairments, and epilepsy, visual defects, hearing, speech or behavioural disorders.
  Other problems which may be increased may include craniofacial, cardiac or other defects; psychiatric disorders; hyperkinesis and stereotyped movements; feeding difficulties; incontinence or pica (the ingestion of inedible substances).

Classification
The intelligence quotient (IQ) represents the quotient between chronologic age and mental age. The average IQ in the population is 100. Borderline patients have an IQ of 70–84. Learning impairment corresponds to an IQ <70. Mild learning impairment corresponds to IQ 50–69, and these people frequently live at home, hold conversations, have full independence in self-care, practical domestic skills and basic reading/writing. Moderate learning impairment (IQ 35–49) causes limited language, needing help with self-care, but individuals can undertake simple practical work (with supervision) and are usually fully mobile. Severe learning impairment (IQ <35) people are often totally dependent on others for care, use words/gestures for basic needs, movement impairments are common, activities need supervision, and they can work only in structured/sheltered settings.

Diagnosis
Clinically based, IQ and learning skills.

Treatment

Learning impairment is so varied in severity and character that generalizations cannot really be justified, but many patients can be cared for adequately at home. Special educational and vocational training is usually required. Special facilities or an escort to facilitate care may be needed.

Informed consent is a fraught issue in patients with learning disability. Drugs to limit any hyperactivity may sometimes be useful. Issues may arise from:

- obesity and its sequelae;
- physical, sexual or drug abuse;
- prolonged use of sedatives, tranquillizers or anticonvulsants.

Communication can be difficult, but can be aided if staff: take time to present information, minimize distractions, use short explanations, simple language, 'tell-show-do', use positive reinforcement/praise.

Main dental considerations

(*See also generic guidance under main dental considerations on page 63 top, and also Section 2).
Guidelines for care are available at www.bsdh.org.uk/guidelines/physical.pdf.

Paralyses (Head and neck)

Bulbar palsy
Definition
Paralysis of tongue, chewing/swallowing and face muscles.

Aetiopathogenesis
Brainstem nuclei lesions, causing lower motor neurone (LMN) dysfunction in:
- Guillain–Barré syndrome (acute polyneuropathy)
- Motor neurone disease
- Poliomyelitis
- Syringobulbia
- Tumours.

Clinical presentation
Weakness and fasciculations of oral muscles, drooling, jaw jerk – may be absent, speech – altered (quiet, nasal or hoarse), tongue – flaccid and fasciculating.

Pseudobulbar palsy
Definition
Upper motor neurone (UMN) paralysis affecting tongue, chewing/swallowing and face muscles.

Aetiopathogenesis

Lesion above mid-pons, caused mainly by:

- Motor neurone disease
- Multiple sclerosis
- Strokes (cerebrovascular events).

Clinical presentation

Tongue – spastic; jaw jerk – exaggerated; speech – like Donald Duck.

Facial palsies

Definition

Either:

- LMN neuropathy affecting the facial (VIIth cranial) nerve alone, usually transitory and self-limiting.
- UMN neuropathy – cerebrovascular events (strokes).

Aetiopathogenesis

LMN neuropathy mostly caused by herpes simplex virus (HSV). Other causes of VII cranial nerve palsy, variously affecting the nerve in pons, skull base, middle ear, parotid or face may include:

- Diabetes mellitus.
- Guillain–Barré syndrome.
- Infections (other herpesviruses, HIV, polio, TB, Lyme disease, leprosy).
- Melkersson–Rosenthal syndrome/Crohn's disease.
- Multiple sclerosis.
- Sarcoidosis.
- Stroke.
- Tumours.
- Trauma.

UMN neuropathy (see Stroke; Section 5).

Clinical presentation

Unilateral facial palsy that includes:

- Loss of nasolabial fold
- Asymmetric smile
- Inability to close the eye on the affected side.

Diagnosis

Clinical and neurologic examination.

Treatment

LMN neuropathy:

- Aciclovir possibly
- Eye pad and ophthalmological consultation
- Corticosteroids (prednisone or prednisolone).

UMN neuropathy (see Stroke, Section 5).

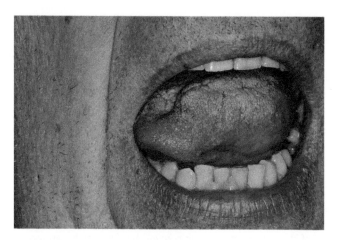

Figure 10.14 Hypoglossal nerve palsy.

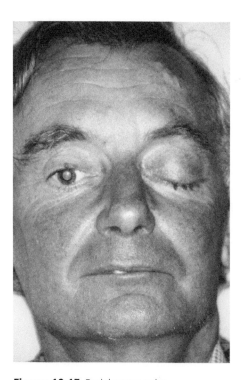

Figure 10.15 Facial nerve palsy.

Spina bifida

Definition
Failure of fusion of vertebral arches.

Aetiopathogenesis
Deficiency of folic acid in pregnancy may predispose.

Clinical presentation and classification
Spina bifida occulta – rarely causes any obvious clinical or neurological disorder, but can be detected by a naevus or tuft of hair over the lumbar spine, and radiographically.
Spina bifida cystica – an extensive vertebral defect through which the spinal cord or coverings protrude as:
- Meningocele: protrusion of the meninges as a sac covered by skin, rarely causing neurological defect but 20% have hydrocephalus.
- Myelomeningocele: ten times as common as meningocele – meninges and nerve tissue protrude and are exposed with severe neurological defects, typically complete paraplegia, patients therefore also suffering from:
  - Inability to walk.
  - Liability to pressure sores.
  - Urinary incontinence.
  - Faecal retention.
  - Liability to infection, particularly meningitis.
  - Other issues (e.g. hydrocephalus, epilepsy, learning impairment), other vertebral or renal anomalies.

In spina bifida there is a high prevalence of latex allergy, the risk increasing with:
- Number of previous surgical procedures.
- Use of bladder catheters.
- Existence of a ventriculo-peritoneal shunt.
- Symptoms when blowing up a toy balloon.
- Family history of atopic diseases.

Diagnosis
Prenatally by amniocentesis (raised alpha-feto protein and acetylcholinesterase).

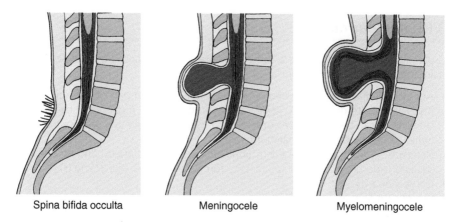

| Spina bifida occulta | Meningocele | Myelomeningocele |

Figure 10.16 Spina bifida types. Adapted from Centers for Disease Control and Prevention. www.cdc.gov/ncbddd/spinabifida/facts.html

Treatment

Patients with myelomeningocele require specialist attention to manage urinary tract, bowel and locomotion. Surgical closure of myelomeningocele and de-compression of hydrocephalus is often carried out in early infancy. Hydrocephalus is typically drained by ventriculo-atrial (VA) or, more frequently, by ventriculo-peritoneal (VP) shunts.

Main dental considerations

(*See also generic guidance under main dental considerations on page 63 top, and also Section 2).
Latex allergy and access for care.

Visual impairment

Visual impairment (VI) can have a range of causes; most is caused by disease, trauma or malnutrition. The main causes include:

- Age-related macular degeneration (ARMD or AMD) – when part of the retina (the macula) starts to degenerate. Appearing after age 65, and predisposed by obesity and smoking, it can be 'dry' (more common and usually a slower loss of vision) or 'wet' (when retinal blood vessels haemorrhage).
- Cataracts – cloudy spots in the lens (irradiation, diabetes, steroids, and excessive sunlight exposure may cause cataracts to form at a younger age in adults).
- Corneal opacity.
- Diabetic retinopathy.
- Genetic defects; visual defects are among the most common genetic disorders and congenital blindness may be associated with other handicaps such as epilepsy.
- Glaucoma – abnormal pressure inside the eye (normal intraocular pressure is 12–21 mmHg).
- Neurological; ocular, optic nerve or cortical damage. A complete lesion of one optic nerve causes that eye to be totally blind, there is no direct reaction of the pupil to light (loss of constriction) and, if a light is shone into the affected eye, the pupil of the unaffected eye also fails to respond (loss of the consensual reflex). However, the nerves to the affected eye responsible for pupil constriction run in the IIIrd cranial nerve and should be intact. If, therefore, a light is shone into the unaffected eye, the pupil of the affected eye also constricts, even though that eye is sightless. Lesions of the optic tract, chiasma, radiation or optic cortex cause various visual field defects involving both visual fields but without total field loss on either side.
- Retinal detachment.
- Retinitis pigmentosa.
- Trachoma.
- Trauma.
- Uveitis.

Visual impairment invariably restricts driving and other activity and can vary from limitations in sight for distance, colour, size or shape to full blindness. Visual impairment may be suspected if a patient has overcautious driving habits; finds lighting either too bright or too dim; has frequent spectacle prescription changes; holds books or reading material close to face or at arm's length; squints or tilts the head to see; has difficulty in recognizing people; changes leisure time activities, personal appearance or table etiquette; moves about cautiously or bumps into objects; or acts confusedly or is disoriented.

An ophthalmological opinion should always be obtained if there is any suggestion of a visual disability. Eye chart – visual acuity testing using the Snellen eye chart or a similar standard eye chart. Normal vision is 20/20, which means that the eye being tested can read a certain size letter when it is 20 feet away. If a person sees 20/40, then at 20 feet from the chart that person can read letters that a person with 20/20 vision could read from 40 feet away. The 20/40 letters are twice the size of 20/20 letters; however, if 20/20 is considered 100% visual efficiency, 20/40 visual acuity is 85% efficient. For people who have worse than 20/400 vision, a different eye chart can be used. It is common to record vision worse than 20/400 as Count Fingers (CF at a certain number of feet), Hand Motion (HM at a certain number of feet), Light Perception (LP), or No Light Perception (NLP).

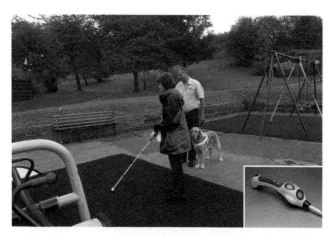

Figure 10.17 UltraCane (Photo courtesy of UltraCane, Sound Foresight Technology Ltd.)

Table 10.2 Types of glaucoma		
Type	**Features**	**Treatment**
Open-angle	Most common. The angle that allows fluid to drain out of the anterior chamber is open, but fluid passes too slowly through the meshwork drain. Optic nerve damage and narrowed side vision develop. Risk groups include people of African heritage over age 40, anyone over age 60 and family history of glaucoma	Drugs or laser trabeculoplasty
Low- or normal-tension	Optic nerve damage and narrowed side vision develop unexpectedly in people with normal eye pressure	Drugs or laser trabeculoplasty
Closed-angle	The fluid at the front of the eye cannot reach the angle and leave, because the angle gets blocked by part of the iris	Without immediate laser therapy, eye can become blind within 48 h
Congenital	Defects in the angle of the eye that slow the normal fluid drainage	Surgery
Secondary	Develops as complication of other medical conditions, cataracts, uveitis, eye surgery, injuries, or tumours	Various

- Ophthalmoscopy – provides a wider, magnified view of the retina.
- Tonometry – measures pressure inside the eye to detect glaucoma.
- A slit lamp examination – allows examination of the front of the eye.
- A phoropter – detects refractive errors.
- Visual field examination (perimetry) – tests the total area where objects can be seen in the peripheral vision while the eye is focused on a central point.

- Confrontation visual field examination – a quick and basic evaluation of the visual field done by an examiner sitting directly in front of the patient who is asked to look at the examiner's eye and tell when they can see the examiner's hand.
- Tangent screen exam – the patient looks at a central target and tells the examiner when an object brought into the peripheral vision can be seen.
- Automated perimetry – the patient sites in front of a computer-driven programme which flashes small lights at different locations, and presses a button whenever the lights in the peripheral vision are seen.

A person is considered blind if they see clearly at 20 feet what someone with very good vision can see at 200 feet, and if glasses or contact lenses cannot make them see better. This is called 20/200 vision. 'Legally blind' indicates that a person has less than 20/200 vision in the better eye or a very limited field of vision (20 degrees at its widest point). Legal blindness in the UK, the statutory definition of 'blind' is: 'so blind as to be unable to perform any work for which eyesight is essential' (the Blind Persons Act 1920).

There is no statutory definition of 'partial sight' although the guideline is 'substantially and permanently handicapped by defective vision caused by congenital defect, illness, or injury' (the National Assistance Act 1948).

'Low vision' generally refers to a severe VI, not necessarily limited to distance vision. Low vision applies to all individuals with sight who are unable to read the newspaper at a normal viewing distance, even with the aid of eyeglasses or contact lenses.

People with low vision use a combination of vision and other senses to learn, although they may require adaptations in lighting or the size of print, and, sometimes, Braille. Totally blind people learn via Braille or other non-visual media. Mostly they use a white walking stick or a tactile wand or UltraCane (Fig. 10.17), which emits ultrasonic waves.

Other assistive technology includes:

- Screen enlargers (or screen magnifiers).
- Screen readers – that present graphics and text as speech.
- Speech recognition systems (voice recognition programmes).
- Speech synthesizers (text-to-speech (TTS) systems).
- Refreshable Braille displays provide tactile output of information represented on the computer screen.
- Braille embossers – transfer computer-generated text into embossed Braille output.
- Talking and large-print word processors are helpful.

Main dental considerations

(*See also generic guidance under main dental considerations on page 63 top, and also Section 2).

It can be helpful to people with VI, if other people:

- Verbally advise them of their presence. They should be told before they are touched. People with VI may have an increased sense of touch.
- When guiding the patient, offer an arm and let them hold, never push them, but describe obstacles.
- Tell the patient before people leave the room.
- Use bright colours for steps, doors and pillars.
- Have notices in large writing.
- Do not touch, pet or interfere with any guide dog.

Vulnerable groups

Vulnerability is the degree to which a population, individual or organization is unable to anticipate, cope with, resist and recover from the impacts of disasters (WHO). It can affect groups that experience a higher risk of poverty and social exclusion than the general population. In UK, the Safeguarding Vulnerable Groups Act 2006 (http://www.legislation.gov .uk/ukpga/2006/47/section/59) defines a person as a vulnerable adult if he/she has attained the age of 18 and is in the following –

(a) is in residential accommodation,
(b) is in sheltered housing,
(c) receives domiciliary care,
(d) receives any form of health care,
(e) is detained in lawful custody,
(f) is by virtue of an order of a court under supervision by a person exercising functions for the purposes of Part 1 of the Criminal Justice and Court Services Act 2000,
(g) receives a welfare service of a prescribed description,
(h) receives any service or participates in any activity provided specifically for persons who fall within subsection (9),
(i) payments are made to him (or to another on his behalf) in pursuance of arrangements under section 57 of the Health and Social Care Act 2001 (c. 15), or
(j) requires assistance in the conduct of his own affairs.

Children and older people are discussed in Section 4. Others vulnerable may include people who are;

- Disabled
- Displaced (internally – people who remain in their own countries) as well as refugees (people who cross international borders) and other migrants
- Ethnic minorities
- Gypsies and travellers
- Homeless
- Ill or Immunocompromised,
- Malnourished
- Poverty stricken
- Pregnant
- Sex workers
- Substance abusers.

Vulnerable people may have poorer health and access to healthcare than the general population. There may also be cultural issues affecting that need to be considered.

Main dental considerations

Access to healthcare is often the main issue. The first dental contact is typically for emergency care. Dental disease, trauma, and infections are the most common challenges. There can be a burden of infectious diseases in certain groups which may impact on oral health and/or healthcare e.g. HIV, HBV, HCV.

Lesbian, gay, bisexual, and transgender (LGBT) or LGBTQ – an acronym that includes Queer

LGBT are a community of people who are non-heterosexual and perhaps with marginalized sexual identities, not conforming to traditional heterosexist assumptions of male and female behaviour, in that they have sexual and emotional relationships with the same sex, and may have shared political and social concerns. However, there are questions whether the various gender groupings currently bracketed together necessarily share the same issues, values and goals.

LGBT adults are estimated to comprise between 3% and 4% of the US adult population. The Caring and Aging with Pride: The National Health, Aging and Sexuality Study (CAP), showed that older LGBT adults will likely more than double over the next two decades.

Whether or not LGBT people openly identify themselves may depend on local political concerns, whether they live in a discriminatory environment, as well as on the status of LGBT rights where they are. Indicators of a hostile climate to LGBT people include homophobic remarks and victimization regarding sexual orientation and gender expression and there may be exclusion from services such as being denied medical and surgical care.

Health related issues may be increased in some LGBT communities and some of these include:

- accessing culturally responsive services
- cardiovascular disease
- childhood sexual abuse (CSA) and adolescent/adult sexual assault (ASA) – strongly associated with women's alcohol use
- disability
- discrimination
- exploitation
- homelessness
- infections, particularly hepatitis (Section 5) and HIV (Section 7). Even those who are not themselves infected have often been affected by experiencing trauma and survivors' guilt through multiple cumulative losses from experiencing the illnesses and deaths of friends or partners
- loneliness
- mental health issues
- obesity
- victimisation.

Ten competencies recommended to healthcare workers are to include to:

1. Critically analyze personal and professional attitudes toward sexual orientation, gender identity, and age, and understand how factors such as culture, religion, media, and health and human service systems influence attitudes and ethical decision-making.
2. Understand and articulate the ways that larger social and cultural contexts may have negatively impacted LGBT older adults as a historically disadvantaged population.
3. Distinguish similarities and differences within the subgroups of LGBT older adults, as well as their intersecting identities (such as age, gender, race, and health status) to develop tailored and responsive health strategies.
4. Apply theories of aging and social and health perspectives and the most up-to-date knowledge available to engage in culturally competent practice with LGBT older adults.

5. When conducting a comprehensive biopsychosocial assessment, attend to the ways that the larger social context and structural and environmental risks and resources may impact LGBT older adults.
6. When using empathy and sensitive interviewing skills during assessment and intervention, ensure the use of language is appropriate for working with LGBT older adults in order to establish and build rapport.
7. Understand and articulate the ways in which agency, program, and service policies do or do not marginalize and discriminate against LGBT older adults.
8. Understand and articulate the ways that local, state, and federal laws negatively and positively impact LGBT older adults, in order to advocate on their behalf.
9. Provide sensitive and appropriate outreach to LGBT older adults, their families, caregivers and other supports to identify and address service gaps, fragmentation, and barriers that impact LGBT older adults.
10. Enhance the capacity of LGBT older adults and their families, caregivers and other supports to navigate aging, social, and health services.

Aging, combined with a history of marginalization and discrimination, increases the potential vulnerability of LGBT older adults, but despite the adversity experienced by many LGBT people, they can display remarkable resilience.

References

https://en.wikipedia.org/wiki/LGBT
http://www.ncbi.nlm.nih.gov/pmc/articles/PMC4091982/

Appendix: Normal test values

Interpretation of blood test results (always check values for the laboratory used).

Full blood count (FBC) examines:

Red cell (erythrocyte) parameters.

Red cell count (RCC) – guideline normal values: $4.5–6.5 \times 1012/L$ in adult males and $3.8–5.8 \times 1012/L$ in adult females.

Mean cell volume (MCV) – guideline normal values: 77–95 fL.

Mean cell haemoglobin (MCH) – guideline normal values: 27.0–32.0 pg.

Mean cell haemoglobin concentration (MCHC) – guideline normal values: 32.0–36.0 g/dL.

White cells (leukocytes).

Total white cell count (WCC)/white blood cell count (WBC) – guideline normal values: $4.00–11.0 \times 10^9/L$.

Neutrophils (polymorphs or polymorphonucleocytes) – guideline normal values: $2–7.5 \times 10^9/L$, comprising 40–75% of WBCs.

Lymphocytes – guideline normal values: $1.3–3.5 \times 10^9/L$, comprising 20–45% of WBCs.

Eosinophils – guideline normal values: $0.04–0.44 \times 10^9/L$, comprising 1–6% of WBCs.

Monocytes – guideline normal values: $0.20.8 \times 10^9/L$. comprising 2–10% of WBCs.

Basophils – guideline normal values: up to $0.01 \times 10^9/L$, comprising 0–1% of WBCs.

Platelets – Platelet count – guideline normal values: $150–400 \times 10^9/L$.

Appendix Table 1 Haematology values

Parameter	Normal range	Level ↑	Level ↓
Haemoglobin	Male 13.0–18.0 g/dL Female 11.5–16.5 g/dL	Polycythaemia (rubra vera or physiological); myeloproliferative disease; dehydration	Anaemia
Haematocrit (packed cell volume or PCV)	Male 40–54% Female 37–47%	Polycythaemia; dehydration	Anaemia
Mean cell volume (MCV) MCV = PCV/RBC	77–95 fL	Macrocytosis in vitamin B_{12} or folate deficiency; liver disease; alcoholism; hypothyroidism; myelodysplasia; myeloproliferative disorders; aplastic anaemia; cytotoxic agent	Microcytosis in iron deficiency, thalassaemia, chronic disease

Continued

Appendix Table 1   Haematology values—cont'd

Parameter	Normal range	Level ↑	Level ↓
Mean cell haemoglobin (MCH) MCH = Hb/RBC	27–32 pg/cell	Pernicious anaemia	Iron deficiency; thalassaemia; sideroblastic anaemia
Mean cell haemoglobin concentration (MCHC) MCHC = Hb/PCV	32–36 g/dL		Iron deficiency; thalassaemia; sideroblastic anaemia; anaemia in chronic disease
Red cell count (RBC)	Male $4.5–6.5 \times 10^{12}/L$ Female $3.8–5.8 \times 10^{12}/L$	Polycythaemia	Anaemia; fluid overload
White cell count (total)	$4–11 \times 10^9/L$	Infection; inflammation; leukaemia; intense exercise; trauma; stress; pregnancy	Early leukaemia; some infections; bone marrow disease; drugs including corticosteroids and chemotherapy; idiopathic
Neutrophils	$2–7.5 \times 10^9/L$	Pregnancy; exercise; infection; bleeding; trauma; malignancy; leukaemia; corticosteroids	Some infections; drugs; endocrinopathies; bone marrow disease; idiopathic
Lymphocytes	$1.3–3.5 \times 10^9/L$	Physiological; some infections; leukaemia; lymphoma	Some infections; some immune defects (e.g. HIV, AIDS); lymphoma; corticosteroids; SLE
Eosinophils	$0.04–0.44 \times 10^9/L$	Allergic disease; parasitic infestations; skin disease; malignancy including lymphoma	Some immune defects
Platelets	$150–400 \times 10^9/L$	Thrombocytosis in bleeding; myeloproliferative disease; chronic inflammatory states	Thrombocytopenia related to leukaemia; drugs; HIV; other infections; idiopathic; autoimmune; DIC
Reticulocytes (Retics)	0.5–1.5% of RBC	Haemolytic states; during treatment of anaemia	Chemotherapy; bone marrow disease
Erythrocyte sedimentation rate (ESR)	0–15 mm/h	Pregnancy; infections; anaemia; inflammation; connective tissue disease; temporal arteritis; trauma; infarction; tumours	–
Plasma viscosity (PV)	1.4–1.8 cp	As ESR and C reactive protein	

Appendix Table 2   Liver function tests

Test	Basis	Abnormalities
Urine bilirubin Serum bilirubin	Red bile pigment from breakdown of haemoglobin. Water-soluble conjugates enter urine	Positive in most jaundice except unconjugated hyperbilirubinaemia rises because of overproduction, or obstruction
Serum alanine transaminase (ALT) or Serum glutamate pyruvate transaminase (SGPT)	Mainly a liver enzyme	Most sensitive marker of any type of hepatocyte damage
Serum alkaline phosphatase	Found in biliary canaliculi, osteoblasts, intestinal mucosa, placenta	Rises in pregnancy, liver disease, gallstones, bone disease, renal or intestinal damage
Serum aspartate aminotransferase (AST) or Serum glutamic-oxaloacetic transaminase (SGOT)	Leaks from damaged liver, heart or muscle	Rises in liver, heart or muscle damage
Serum 5′ nucleotidase	Found in liver, thyroid and bone	Rises mainly in biliary obstruction
Serum gamma glutamyl transpeptidase (GGT or GGTP)	Found in liver, kidneys, pancreas, prostate	Alcohol is the main cause of a rise. Most liver diseases, pancreatitis, diabetes, and myocardial infarct can increase levels
Serum albumin	Synthesized by the liver	Low albumin (hypoalbuminaemia) may indicate severe liver damage. Falls also in malnutrition, nephrotic syndrome, gastrointestinal disease
Prothrombin time	Affected by clotting factor proteins synthesized by the liver using vitamin K metabolites.	Prolonged in liver disease, and malabsorption (decreased vitamin K ingestion).

Appendix Table 3 Interpretation of biochemical results (always check values for the laboratory used)

Parameter	Level ↑	Level ↓
Acid phosphatase	Prostatic malignancy; renal disease; acute myeloid leukaemia	–
Alanine transaminase (ALT)	Liver disease; infectious mononucleosis	Hypothyroidism; hypophosphatasia; malnutrition
Alkaline phosphatase	Puberty; pregnancy; Paget disease; osteomalacia; fibrous dysplasia; malignancy in bone; liver disease; hyperparathyroidism (some); hyperphosphatasia	–
Alpha1-antitrypsin	Liver cirrhosis	Congenital emphysema
Alpha-fetoprotein (AFP)	Pregnancy; gonadal tumour; liver disease	Fall in level in pregnancy indicates fetal distress
Amylase	Pancreatic disease; mumps; some other salivary diseases	–
Angiotensin-converting enzyme (ACE)	Sarcoidosis	–
Antistreptolysin O titre (ASOT)	Streptococcal infections; rheumatic fever; drugs	–
Aspartate transaminase (AST)	Liver disease; biliary disease; myocardial infarct; trauma; drugs	–
Bilirubin (total)	Liver or biliary disease; haemolysis	–
Brain natriuretic peptide	Cardiac failure	–
Caeruloplasmin	Pregnancy; cirrhosis; hyperthyroidism; leukaemia	Wilson disease
Calcium	Primary hyperparathyroidism; malignancy in bone; renal tubular acidosis; sarcoidosis; thiazides; calcium supplements; excess vitamin D	Hypoparathyroidism; renal failure; rickets; nephrotic syndrome; chronic renal failure; lack of vitamin D; low magnesium levels; acute pancreatitis
Cholesterol	Hypercholesterolaemia; pregnancy; hypothyroidism; diabetes; nephrotic syndrome; liver or biliary disease	Malnutrition; hyperthyroidism
Complement (C3)	Trauma; surgery; infection	Liver disease; immune complex diseases (e.g. lupus erythematosus)
Complement (C4)	–	Liver disease; immune complex diseases; HANE (hereditary angioneurotic oedema)

Appendix Table 3   Interpretation of biochemical results (always check values for the laboratory used)—cont'd

Parameter	Level ↑	Level ↓
Cortisol (see Steroids)	–	–
Creatine kinase (CK)	Myocardial infarct; trauma; muscle disease; rhabdomyolysis; statins	–
Creatinine	Renal failure; urinary obstruction	Pregnancy
C-reactive protein (CRP)	Inflammation; trauma; myocardial infarct; malignant disease	–
C1 esterase inhibitor	–	Hereditary angiodema
Cyclic citrullinated peptide (CCP)	Rheumatoid arthritis	–
Erythrocyte sedimentation rate (ESR)	Inflammation; trauma; myocardial infarct; malignant disease	–
Ferritin	Liver disease; haemochromatosis; leukaemia; lymphoma; other malignancies; thalassaemia	Iron deficiency
Fibrinogen	Pregnancy; pulmonary embolism; nephritic syndrome; lymphoma	Disseminated intravascular coagulopathy (DIC)
Folic acid	Folic acid therapy	Alcoholism; dietary deficiency; haemolytic anaemias; malabsorption; myelodysplasia; phenytoin; methotrexate; trimethoprim; pyrimethamine; sulfasalazine; cycloserine; oral contraceptives; pregnancy
Free thyroxine index (FTI; serum T4 and T3 uptake)	Hyperthyroidism	Hypothyroidism
Gamma-glutamyl transpeptidase (GGT)	Alcoholism; obesity; liver disease; myocardial infarct; pancreatitis; diabetes; renal diseases; tricyclics	–
Globulins (total; see also Protein)	Liver disease; multiple myeloma; autoimmune disease; chronic infections	Chronic lymphatic leukaemia; malnutrition; protein-losing states
Glucose	Diabetes mellitus; pancreatitis; hyperthyroidism; hyperpituitarism; Cushing disease; liver disease; post-head injury	Hypoglycaemic drugs; Addison disease; hypopituitarism; hyperinsulinism; severe liver disease
Hydroxybutyrate dehydrogenase (HBD) immunoglobulins	Myocardial infarct	–

Continued

Appendix Table 3   Interpretation of biochemical results (always check values for the laboratory used)—cont'd

Parameter	Level ↑	Level ↓
Total immunoglobulins	Liver disease; infection; sarcoidosis; connective tissue disease	Immunodeficiency; nephrotic syndrome; enteropathy
IgG	Myelomatosis; connective tissue disorders	Immunodeficiency; nephrotic syndrome
IgA	Alcoholic cirrhosis; Berger disease	Immunodeficiency
IgM	Primary biliary cirrhosis; nephrotic syndrome; parasites; infections	Immunodeficiency
IgE	Allergies; parasites	–
Lactate dehydrogenase (LDH)	Myocardial infarct; trauma; liver disease; haemolytic anaemias; lymphoproliferative diseases	Radiotherapy
Lipase	Pancreatic disease	–
Lipids (triglycerides)	Hyperlipidaemia; diabetes mellitus; hypothyroidism; hyper-vitaminosis D	–
Magnesium	Renal failure	Cirrhosis; malabsorption; diuretics; Conn syndrome; renal tubular defects
Nucleotidase	Liver disease	–
Percent carbohydrate-deficient transferrin	Alcoholism	–
Phosphate	Renal failure; bone disease; hypoparathyroidism; hyper-vitaminosis D	Hyperparathyroidism; rickets; malabsorption syndrome
Potassium	Renal failure; Addison disease; ACE inhibitors; potassium supplements	Vomiting; diabetes; Conn syndrome; diuretics; Cushing disease; malabsorption; corticosteroids; salbutamol
Protein (total)	Liver disease; multiple myeloma; sarcoid; connective tissue diseases	Pregnancy; nephrotic syndrome; malnutrition; enteropathy; renal failure; lymphomas
Albumin	Dehydration	Liver disease; malnutrition; malabsorption; nephrotic syndrome; multiple myeloma; connective tissue disorders
Alpha1-globulin	Oestrogens	Nephrotic syndrome
Alpha2-globulin	Infections; trauma	Nephrotic syndrome
Beta-globulin	Hypercholesterolaemia; liver disease; pregnancy	Chronic disease
Gamma-globulin	(see Immunoglobulins)	Nephrotic syndrome; immunodeficiency

Appendix Table 3 Interpretation of biochemical results (always check values for the laboratory used)—cont'd

Parameter	Level ↑	Level ↓
SGGT (see GGT)	–	–
SGOT (see AST)	–	–
SGPT (see ALT)	–	–
Sodium	Dehydration; Cushing disease	Cardiac failure; renal failure; SIADH (syndrome of inappropriate antidiuretic hormone); Addison disease; diuretics
Steroids (corticosteroids)	Cushing disease; some tumours	Addison disease; hypopituitarism
Thyroxine (T4)	Hyperthyroidism; pregnancy; oral contraceptive	Hypothyroidism; nephrotic syndrome; phenytoin
Troponin	Myocardial infarction	–
Urea	Renal failure; dehydration; gastrointestinal bleed	Liver disease; nephrotic syndrome; pregnancy; malnutrition
Uric acid	Gout; leukaemia; renal failure; multiple myeloma	Liver disease; probenecid; allopurinol; salicylates; other drugs
Vitamin B_{12}	Liver disease; leukaemia; polycythaemia rubra vera	Pernicious anaemia; gastrectomy; Crohn's disease; ileal resection; vegans; metformin

Appendix Table 4 Urinalysis: interpretation of results

	Colour	Protein	Glucose	Ketones	Bilirubin	Urobilinogen	Blood
Comment	–	Tetrabromphenol blue dye binds to some proteins in urine – mainly albumin. Not all proteins are detected and the sensitivity is not high	–	–	–	–	Tests for intact red cells and free haemoglobin (Hb)
Health	Yellow	Usually no protein, but a trace can be normal in young people	Usually no glucose, but a trace can be normal in 'renal glycosuria' and pregnancy	Usually no ketones but ketonuria may occur in vomiting, fasting or starved patients	Usually no bilirubin	Usually present in normal healthy patients, particularly in concentrated urine	Usually no blood
False positives	Red: beet	Alkaline urine. Container contaminated with disinfectant (e.g. chlorhexidine). Blood or pus in urine. Polyvinyl pyrrolidone infusions	Cefamandole. Container contaminated with hypochlorite	Patients on L-dopa or any phthalein compound	Chlorpromazine and other phenothiazines	Infected urine. Patients taking ascorbic acid, sulfonamides or paraminosalicylate	Menstruation. Container contaminated with some detergents
Disease	Brown: homogentisic acid, bilirubin, urobilin, porphyrins Red: Hb Milky in chyluria	Renal diseases. Also cardiac failure, diabetes, endocarditis, myeloma, amyloid, some drugs, some chemicals	Diabetes mellitus. Also in pancreatitis, hyperthyroidism, Fanconi syndrome, sometimes after a head injury, other endocrinopathies	Diabetes mellitus. Also in febrile or traumatized or starved patients on low carbohydrate diets	Only where conjugated bilirubin is increased – hepatocellular and obstructive liver disease	Haemolytic or hepatic, hepatocellular or obstructive disease. Prolonged antibiotic therapy	Genitourinary diseases. Also in bleeding tendency, haemolysis, rhabdomyolysis, some infections where bacteria contain hydroperoxidase, some drugs, endocarditis

Index

Page numbers followed by "*f*" indicate figures, "*b*" indicate boxes, and "*t*" indicate tables.